# Physicians, Peasants, and Modern Medicine

# CEU Press Studies in the History of Medicine
## Volume XI

Series Editor: Marius Turda

# Physicians, Peasants, and Modern Medicine

*Imagining Rurality in Romania, 1860–1910*

## Constantin Bărbulescu

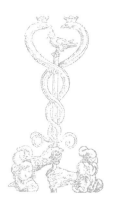

Central European University Press

Budapest—New York

First published in Romanian as *România medicilor. Medici, țărani și igienă rurală în România de la 1860 la 1910* © 2015 Humanitas

Published in 2018 by
Central European University Press
Nádor utca 9, H-1051 Budapest, Hungary
*Tel*: +36-1-327-3138 or 327-3000
*E-mail*: ceupress@press.ceu.edu
*Website*: www.ceupress.com

224 West 57th Street, New York NY 10019, USA

Translated by Angela Jianu

Financial support for the translation was granted by the Romanian Cultural Institute, Bucharest

INSTITUTUL
CULTURAL
ROMÂN

ISBN 978-963-386-267-4
ISSN 2079-1119

### Library of Congress Cataloging-in-Publication Data

Names: Barbulescu, Constantin, 1969- author.
Title: Physicians, peasants and modern medicine : imagining rurality in Romania, 1860-1910 / by Constantin Barbulescu.
Other titles: Romania medicilor. English | Imagining rurality in Romania, 1860-1910
Description: Budapest : New York : Central European University Press, [2018] | Series: CEU Press studies in the history of medicine ; volume XI | Includes bibliographical references and index.
Identifiers: LCCN 2018026384 (print) | LCCN 2018029609 (ebook) | ISBN 9789633862681 | ISBN 9789633862674 (alk. paper)
Subjects: LCSH: Rural health--Romania--History--19th century. | Rural health--Romania--History--20th century. | Medicine, Rural--Romania--History--19th century. | Medicine, Rural--Romania--History--20th century. | Social medicine--Romania--History--19th century. | Social medicine--Romania--History--20th century.
Classification: LCC RA771.7.R6 (ebook) | LCC RA771.7.R6 B3713 2018 (print) | DDC 362.1/0425709498--dc23
LC record available at https://lccn.loc.gov/2018026384

Printed in Hungary

*For my wife, Ena*

# TABLE OF CONTENTS

# ACKNOWLEDGEMENTS

This volume, as it is presented to you today, owes a great deal to individuals who have been there for me, supporting and advising me along the way. Without their contributions this would be an entirely different book. I would like to acknowledge this support and thank them all. Special thanks are due to Constanța Vintilă-Ghițulescu, who read the Romanian version of this manuscript attentively and accepted it for publication in the series "Society and Civilization" which she coordinates for Humanitas Publishers in Bucharest. I am grateful for the time and effort she invested in this project. The second reader of the manuscript was my colleague Alin Ciupală, whose friendship and support I have enjoyed since the moment we met. Last but not least, I would like to thank a third reader, my colleague Sorin Mitu, whose advice, support and faith have been crucial.

I am also grateful for support I received from the staff at the "Lucian Blaga" Central University Library in Cluj-Napoca, where I completed most of my preliminary research. A few members of the library staff there made my life significantly easier. I would like to express my special thanks to Alina Ioana Bogătean, Agnota Pop, Eliza Man and Mariana Falup, whose friendly and collegial support has been invaluable.

Finally, I would like to acknowledge my chief source of inspiration, my wife Ena. Without her encouragement, this book would not exist.

\*\*\*

The English-language edition of this book was made possible through the support of my friend and colleague Marius Turda, who accepted it for the series he coordinates at Central European University Press in Budapest. I would like to thank him for this opportunity. I also wish to offer my sincere gratitude to the two institutions that sponsored the English-language edition: Central European University Press, which took on the project, and the Romanian Cultural Institute, which awarded the translation grant. Last but not least, I would like to thank Angela Jianu for a tactful, professional translation.

# INTRODUCTION

A book should always start with a story—its own story. What could be, after all, of greater interest to the reader than an introductory answer to a simple query: how did this book come to be? But when you talk about a book, you ultimately talk about a person—the author—about his or her ideas and life, both of which are normally kept invisible in what we generally think of as scientific literature. In this introduction, I decided to break this taboo.

First, I shall attempt an explanation of how I chose the theme of this book. For this, we need to go back in time, to the mid-1990s to be more precise, when I decided upon the general subject of my doctoral research: the imaginary of the human body in the rural world. I started by envisaging a purely ethnological endeavor: I intended to visit some of the country's villages armed with a questionnaire and collect oral testimonies about the ways in which peasants viewed the body. The responses were going to be the empirical basis for my doctoral thesis. Since I was about to embark on post-graduate research in a department of history, it was inevitable that someone in the doctoral panel, perhaps overly protective of their discipline, should inquire into the historical relevance of my chosen topic. The topic itself and the methodological approach were further breaches of entrenched disciplinary taboos. It became obvious that I had to add a historical dimension to my research on representations of the body. I had to provide an answer to a question that was as simple as the ethnological premise from which I started: in what ways did the modern state attempt to equip Romania's rural population with a modern and scientific conception of the body? More precisely, why did such attempts fail? I already intuited that the views of the human body that I was about to collect during my fieldwork at the end of the twentieth century differed in significant ways from conventional, modern representations. An attempt to answer this question involved a partial detour away from my main interests: during the next few years, I immersed myself in the medical literature relating to the rural world of the nineteenth century. The endeavors of those years resulted in a doctoral thesis and two books: one was a study of images of the body in the peasant world, and the other a monograph on medical modernization in the village. What in the dissertation had been a rather forced fusion of the two themes ultimately proved an enduring union: from that moment on I was never able to fully disentangle field research from history, at least not on this particular topic.

In time, this two-pronged approach led to an intellectual shift with relevance for the present volume: I was gripped by the history of the nineteenth century and could no longer disengage myself from its spell. And even though my relationship to this period has had its moments of doubt and fatigue, I keep returning to it with renewed intellectual pleasure and curiosity. The present volume is, obviously, the outcome of this relationship and I would hope that it is a success. For several years after the completion of my doctoral studies, I combined research into the rural world, which has remained a constant interest, with occasional forays into an older passion of mine: the social history of medicine in the nineteenth century. This work resulted in studies published in periodicals, on topics that, I hoped, would one day yield their potential.

A few texts, originally conceived and published as independent studies, have made their way into the present volume with either small changes or after significant re-writing. However, most of the texts comprising the second half, which is also the core of the volume, were written especially for this book. As I tried to imagine the outline of the book, I was pleasantly surprised by the realization that the small-scale case studies I had published over the years fitted quite well into the whole, not unlike the pieces of a jigsaw puzzle. In other words, I discovered that my partial findings on the doctors and villagers of nineteenth-century Romania had a certain cohesiveness, which held great promise for the creation of a book: the book you now have in front of you. It brings together all the insights I gained and all the answers I found after more than a decade of pouring over the available literature on health care provision and hygiene in the nineteenth century. Now you know almost everything about the origins of this book.

If I were to summarize the subject in a single phrase, I would say that it is a study of social imagology. In other words, the research focuses primarily on a section of the Romanian elites of the late nineteenth century, namely the health professionals, and on the imagery they constructed as they interacted with the peasant and his world. More broadly, however, this research also looks beyond the village to wider modernizing processes and their effects on the peasants' way of life. But why should it be important or relevant to look at the past through the eyes of a specific socio-professional group, albeit an elite one? Looking at the past from as many perspectives as possible should be every historian's dream. In my case, it was, I think, a happy accident that I ended up looking at the nineteenth century through the gaze of doctors. My dream would have been complete if I had been able to have the peasants' perspective: alas, it was not to be… But writing the history of the nineteenth century from the doctors' angle presents major advantages: first of all, this angle places us on a level with ordinary people in the cities, primarily because, at least initially, medicine was an eminently urban profession. However, increasingly, in the last decades of the nineteenth century, doctors ventured out of cities and became a more or less familiar sight on dusty country roads. This was as much due to obligation as to a charitable impulse, because new health legislation required the district general practitioner (in Romanian: *medicul de plasă*) to visit the villages in his catchment area twice a month. The chief county medical officer (in Romanian: *medical primar de judeţ*) was required to perform at least an annual tour of the villages in his county. Between 1885 and 1893, even officers of the Higher Medical Council (in Romanian: *Consiliul Sanitar Superior*) had to inspect circumscriptions of four villages each. All these people, situated at different levels of Romania's health care system, would travel across the country from village to village and from town to town, escorted by junior officials, mayors, deputy prefects and even prefects, to inspect health care institutions, the services they provided, and to measure the health of the nation. Most often, they wrote desperate reports on the disastrous state of health care provision, in which they tried valiantly to offer suggestions for "steps to be taken to improve the situation." And one should not overlook the frequent and dramatic rural epidemics that stretched the capacity and skills of district and county medics to their limits. Gradually, all the sectors of the health system became involved with the rural world, as the latter's position within the national ideology became ever more prominent. Health care providers at all levels engaged fully with the period's major struggle against morbidity and mortality. In a famous text, Claude Lévi-Strauss noted that the last two centuries of the modern age are essentially defined by the rise of expertise and of technologies for the maintenance and extension of human life.[1] In nineteenth-century Romania, the medical profession rose rapidly to become one of the most prestigious careers precisely because its practitioners were perceived as specialists in the improvement of life. However, it is equally true that, as the modern Romanian state emerged, the most popular of the liberal professions was law rather than medicine. The modern state in Romania is still widely perceived, not without some exaggeration, as a creation of the lawyers. However, it was equally a creation of the doctors, engineers and men of letters who worked together, throughout the long nineteenth century, to transform the Romanian Principalities from Ottoman vassals into the Kingdom of Romania.

Before moving on, let's look briefly at this body of professionals. The Principalities did not have a large number of doctors, but they were significant enough for the historian Alexandru-Florin Platon to include them among the socio-professional groups, such as teachers, lawyers and civil servants, which formed a weighty section of the country's nascent bourgeoisie in the first half of the nineteenth century.[2] In 1862, Doctor Carol Davila proceeded to streamline the Health Services (in Romanian: *Serviciul Sanitar*) of the Principalities, as we shall see in greater detail in a later chapter. This attempt involved maintaining a register of doctors and imposing strict guidelines of professional conduct. It is due to his efforts that today we know that, as of February 1, 1862, the "Romanian state" had 99 practicing doctors, which was not a lot. More than a third of these (34) had completed their medical studies in Austria; if to these we add the 22 who had graduated from German universities, it becomes clear that the majority of doctors in the Principalities had been trained in the German-speaking world. France as a place of study came a modest fourth, with 14 doctors, just below to Italy, which had trained 18 doctors.[3] By the mid-century, most medical professionals were foreigners, with a few isolated ethnic Ro-

---

1   Lévi-Strauss, "Rasă și istorie," 29.
2   Platon, *Geneza burgheziei în Principatele Române*, 309–11.
3   *Monitorul. Jurnal Oficial*, February 3, 1862, no. 25, 103.

manians, which was comparable to the other liberal professions. In the 1860s, the number of doctors rose rapidly, reaching 366 in 1866, a number which included licensed doctors as well as graduates of medical schools.[4] More than thirty years later, on October 1, 1898, the "art" of medicine was practiced by no less than 966 licensed doctors and 34 medical graduates. Importantly, more than two thirds of these (679 licensed doctors and 25 graduates) were Romanians.[5] Thus, by 1898, the medical corps had become comprehensively Romanianized, a fact that had an overwhelming impact on the medical discourse, the topic of the second part of this book. And while sheer numbers were unimpressive, doctors played an active part in the creation of modern Romania.

Looking at Romania through the eyes of doctors also means seeing it from the vantage point of the elites, as many of the medical practitioners considered themselves. This vantage point was informed by the most radical variant of the state's modernizing ideology, hence the hypercritical tone of this discourse. Doctors had extremely negative appraisals of contemporaneous Romania: they despaired at the mud-drenched towns, the derelict, unfenced cemeteries, the markets teeming with vegetable and animal debris. Not to mention the villages, pictures of sanitary hells where pale, ghostly figures, weakened by illness and malnutrition, lived in small, damp and inadequate habitations. The way doctors saw it, Romania was modern solely in its aspirations.

Part One of this book is primarily an introduction to the sources. The two main categories of sources selected for analysis were public health reports and the memoirs of doctors. Although used extensively, they do not completely exclude other types of materials, such as medical articles published in specialized journals, pamphlets and individual studies, all of which are like pixels in a high-resolution picture. The medico-social literature of the latter half of the nineteenth century is an extremely rich source-base for the study of the medical discourse as a discourse on society as a whole.[6] This richness, however, does not preclude a certain limitation in the range

---

4   This calculation is based on adding those licensed to practice by 1866 to Carol Davila's original list. See Obregia, *Raport general asupra igienei publice și asupra serviciului sanitar*, XLI–XLIV.

5   Felix, *Raport general asupra igienei publice*, 340.

6   To form an idea of the richness of this literature, one can consult, for instance, the monograph of Crăiniceanu, *Literatura medicală românească. Biografii și bibliografie*, as well as the study by Gomoiu, *Istoria presei medicale în România*.

of themes as well as of style. Part Two, which forms the nucleus of the book, is devoted to an analysis of the themes in the period's medical discourse. Separate chapters look at individual themes in the medical discourse on the peasant and the rural world, with occasional forays, when necessary, into the opposite camp, the urban realm. Readers may wonder, and rightly so: why limit ourselves to the world of the village, why not look at Romania as a whole? Part of the explanation lies in my own personal and intellectual history and my twin training as a historian and an ethnologist, which means that I am irresistibly biased in favor of the rural world. In this respect, I am a "ruralist," someone who never reached the "anthropological stage of contemporary social research" as defined by Vintilă Mihăilescu.[7] Fortuitously, my interest in the peasant overlapped with the interest of the Romanian elites, as expressed in their almost obsessive focus on the so-called "rural question" and all its facets in the late nineteenth century. In the nineteenth century, the peasant became a historical figure of the first order, but his role as an historical agent was often obscured by the historiography of the second half of the twentieth century, and, may one add, of the last two decades. Romanian historiography lacks a serious, institutionally-supported sub-discipline of rural history. The only two moments when the peasant emerges into the limelight of historiography are when he is the recipient of land or when he revolts. The Marxist origin of this approach is obvious. However, the life of the peasant and the rural world in the long nineteenth century is multi-faceted, and I hope that the present study will shed light on this complexity. I also hope that this enquiry into the social history of the village, albeit from a medical viewpoint, will encourage other researchers to join this promising field of research.

Finally, Part Three of the volume goes beyond imagology to look at the interactions of the two Romanias: the urban world of the elites and the world of the village. The two chapters present two case studies illustrating the interactions between the hegemonic, mainstream culture of modernity and the subaltern rural culture. The focus in these chapters is different: the first chapter, devoted to health legislation, explores attempts by the elites to impose the dominant medical culture on society as a whole; the second chapter leaves the macro-scale of analysis behind to look at the micro-scale

---

7    Mihăilescu, *Etnografii urbane. Cotidianul văzut de aproape*, 7–29.

realities of social life and the challenges they pose to the dominant culture. The structures and rhythms of the modernization process were embedded then—as they are today—in entanglements of the archaic and the new, the rural setting and the city. Ultimately, therefore, this book is not simply a study of social representation and imagology, but also an enquiry that charts the modernization of the rural world in Romania.

A few explanations on the methodology and theoretical approaches are in order. As the main section of the study is concerned with the medical discourse about the rural world, what is attempted here is both a description and an analysis of this discourse. As already mentioned, one of the early findings of this study is the rather surprising fact that the medical representations of the peasantry—scattered across the dusty pages of old medical journals and monographs—was rather more standardized than expected. Consequently, the first operation performed on this body of texts was a classification of themes, an operation that, in the early stages, was meant to make these sources more intelligible and easier to study. Naturally, this thematic "slicing" implies some arbitrary selection, but I do not think that, by doing this, I strayed too far from the intellectual mindset of the period's doctors. If you pay close attention to a text, you will find that it easily unlocks the link between the computer keys and the original ideas of the text's author. Sometimes, things get a little more complicated, as we shall discover when looking at the theme of racial degeneration.

Next is a chronological outline of each individual theme, discussed in a separate chapter in Part Two: as a rule, I started from early nineteenth-century sources and proceeded to the eve of World War I. When I deemed it necessary, I progressed into the interwar period. At the last stage, and for almost each of the themes, I rounded up by citing contemporary sources, because the medical discourse on the Romanian peasant and the village continues well into the modern and contemporary age.

Part Three of the book is unlike Part Two, which means that the approach and methodology had to be adapted. The aim of the first chapter is to demonstrate to what extent the period's health legislation translated into social reality. There was only one way of doing this, namely, by juxtaposing two categories of sources: legislative sources and health reports, which often made references to the enforcement of the law *in situ*. In Chapter Two, we leave the literary arena behind to delve into the archives. Archival "hardliners" will say that a historical study worth its salt must use archival sources. Personally, I have my reservations, because I have seen far too many mediocre studies based on archival material. However, if you know where to look—no easy task—archival documents are likely to bring you closer to the people of the past. Therefore, in Chapter Two of Part Three, I discuss two popular healers from the year 1860: one attempted to cure rabies two decades before Pasteur, the other tackled mental illness; both were subjected to enquiries into their activities by the Health Service. I decided to try to unpack their stories to understand the interactions between the dominant medical culture of the mid-nineteenth century and the subaltern peasant culture.

While writing this book, I would have loved to be able to read historical overviews of the doctors and medical practices of nineteenth-century Romania. Such a synthesis exists: a 2011 study by Lidia Trăuşan-Matu,[8] but its coverage ends in 1869, a date which is fairly close to my starting point. A survey of the medical corps along the lines of Andrei Florin Sora's study of prefects from 1866 to 1940[9] is still sorely lacking. This does not mean that nothing has ever been written about the nineteenth-century medical profession in Romania. While there is no space here for a serious discussion on medical historiography in Romania,[10] a few recent contributions must be highlighted. One thing is certain: the social history of nineteenth-century medicine in Romania is about to take off. Academic circles in Bucharest and Cluj, notably, organize workshops and study groups devoted to the history of medicine and researchers who at least nod towards medical topics. Recent years have seen the publication of studies on relevant themes. While writing my own book, I received the latest study by Ligia Livadă-Cadeschi on a related theme: the medico-social discourse of Romanian hygienists.[11] Around the same period, I read Constanța Vintilă-Ghițulescu's book *Evgheniți, ciocoi, mojici*,[12] which has a substantial section on the early stages of Romania's modernization, including the medico-social aspects of changes in the ru-

---

8   Trăuşan-Matu, *De la leac la reţetă. Medicalizarea societăţii româneşti în veacul al XIX-lea (1831–1869).*

9   Sora, *Servir l'État Roumain. Le corps préfectoral, 1866–1940.*

10  On this topic, see the useful survey by Popovici, "Istoriografia medicală românească (1813–2008)," 463–80.

11  Livadă-Cadeschi, *Discursul medico-social al igieniştilor români. Abordarea specificităţilor locale din perspectiva experienţelor occidentale europene, secolele XIX-XX.*

12  Vintilă-Ghițulescu, *Evgheniți, ciocoi, mojici: despre "obrazele" primei modernităţi româneşti (1750–1860).*

ral world. 2013 was a productive year for the history of medicine in Romania. It is perhaps useful to mention a slightly older volume,[13] which comprises studies on medicine-related topics by researchers in Bucharest and Cluj, thus joining the early efforts of the two emerging academic "schools." The publication of original research went hand in hand with the publication of sources, for example Octavian Buda's edited collection of medical inaugural speeches from the reign of King Carol I,[14] as well as collections of health legislation[15], and health reports.[16] All these studies were published in an interval of only five years—this bodes well for the future of medical historiography. I hope that the present study will make a contribution to this growing research area.

Whereas, as mentioned above, the themes of this book are relatively new to Romanian historiography, they are not so in other scientific communities, for instance in French or Anglo-American historical literature. Here, research in these areas has resulted in a significant body of published studies. For instance, in Britain, we have the comprehensive, and now classic, study by William F. Bynum, *Science and the Practice of Medicine in the Nineteenth Century*,[17] and a more recent survey of the "Western medical tradition."[18] *The Oxford Handbook for the History of Medicine*,[19] edited by Mark Jackson, is a very informative survey of the main trends in the history of medicine, which references a considerable body of research.

My research is part of a more recent effort in embedding emerging scholarship on the history of medicine in South-East Europe within this vast bulk of Western research. It follows in the footsteps of studies by such authors as Christian Promitzer, Sevasti Trubeta, Marius Turda,[20] Heike Karge, Friederike Kind-Kovács and Sara Bernasconi.[21] However, the present study addresses two themes that are new to Romanian historiography: the theme

---

13 Bărbulescu and Ciupală, *Medicine, Hygiene and Society from the Eighteenth to the Twentieth Centuries.*

14 Buda, *Despre regenerarea și degenerarea unei națiuni. Discursurile inaugurale medicale în vremea lui Carol I, 1872–1912.*

15 Șuta, Tămaș, Ciupală, Bărbulescu, and Popovici, *Legislația sanitară în România modernă (1874–1910).*

16 Gudin, Tămaș, Mehedinți, Ciupală, Bărbulescu, and Popovici, *Rapoarte sanitare în România modernă (1864–1906).*

17 Bynum, *Science and the Practice of Medicine in the Nineteenth Century.*

18 Bynum et al., *The Western Medical Tradition: 1800 to 2000.*

19 Jackson, *The Oxford Handboock for the History of Medicine.*

20 Promitzer, Trubeta, and Turda, *Health, Hygiene and Eugenics in Southeastern Europe to 1945.*

21 Karge, Kind-Kovács and Bernasconi, *From the Midwife's Bag to the Patient's File. Public Health in Eastern Europe.*

of racial degeneration in nineteenth century medical discourse, and the "medical" practices of empirical healers. Internationally, the 1980s saw an emerging interest in the topic of racial degeneration, with the publication of at least three studies addressing the theme from different perspectives. The classic 1984 study by Robert A. Nye examines one of the sources of the theme: an intense concern for national decline in late nineteenth-century France.[22] One year later, a volume edited by J. Edward Chamberlin and Sander L. Gilman[23] presented an overview of several lines of enquiry into these topics. At the end of the decade, Daniel Pick offered a monograph on "national" variants of racial degeneration in France, Italy and Britain.[24] Interest in my second theme, the "medical" practices of empirical healers, was spurred by Matthew Ramsey's study *Professional and Popular Medicine in France, 1770–1830,*[25] which presents a comparative analysis of groups of professional medical practitioners and empirical healers (often viewed as "charlatans") in one of the most troubled periods of French history. Roy Porter has studied the latter group, the "quacks," operating in Britain in the period 1660–1850.[26] My aim in the present study is more modest: to make a few forays into the vast and highly complex field of research that is the history of nineteenth-century Romanian medicine.

---

22  Nye, *Crime, Madness and Politics in Modern France: The Medical Concept of National Decline.*
23  Chamberlin and Gilman, *Degeneration: The Dark Side of Progress.*
24  Pick, *Faces of Degeneration: A European Disorder, c.1848 – c.1918.*
25  Ramsey, *Professional and Popular Medicine in France, 1770–1830.*
26  Porter, *Health for Sale: Quackery in England, 1660–1850.*

# PART ONE

# ROMANIA THROUGH THE EYES OF DOCTORS

## 1
### "Minister, I submit this report…"

Doctors—a socio-professional group who regarded themselves as an elite within an elite—were never silent. Throughout the long nineteenth century, they produced written testimonies on the nation's health, which show that, far from simply doing their jobs, they considered it their *duty* to reflect on the realities they encountered. The picture resulting from these narratives—often written as memoirs in old age—is of "their personal Romania," to paraphrase Sorin Mitu's title,[1] a Romania of squalor and suffering, of illness and death, in villages and towns and cities alike. It was often a hideous picture—much like a grim, grainy photographic negative—capturing a situation they abhorred and wished to change. In this book, we shall uncover the rationale for such negative constructions. In Part One, I focus on two categories of medical sources generally neglected by the historiography: public health reports and doctors' memoirs. Both are extremely rich in information and data about the world of the past, and as such essential, I would say, for the historian of nineteenth-century Romania, especially for the historian who looks at history from below, from the ground level, where major and lesser historical agents act out their roles.

Let us turn our attention to the health reports, their emergence, typology and development, and their role in the reconstruction of the rural and

---

1    Mitu, *Transilvania mea. Istorii, mentalități, identități.*

urban worlds of the latter half of the nineteenth century and the beginning of the twentieth. I believe that we must define our terms from the outset: public health reports are a type of administrative document that is very specific in terms of both the issuing authority and the target audience. The issuers are doctors, who write the reports according to strict guidelines and address them as a rule to the top echelons of the medical hierarchy. In terms of content, the reports describe the state of hygiene and health in the issuing doctor's catchment area. In other words, health reports are generally descriptive and only rarely, if at all, normative. Moreover, they have the advantage of describing Romania through the doctors' eyes. In some instances, the reports outline, for the attention of the medical authority, the specific action taken by the author on well-defined missions. This category includes, for instance, the beautifully written reports of members of the Institute of Bacteriology, who had been sent to various parts of the country to study and contain epidemics, as well as reports by top medical officials participating in medical congresses held across Europe during the last decades of the nineteenth century. These officials reported directly to the Home Ministry about the participation of the Romanian delegations.

My analysis will consider mainly published reports, and therefore this study cannot make claims of comprehensiveness: I have not aimed at identifying and analyzing all the medical reports ever written in the period—which would have been ideal, but not realistic. I have focused instead on the reports already available as I attempted to establish typologies and to highlight the utility for the historian of this important source of information about nineteenth-century Romanian society.

### The Earliest Public Health Reports

The earliest public health reports were issued prior to the introduction of modern health legislation in 1874. A rudimentary health system that did not, however, cover all the country's provinces existed before 1874. Some of the earliest health reports—even though they did not always carry this title—were published in the Public Health Service's newsletter *Monitorul Sanitar* between 1863 and 1866.[2] One question immediately arises: do these

---

2    Coridaly, "Studii phisice asupra districtului Ismail," 182–83, 186; Niculescu, "Memoriu asupra stărei

earlier reports bear any resemblance to those issued after 1874? Do they observe the norms of the genre? Or do they have a different template? The first discernible feature of these earlier reports is their brevity, which distinguishes them from their later counterparts. It is easy to see at a glance that they were written in a rush, as a response to some official demand from above. On the other hand, despite their modest size, these early reports are thematically rich and overlap significantly with the post-1874 reports. They contain information about the way hygiene was observed among the population, about the main illnesses and conditions, as well as demographic data (a constant feature after 1874) and geographical descriptions of the areas covered. This latter characteristic links them to the early nineteenth-century medical monographs, which were undoubtedly a model for the authors of the health reports.

In terms of content, one general characteristic distinguishes these early health reports from subsequent reports: they include many positive observations about the hygiene of the peasant world. Thus, doctor I. Niculescu noted that the "hygiene levels among the locals" were "generally adequate."[3] And—in stark contrast to later comments—doctor Coridaly described the peasants in the district of Ismail as hard working: "The peasant works hard and does not shirk hard labor. [...] The peasant women work as hard as their men."[4] It is difficult to reconcile such views with the older stereotypes of peasant indolence and sloth.[5] Should we recognize here the echoes of a polarization, which took place in public opinion around the time of Al. I. Cuza's agrarian reforms, between views of the peasant as good and the landowner as bad?[6] Future research could establish whether the overwhelmingly negative representations of the rural world became more firmly entrenched in health reports in the later nineteenth century.

However, not all medics were as happy as the doctors Niculescu and Coridaly with the health and hygiene situation in their circumscriptions. For example, doctor Robert Hintz, the chief medical officer of the district

---

arondismentului Fundu," 381–84; Michelstaedter, "Raportul D-lui Michelstaedter," 35–37, 44–45; Kopeţki, "Raport general a serviciului sanitar," 99–101; Hintz, "Raport statistic de serviciul sanitar," 115.

3    Niculescu, "Memoriu asupra stărei arondismentului Fundu," 382.
4    Coridaly, "Studii phisice asupra districtului Ismail," 183.
5    For this stereotype, see the study by Popovici, "Autopsia unei imagini: 'lenea ţăranului român' între stereotip etnic şi social," 105–70.
6    This suggestion belongs to Alin Ciupală.

Vlaşca—a man we shall encounter again in this book—described the villages in his catchment area as follows: they were generally in a "good state, few [above-ground, *author's note*] houses, many [underground] damp shacks, and much uncleanliness both among the humans and the cattle."[7] Therefore, despite doctor Hintz's positive opening, the general health situation he reported was far from good. Equally alarming was the situation of the Jewish population of Roman county, as reported in 1864 by doctor Niculescu: "The majority of the Jewish inhabitants know nothing but suffering caused by anaemia, hypertrophic liver and spleen, scurvy and scurvy-induced stomatitis. In the market town of Băceşti I saw two families living in one and the same room; these families, and all the other Jewish families, had 3–6 children each; one cannot imagine the foul air and the gross odors in those rooms."[8] These were images of decay in the body and the habitat that later re-emerged in the doctors' descriptions of the Romanian rural population. It would appear that during the reign of Cuza, the medical perception of the peasants and the rural world was marginally more positive than in the long decades of the reign of Carol I. The mid-1860s seems to be the period when peasant prosperity peaked—a period on which the doctors of the later nineteenth and early twentieth centuries looked back with nostalgia. I personally have always believed, without being able to verify, that this nostalgia was enhanced by a perception of contemporary "ills." Or perhaps the difference is due to the gap—greater in 1900 than in 1865—between the expectations of a medical corps that was increasingly modern and well trained, and a rural world that appeared to be largely stuck in a previous century. It is hard to say.

For reasons that have much to do with the discursive logic of my own text, I have opted for an analysis of the public health reports that links typology to content. In other words, content analysis calibrated on each type of report seemed to yield the most appropriate structure. And, because the health system was hierarchic, in practice every doctor had to compile such reports, published abundantly in the period's press, in *Monitorul Oficial*, in pamphlets and even in volumes, or simply filed away at the National Archives in the document collections of the Health Authority (in Romanian: *Administraţia Sanitară*). For today's historian, the amount of such documents can be over-

---

7    Hintz, "Raport statistic de serviciul sanitar din Districtul Vlaşca pe anul 1864," 115.
8    Niculescu, "Memoriu asupra stării arondismentului Fundu," 383.

whelming. Let's consider them one by one and see to what extent the data they yield creates a picture of late nineteenth-century Romania.

### The Reports of District Health Practitioners

A first category of medical reports derives from the very hierarchical structure of what the health legislation called "medical bodies" (in Romanian: *organe sanitare*).[9] The lowest rank in the health system was that of the district general practitioner (in Romanian: *medic de plasă*). In accordance with the law of 1874, the district practitioner was required to "forward to the county's top medical officer (in Romanian: *medic primar*) regular reports and statistics about public health and the policing of health services."[10] Unfortunately for the historian, these reports by district doctors—those who lived among peasants and were called "the peasants' doctors" by Iacob Felix— are the most difficult to locate. Apart from those that have been published so far,[11] it has been impossible to find any in the Fonds of the General Directorate of the Health Services (in Romanian: *Fondul Direcției Generale a Serviciului Sanitar*), held at the National Archives in Bucharest. Likewise, searches at the Olt County Archives[12] and the Suceava County Archives[13] have yielded no results. The hope that further sources might have helped could be an illusion, because the legislation in this area is imprecise: the reports are said to be required "periodically," which can mean anything or nothing. In addition, district practitioners had a precarious position, which did not attract young doctors. Here is how doctor Felix described the situation:

These young men, who lived in relative comfort during their studies and military service, are reluctant to take up positions that entail a basic lifestyle in rural villages with little comfort and a shortage of rented accommodation;

---

9   For a historical outline of health legislation after 1874, see Felix, *Istoria igienei în România în secolul al XIX-lea și starea ei la începutul secolului al XX-lea*, 54–64.

10   Pârvulescu, *Culegere de legile, regulamentele, instrucțiele, decretele și ver-ce alte dispozițiuni sanitare civile și militare*, 81.

11   Bianu, "Serviciul sanitar al Plasei Bistrița de Sus jud," 333–38, 365–69; Ionescu-Trifan, "Dare de seamă asupra unui arondisment medical," 553–60; Hârsu, "Fragmente din raportul unui medic de plasă," 213–16, 249–52, 278–83, 315–17; Pitișteanu, "Raport general pe anul 1899. Starea sanitară a Plășei Snagov," 204–10; Antonescu, "Din raportul unui medic de circumscripție," 381–85.

12   Searches conducted by Nicolae Dumitrana.

13   Searches conducted by Vlad Popovici.

especially affected are those doctors who do not receive accommodation at the sub-prefecture or the headquarters of the district law court and thus lack a company suitable to their degree of education, and those who have a large catchment area, which forces them to work long, arduous hours, which prevents them from pursuing their studies [...]. Many of the district practitioners do not provide a real service to the population; for them, this position is nothing but a temporary setback, which they wish to leave behind as soon as they can; they do not even buy a carriage, using rented horses instead and going out and about as little as possible. Our ideal of a district practitioner is represented by a few doctors who have grown old in service, who, having spent all their life among peasants and sympathized with their beliefs and their sufferings, have earned their complete trust.[14]

Future research in County Archives might uncover reports by such doctors "grown old in service." It is quite possible that doctor M. Hârsu is one of them, because his report is one of the longest, and it suggests a deep knowledge of people and places. Which leads to the question: what is the value of these reports for the historian? What knowledge do we derive from them? Judging from his detailed descriptions of the locals' occupations, dress and houses, doctor Hârsu is an excellent ethnographer:

The houses are made of timber and covered with wood slices (*margini*) or with clapboard (*draniță*). Usually, they comprise a spacious room, a porch (*sală*) and a storage room; houses with two rooms are very rare. The walls are bound with clay and whitewashed with lime or slurry (*mal*, a type of shiny, white clay) or with kaolin (a type of ashen-grey earth). Repairs are usually made ahead of special occasions such as Easter, or a saint's day, etc. The windows are always very narrow, almost microscopic; it is rare to encounter a bigger house with large, luminous windows."[15]

The doctors' reports are replete with such descriptions, which offer invaluable data on the past realities of the rural universe, otherwise inacces-

---

14   Felix, *Raport general asupra igienei publice și asupra serviciului sanitar al Regatului României pe anul 1895*, 28–31.

15   The terms in italics are given as alternatives by the author of the original report. Hârsu, "Fragmente din raportul unui medic de plasă," 215–16.

sible to today's ethnographer or historian. In fact, even the doctors who wrote the earliest monographs on the hygiene of the peasant environment in the late nineteenth century—such as Gheorghe Crăiniceanu and Nicolae Manolescu[16]—made good use of the public health reports as primary sources. Sometimes, the reports included representations of the body and its ills, which were unique to the peasant mentality. Here, for example, is doctor Hârsu on representations of syphilis in the rural world: "The people call syphilis *frenţe*,[17] bad scabs (*bube rele*), the goner (*cel perit*), worldly disease (*boale lumeşti*). They believe that 'all men are born with the goner'; it is enough to eat hot, salty food or pickles to trigger it. Hot chilli in particular, as well as salted carp, are foods that bring it out."[18]

Smallpox vaccination is another aspect of health provision that reveals specific attitudes among the doctors. In a mountainous, scattered habitat and among a population that had its own traditional practices, vaccination was difficult to enforce. "[M]any of those who receive the vaccine," doctor Hârsu wrote, "rub their arm clean behind the doctor's back; infants have their arms wiped clean by their mothers, their aunts and other womenfolk, who are unwilling to face the after-effects of the jab in inoculated children."[19] This is just one of many testimonies about the peasant's lack of faith in modern doctors and medicine. In 1882, doctor Vasile Bianu was district practitioner at Bistriţa de Sus in the county of Bacău. He, too, had to face the peasants' lack of trust and their reluctance to receive the smallpox vaccination, noting that the peasants in his district "used every means possible to prevent their progeny from being immunized."[20] Communal officials themselves—who should have been the first to set an example and endorse vaccination—kept their own children away from the procedure. When immunization started in the village Luizi Călugăra, for instance, and to the great chagrin of the good doctor, the mayor "ordered all children to be brought to the village hall, while sending his own wife and children scampering off like rabbits!"[21]

---

16 Crăiniceanu, *Igiena ţăranului roman*; Manolescu, *Igiena ţăranului.*

17 Similar terms were used in other European languages from the early modern period onwards to denote what was essentially seen as a French disease: *mal francese* in Italian, for example. [Translator's note]

18 Hârsu, "Fragmente din raportul unui medic de plasă," 281.

19 Ibid., 251.

20 The term used in the Romanian original is "*hultuire*," meaning grafting. Like the term "inoculation" itself, the word was borrowed from horticulture, where it means "implanting a bud into a plant." [Translator's note] Bianu, *Serviciul sanitar al Plasei Bistriţa de Sus jud*, 337.

21 Ibid., 338.

Doctor Bianu also talks about the impossibility of isolating patients suffering from contagious conditions in the overcrowded, one-room houses of the
rural environment: "Where shall we have the patient, and where the rest,
the fit individuals?"[22] This was a dilemma for which doctors had no solution.
The alternative was to isolate the contaminated house, but this did not work
either, because no peasant would restrict his freedom of movement for the
sake of a "gentleman," district doctor or not. However, one Sunday in the village Flipeni, doctor Bianu scored a minor victory: he managed, "not without
some difficulty" and only after "enlisting the help of a junior local official, to
send home a woman with her child, who suffered from the later, resolving,
stages of smallpox, away from the pub, which was full of people with their
children!"[23] One should not imagine that the fear of vaccination and the resulting attempts at absconding were new attitudes emerging out of the blue in
the mid-nineteenth century. The avoidance of this prophylactic measure was
as old as the procedure itself. As early as the first half of the nineteenth century, the state and church authorities did their best to promote vaccination
among the population.[24] Despite their relatively small number, the reports of
district practitioners are an extremely valuable source of information about
Romania's rural world in the second half of the nineteenth century.

### The Reports of County Medical Officers

Unlike the district practitioners' reports, the reports issued by their superiors, the county medical officers, are abundant. This is due to changes in
health legislation, which, from 1885 onward, required the publication of all
reports in the official state periodical *Monitorul Oficial*.[25] Consequently, between 1885 and 1893, *Monitorul Oficial* issued the complete series of reports
by county medical officers.[26] After 1893, *Monitorul Oficial* continued to publish the medical reports, but only in excerpts instead of the entire text.[27] This

---

22  Ibid., 337.

23  Bianu, *Serviciul sanitar al Plasei Bistrița de Sus jud,* 337.

24  Vintilă-Ghițulescu, *Evgheniți, ciocoi, mojici. Despre obrazele primei modernități romanești (1750–1860),*
    322.

25  See art. 35 of the Health Act of 1885, in *Legislația sanitară în România modernă (1874–1910),* 78.

26  For the complete series of medical reports covering the period 1886–1890 published in *Monitorul Oficial,*
    see Colceriu, *Imaginea lumii rurale în rapoartele medicale din România (1860–1914),* 67–83.

27  See art. 48 of Legea sanitară [Health act], in *Buletinul Direcțiunei Generale a Serviciului Sanitar,* year V,
    1893, no. 12, 190.

marked the birth of the massive collection of published health reports available today.

Unlike the district practitioners' reports, those issued by the county chief doctors were published annually and addressed to the Higher Medical Council (in Romanian: *Consiliul Sanitar Superior*). Their structure was largely dictated by the roles of the county medical officer. In other words, these public health reports are directly linked to the health legislation both in terms of the context of their publication and in terms of content.[28] They cannot be dissociated from the health legislation. One of the outcomes of the emergence of modern health legislation in Romania was precisely the collection of vast amounts of data on the levels of hygiene and health among Romania's population.

The reports by the county medical officers have a very specific structure and cover a limited number of topics. They include for instance:

Statistical data

Information on health personnel

Data on the levels of hygiene among the population, with an emphasis on the hygiene of dress, domestic areas and food

Data on the hygiene of "public venues" such as prisons, schools, public houses, etc.

Minutes of the sessions of the Hygiene Council

Suggestions for improvements in the country's health services

With respect to content, I shall give only one example, the report for the year 1887 by the head doctor of Vâlcea County, Gheorghe Sabin. This is, indeed, an exemplary report, because the doctor added his own observations, narratives and personal comments, which enhance the value of this document. For instance, he describes with disarming ingenuity the malfunctions of the public health system in the county as well as those of the entire health system in rural areas in 1887. The difficulties were huge: it would appear that the health system was not healthy at all. For instance, there was a massive shortage of doctors: of the five districts in the county, only two

---

28  In this context, by health legislation I mean not only the health acts as such, but also their appendices, i.e. the additional public health regulations.

had their own doctors, which means that three districts comprising 106 villages lacked medical provision altogether. The vaccination programs were largely unsuccessful, as the inhabitants absconded during the winter vaccination periods, "fearing that the cold weather might harm them."[29] There were areas where the cooperation between doctors and local authorities, as demanded by the legislation, was impossible to enforce. The case of the village of Orleşti is a good illustration:

> [M]any times, the mayor, who lived in the village, refused to accompany me to the houses which had ill residents in them, was unwilling to make lists of all those affected by illness in the village or show me where they lived. [...] If, as I went from house to house, I gave the villagers advice on how to maintain cleanliness, how to stop their children getting colds and left medicine for them along with guidelines on how to take them, the mayor often visited after me, making jests about everything I had said, so that quite often they lost all respect for me. When I left the medicine with the mayor for him to distribute to the sick, he, in order to make a laughing stock of me, stormed out onto the village hall balcony and gave orders to some junior clerks to go out at crossroads, stop passersby and bring them over to the village hall: there, they were treated to a spoonful of castor oil or quinine powder, or maybe a cup of guarana tea, until all the stock was gone. If those forced to take these remedies protested, he explained that this was done on order from Mr. Chief County Doctor."[30]

The doctor had trouble with some peasants from the village Fişcălia, who, he wrote, "treated me with disrespect."[31] Whereas many doctors complained of a lack of support from the local authorities, there were fewer who complained about the lack of respect shown by peasants to a doctor. It could well be that doctor Sabin was an exception, as he seems to have never avoided direct confrontation with the peasants in the areas in which he was supposed to enforce public health legislation. Thus, for example, in cases of epidemics that resulted in fatalities, he confesses that on many occasions, he disrupted "gatherings of people who attended wakes."[32] This may have been

---

29   Sabin, *Raport general asupra serviciului sanitar al județului Vâlcea pe anul 1887*, 2878.
30   Ibid., 2881.
31   Ibid., 2881.
32   Ibid., 2883.

the right thing to do from a medical, preventative angle, but from the perspective of peasant tradition and belief it was an act that risked compromising the afterlife of the deceased. It was an attitude that peasants were bound to find offensive and it is no surprise that doctor Sabin became *persona non grata* in the villages where such incidents occurred.

Nevertheless, such testimonies are reminders that the social and symbolic capital of doctors and medicine was not acquired overnight in the nineteenth century, and certainly not in the rural world. But why should the peasant in 1880 have had faith in doctors and their medical practices? After all, in 1880, the great majority of the peasantry practically had no access to modern health care and services. The first district doctors were appointed in 1862, and the earliest rural hospitals appeared in 1881. For centuries, peasants had dealt with health issues in their own traditional ways before the modern health system emerged, offering different types of health assistance based on new principles. Why should medicine be any better than the plant infusions and incantations of the rural healers? Why should the trained doctor be trustworthier than the local witch? These are questions that must have crossed the minds of peasants when suddenly a gentleman calling himself a "doctor" appeared in their midst every few months on horseback or in a cabriolet, claiming to have a cure for all ailments. It took much more than this claim to win the peasants' hearts and minds, and it happened much later.

But let's return to doctor Sabin, who, as we have seen, outlined in his report all the shortcomings of the health system: the avoidance of vaccination, the shortages of middle-level medical and nursing staff, the lack of support from local authorities, and the peasants' own reservations. One might wonder whether things were perhaps better in an urban environment. Judging from doctor Sabin's description of the hospital in the town of Râmnic, they were not. There, the doctor wrote, "in the winter or in the summer, dozens of patients lying on floors, in the kitchen and other annexes of the hospital, received treatment and food that was being paid for from the same allocations covering the patients in beds."[33] Such descriptions were frequent in the health reports.

In conclusion, doctor Sabin's report offers a very negative picture of the health services in the county of Vâlcea in 1887. There is little doubt that he exaggerated. However, looking at the entire body of available reports, one is

---

33  Ibid., 2878.

21

struck by the disastrous overall picture of the levels of hygiene and health care in rural and urban Romania alike. These representations were ultimately incorporated into what we referred to earlier as a negative image of the peasant and the rural world. Nothing is idealized in the reports: the entire discourse is dominated by a story of unmitigated and hopeless misery. Why is it that the more positive aspects of peasant life took so long to enter the medical literature? There is no easy or simple answer. But I do believe that this relentlessly dark picture was produced by a distorting, powerfully ideologized mirror, one that is a hidden trap for the historian studying Romanian health reports. They are, after all, official, administrative documents, and as such they had to highlight the shortcomings and failures of the system and the inadequacy of the agents, because *these needed to change.* Successes rarely, if at all, made the headlines.

## *The Reports of the Higher Medical Council*[34]

In contrast to the reports of district and county doctors, which only had local, partial coverage and could only aspire to offer a global view if considered serially, the reports compiled by the Higher Medical Council are comprehensive sources par excellence. This is the top of the medical hierarchy and, in fact, these reports were invariably compiled by the Director-General of the Health Service. Even though the Health Act of 1874 required that these reports be issued annually, in reality this was not the case. The earliest general reports were compiled by doctor D. Sergiu for the years 1886 and 1887.[35] The series continued in 1892 with the beautifully written reports by doctor Iacob Felix,[36] followed by the report of doctor Al. Obregia for the period 1899 to 1904.[37] It was only after World War I that doctor Ioan Bordea published a general report for the years 1905 to 1922.[38] Such multi-year reports have the advantage of offering synthetic data and overviews across the entire Kingdom of Romania, but their weakness is the lack of direct information, first-hand observations and local detail on what was a multi-faceted and complex reality.

---

34  In Romanian: Consiliul Sanitar Superior.
35  Felix, *Raport general despre igiena publică și despre serviciul sanitar ale Regatului României pe anul 1892*, v.
36  Doctor Felix wrote and published general reports for the period 1892 to 1897.
37  Obregia, *Raport general asupra igienei publice și asupra serviciului sanitar al Regatului României pe anii 1898-1904.*
38  Bordea, *Serviciul sanitar al României.*

The reports in this category, as the ones I discussed above, are formulaic documents that offer standardized images about, for example, the "salubriousness of villages." This is one of them, written by doctor Iacob Felix: "In general, our peasant will not keep his yard clean, nor collect dung in a corner to use as manure; in a word, many of our villages are still in a barbarous state."[39] As for the urban areas, the same doctor noted in 1895 a state of affairs that is still a familiar sight in today's Romania. "In all towns, without exception," wrote the doctor, "outlying suburbia are neglected, side streets remain unpaved, whereas the city center is usually groomed with some care, even with some sense of luxury. There is no available funding for marginal suburbia, which are left languishing in the barbarous state they are in. This is because budgets are also allocated with a sense of luxury, with new projects being created incessantly and no money left for the materials and labor needed for public works." For example, the municipality of Iaşi arranged for an "elegant bath establishment" to be built, which, however, could not function because there was no running water. Craiova, an unhealthy town that lacked basic services such as water supply, a sewage system and street paving, acquired electric illumination ahead of all of these as a priority.[40] Such examples are part of a long-term pattern in the administration of towns and counties in Romania.

## The Reports of Public Health Inspectors

1885 was a good year in terms of the volume of sources that concern us here. As we have seen, changes to the Health Act required the publication of county doctors' reports in *Monitorul Oficial*. In addition, changes to Art. 22[41] of the Health Act required members of the Higher Medical Council to perform annual inspections and compile reports for publication in the *Monitor*

---

39  Felix, *Raport general despre igiena ... pe anul 1892*, 91.
40  Ibid., 179.
41  "Art. 22. The members of the Higher Medical Council will inspect the entire civilian health system, as well as public and private medical establishments, and will make suggestions to the minister for addressing the shortcomings they observe in their circumscriptions. Each member of the Higher Medical Council will inspect all the health services in his circumscription once a year; any member who fails to perform the inspection and draw up a report within a month from the end of the year, will have his membership terminated. The report on the inspection will be published in Monitorul Oficial. There will be specific regulations on the catchment area of each circumscription and guidelines for the inspection." *Monitorul Oficial*, April 3, 1885, 35.

*Oficial.*[42] Each doctor had four counties allocated to him, which he had to in-spect during the summer. Each report had its own individual tone, imparted by the issuers, who were the period's most prominent health practitioners. Accompanied by the prefect and the county medical officer, these eminent doctors, the *crème de la crème* of Romanian medicine in the late nineteenth century, went from town to town and from village to village: for exam-ple, the doctors Iacob Felix and D. Sergiu, Nicolae Măldărescu and Nico-lae Kalederu, Grigore Romniceanu and Iuliu Theodori. The outcomes were commensurate to their prestige: the reports were replete with abundant in-formation on the functioning of the health system and the levels of salubri-ousness and public health in villages and cities. For example, in the summer of 1886, doctor Sergiu, the director of the Health Services of the Romanian Kingdom, visited the village of Batogu in Brăila county, which he found gen-erally "impoverished, [with] badly constructed and unhygienic houses, and untidy streets and courtyards."[43] Not all the villages in Brăila county dis-pleased doctor Sergiu, who also reported on visiting villages with a "clean and pleasant" aspect, with "straight and well-maintained" streets and "solid, healthy" housing.[44] It is difficult to ignore the binary categorial oppositions used by the doctor in his description. The general aspect of the village is good/bad, the streets are straight/irregular, clean/dirty, the houses good/bad and the courtyards clean/dirty; hence the rather stereotypical format of the descriptions.

Whereas the town of Brăila by and large receives a positive appraisal, Călăraşi does not fare so well. The doctor notes that there, "as in most of our towns, public hygiene leaves much to be desired."[45] The town has unpaved and pot-holed streets, dusty in the summer and clogged by mud in the au-tumn. The rudimentary street-cleaning equipment means that only "two of the main streets are clean," the rest being left to suffer from the inhabitants' unhealthy habit of dumping "the debris and rubbish from their courtyards" out into the streets.[46] It was by all accounts a public health and sanitary di-

---

42  Another change in the Health Act of 1893 would eliminate both the inspections and the resulting reports. See "Lege Sanitară," in *Buletinul Direcţiunei Generale a Serviciului Sanitar,* year V, 1893, no. 12, 177–218.

43  Sergiu, *Raportul D-lui dr. Sergiu,* 1306.

44  Ibid.

45  Ibid., 1307.

46  Ibid.

saster. The grim picture is reiterated for every village and every town visited. Although all doctors by and large observed the algorithm of the report format, occasionally there are significant discrepancies. For example, as we have seen, doctor Sergiu used the typical formula for between twelve and twenty-two villages in every county he inspected, while doctor Felix offered only a general overview of hygiene levels and public health among the rural population.[47] It is in the latter type of report that the subjectivity of the writer comes to the fore. To mention doctor Sergiu again, he gives a fairly positive account of the work of district doctors. In stark contrast, doctor Felix would rather see this role, which he deems rather useless, abolished. His comments are worth quoting in full: "The services of district practitioners leave a lot to be desired; in many places, the role has degenerated into a mere formality with no content. The doctor reports to the village hall, asks the mayor whether there are any known ailments in the village, and the complacent mayor answers most of the time that all inhabitants are healthy. The doctor then fills in a form which certifies that he was present in the village and leaves without visiting the hamlets that comprise the village."[48] Without exception, all members of the Higher Medical Council were horrified by various aspects of public health and hygiene encountered during their inspection. Thus, doctor Iuliu Teodori noted in 1887 that at the "county-communal hospital in Huși"—a misnomer, certainly, as it had been built as "private accommodation"—the lavatories were "badly built, old, inadequately cleaned and clogged with decomposing matter which causes mephitic pollution; they are used by both sexes. There is no evidence of the use of disinfectants. [...] As the lavatories open directly onto the hospital's main corridor, the air in the wards and in the entire establishment is polluted by the mephitic odors emanating from the latrines every time the door opens."[49] In other words, the odors of excrements filled the "atmosphere" of the Huși hospital.

Doctor A. Fotino used a mildly ironic tone to paint a profoundly negative picture of hygiene standards in the harbor town of Brăila. His unforgiving gaze noticed everything:

---

47  Ibid., 965–66.
48  Ibid., 964.
49  Teodori, *Raportul*, 1805–6.

Considering Brăila without its spacious boulevards and its straight, wide streets, but only in terms of public—and to a large extent private—hygiene, it would be an extraordinary city indeed. Even King Street, the city's main street, is kept clean only along a small segment. Wherever there are stores, the pavements have been transformed in Eastern bazaars, where piles of merchandise block the traffic and cleanliness is totally ignored. On the more peripheral streets, people choke in dust in the summer, and drown in mud when it rains or when the winter snows thaw. The streets everywhere, and particularly in front of inns and taverns, are covered in unwholesome refuse. Public marketplaces, and the so-called people's market in particular, are dirty, a sad icon of official concern for the health of the nation. Fisheries are a real threat to the town's general hygiene and it is to be wondered why the communal authority should allow the building of fish warehouses close to the city center."[50]

This sounds like a profoundly disillusioned picture of the state of the town of Brăila in the summer of 1891.

The reports of these high medical authorities are scathing condemnations of the unimaginable levels of squalor in Romania's villages and towns in the late nineteenth century.

### The Reports of the Metropolitan Health and Sanitary Services

With the annual reports of the health and sanitary services of the city of Bucharest, we enter the realm of public health in the urban environment proper. Fortunately for us, for a long period the "head medic of the village" was doctor Iacob Felix, who, from 1868 to 1891, published detailed reports almost on an annual basis.

As already noted, modernization in the area of hygiene, sanitation and public health is a long-term process, still continuing today. Progress in this area is easier to measure over a half-century period rather than over a mere decade. Because of specific patterns of modernization in the region, any progress in terms of modernizing the sanitary and public health services in urban Romania was first visible at the center, the capital city Bucharest. However, Bucharest underwent significant change between 1869 and the early twenti-

---

50    Fotino, *Raportul d-lui dr. Fotino… în anul 1891*, 337.

eth century. First of all, there was a demographic growth of 100 per cent during this interval. According to doctor Felix's statistics, the population of the city stood at 150,000 in the last year of the seventh decade,[51] whereas doctor Gh. Orleanu estimated that the city's population in 1906 was 292,395.[52] One of the measures of progress in sanitation is the quality of the street hygiene services. When reviewing the street cleaning services in 1869, doctor Felix noted that residents threw out domestic refuse in the streets "wherever it pleases [them]," and that street-sweepers in their turn dumped the collected rubbish "wherever it suits them best."[53] Forty-seven years later, the city of Bucharest was equipped with two rubbish incinerators.[54] While progress was visible, the results were patchy: the city center was hygienized by 1891, but the peripheries remained insalubrious.[55] The year 1891 also saw the experimental introduction in twenty residential buildings of the modern sewage disposal system still in use today. And it worked.

## The Reports of Doctors from Rural Hospitals

In 1881, the national health care system acquired a new institution: the rural hospital. In the new system, any peasant who got sick could resort to the services of the district practitioners or go to a rural hospital, if there was one in the area. An ambitious building programme launched in the last two decades of the nineteenth century resulted in each county having one rural hospital by the century's end. The doctors in these establishments, too, had the obligation of issuing annual reports, some of which were published in the period's medical journals. These reports focus on the "movements of patients within the hospital" and the clinical aspects of the conditions being treated. In other words, at first sight they might appear to be of lesser interest to the historian. However, they should not be dismissed as entirely irrelevant. We shall try to demonstrate this relevance with two examples of reports from the rural hospital of Horezu, compiled by two doctors who went on to build distinguished careers in the Kingdom's health service: doctors Vasile Bianu and I.V. Ştefănescu. For the historian of the nineteenth century, the most inter-

---

51 Felix, *Serviţiul sanitar al comunei Bucuresci*, 19.
52 Orleanu, *Raport general asupra igienei*, 147.
53 Felix, *Serviţiul sanitar al comunei Bucuresci*, 24.
54 Orleanu, *Raport general asupra igienei*, 126.
55 Felix "Ordinul circular sub no. 10850," 12.

esting aspect of doctor Bianu's report is his description of the hospital building itself. It was one of the earliest rural hospitals to be created and as such it did not have a dedicated building but was accommodated in a former monastery. Hence the many shortcomings of the venue, which doctor Bianu lists in some detail. The lavatories had doors that opened onto the wards, preventing natural ventilation in the summer. The bathrooms were conspicuous by their absence: "[O]ne cannot call *bathroom* a small room without sufficient space to accommodate a tub and a bed. Well, our hospital has only one small, dark room, without heating and containing one single wooden bathtub, serving a hospital with fifty-six beds."[56] This was hardly adequate, considering that each patient had to be washed and undergo disinfestation when admitted.

Whereas doctor Bianu offered a near-photographic account of a rural hospital in 1888, doctor Ştefănescu claimed that, two years earlier and in the same hospital, he had had an experience of ultimate alterity, and as a result he constructed his entire report around representations of otherness. Doctor Ştefănescu left his readers in no doubt that he was confronted with a habitat of unmitigated barbarity. Agriculture was performed "with primitive means," the roads were "in a rudimentary state and trade was basic."[57] As for his depiction of the "natives," the doctor's palette is dark: they spoke a "rough, impoverished" language, and their gestures for affirmation and negation were the opposite of the established ones: they nodded when they meant "no" and shook their heads to indicate "yes."[58] In a word, the peasants he treated at the rural hospital were not too different, he commented, from the Fuegians "whom anthropologists place within the lowest order of humanity."[59] Doctor Ştefănescu needed no further proof that the peasants were strange, primitive, barbarous beings. He believed that they differed profoundly from individuals like himself and, by extension, from the "educated classes," because they had features contravening commonly accepted core values of "Civilization," for example their "aberrant affective faculties such as: lack of shame, proclivity to bestial amorous relations [...], and vices such as: drunkenness, sloth, stealing, lying and, in women especially, a love of luxury."[60] There was no empathy between doctor Ştefănescu and his rural patients: the doctor did not

---

56  Bianu, "Spitalul rural Horezu," 278.
57  Ştefănescu, "Raport asupra mişcării bolnavilor," 362.
58  Ibid., 363–64.
59  Ibid., 378.
60  Ibid., 379.

understand them and only had a profound contempt for them—as suggested by the derisive and ironic tone of his narrative. One can easily imagine that the peasants in their turn responded in kind.

What is certain is that doctor Ştefănescu's views on the peasants and the rural world were not exceptional in this period, and there are other examples. Even in today's culture and language, "peasant" and "rural" are not deemed to be attributes of modernity. And let's not forget that to be called a "peasant", then as now, carried with it negative connotations.

### The Reports of Regimental Medical Personnel

A special sub-category were the reports of regimental medics, a small portion of which were published in the only periodical of the army's medical services, *Revista Sanitară Militară* [Army medical review]. Here, too, we are faced with the over-arching question that informs this study: what is the utility of these documents as historical sources? A possible answer is offered by the analysis of the thirteen such reports available to us: they contain data about many aspects of sanitation and health in army barracks and the enforcement of army regulations in the realm of hygiene. The vast majority of the recruits were young peasants who needed to be trained to observe the comparatively modern prescriptions on health and hygiene at the barracks.

Generally speaking, the discourse of the public health reports as a whole is predominantly negative and focuses on failures to observe sanitary norms rather than on compliance. The regimental health reports are no exception. For example, we learn that in 1897, the new barracks of the 34th Regiment in Constanţa had lavatories fitted in the soldiers' quarters, in place of the older, outdoor privies. Surely this was a good sign, one might say, but let's not jump to conclusions, because the new toilets were "locked and had a sentinel at the door, so they were opened only exceptionally at night if needed by a soldier who was ill."[61] We do not know why this was done in Constanţa, but we are given more details for the barracks of the 1st Regiment in Mehedinţi, where the indoors latrines were "locked during the day and the night" because they were flooded by water infiltrating from the surrounding marshy terrain.[62]

---

61  Crăiniceanu, *Dare de seamă asupra stărei sanitare*, 361–62.
62  Carp, *Dare de seamă asupra stărei sanitare*, 381–82.

Regarding soldiers' personal hygiene, army regulations prescribed one weekly bath. But we know from some of the regimental medics' reports that this was still not possible in all the barracks in late nineteenth-century Romania. In fact, the weekly ablutions of the troops posed huge problems: at Ploieşti, for instance, the garrisoned men "were sent to some old public baths, because the municipal baths did not accept soldiers; an order was then sent from the top to authorize regiments to send the men to use the baths of the military hospital [...] in Bucharest."[63] However, there remained one tiny problem to solve: at the time, the entire Bucharest garrison sent its troops to have their weekly bath at the Military Hospital!

*\*\**

It has probably become apparent by now that the medical reports as historical sources are important for several reasons and research areas. Of these, I would single out the modernization of the Romanian rural world as a major—and still under-researched—line of enquiry. As all the public health reports cover the rural environment, they are indispensable sources for many aspects of peasant life and culture. For instance, the foods and dietary habits of peasants in the latter half of the nineteenth century have been largely left aside in ethnographic studies. As a result, ethnographic bibliographies mainly cite medical sources in their sections on "alimentation."[64] The reports are authored by doctors who were in close contact with the peasants and thus gained first-hand knowledge of rural lifestyles, a knowledge which can be used by historians to complement the data from other types of sources. However, one should guard against imagining that the contact and the gaze are innocent, that *the doctors see and describe factual reality*. The medical discourse was strongly ideologized and informed by the cultural and educational backgrounds of the doctors, as well as by the Romanian elites' stereotypes of and prejudices against the peasants. Throughout the nineteenth century, these elites constructed and drew on a two-tiered body of representations of the peasant and the rural world: one type of imagery depicted the peasant as the native representative of the nation's true

63    Crăiniceanu, *Raport General asupra stărei sanitare*, 48.
64    See Fochi, *Bibliografia generală a etnografiei şi folclorului românesc*, vol. I (1800–1891), 86–90.

identity,[65] while the other saw the peasant as the savage within society in acute need of civilizing. Within the "indigenous noble paradigm," the peasant is the country's foundation (in Romanian: *talpa ţării*, meaning, literally, the "country's feet," its foothold), the base of the national body, ultimately signifying that *the peasants are us, we are all peasants*. However, the medical discourse on the peasant and his world as it appears in the health reports derives from the opposite paradigm, namely, that of the peasant as "savage."

These reports also reveal in exemplary fashion the divergence between health legislation and its actual implementation. The lawmaker is chiefly interested in producing a coherent and modern medical discourse and only marginally in the applicability of the law. This is especially obvious for the health regulations aimed at the rural population.[66]

One of the greatest virtues of the health reports is the level of detail the descriptions contain about the workings of the health system at all levels and their unsparing attention to its failings. They show, for example, the district doctor on his perpetual health rounds in the countryside; we see doctor Sabin, the chief medical officer of Vâlcea county, in open conflict with the mayor of Orleşti, a conflict which worked against him until 1887, when he finally refused to continue his inspections in the village; we see members of the Higher Medical Council doing the annual summer rounds of villages, chaperoned by the county medical officer and the prefect. Here is a comprehensive professional corps inspecting, studying and attempting to modernize the huge peasant masses, obviously with the declared purpose of supporting the period's national ideological programme of reducing morbidity and mortality among the rural population. Making a contribution to demographic growth in the countryside meant implicitly encouraging general population growth in Romania.

The health reports focus mainly on the negative aspects of public hygiene and are informed by an undisguised agenda for "improvement." Health and hygiene conditions in the towns and villages of nineteenth-century Romania were probably not much better than suggested by the reports, and I am not claiming that they were. Nevertheless, the documents in this category

---

65  See Mihăilescu, *Antropologie. Cinci introduceri*, 18–19.
66  See, for example, Bărbulescu and Popovici, *Modernizarea lumii rurale*, 56–60, for the application of the "Regulamentul pentru alinierea satelor şi pentru construcţia locuinţelor ţărăneşti" [Regulations on the alignment of village streets and the construction of peasant dwellings].

must be read critically, and in the context of their production and reception. The higher up the authors were in the health system hierarchy, the more negative the reports. The reason for this was because the gap between expectations and the reality on the ground increased in proportion with the rank and position of the observer. A district doctor was far less critical of the levels of pubic hygiene and health than a member of the Higher Medical Council on his annual summer inspection, and the reports visibly display this difference in perspective. In addition, because the reports offer a static image of public health, a snapshot captured at circumscription level, the only way to make sense of them historically is by studying them serially. For example, looking at annual county-level reports, you may get the impression—just like the authors themselves—that nothing ever changed here and there was no progress: you encounter the same reluctant peasants, the same complacent communal authorities, the same squalor everywhere. The shifts in personnel meant that, as doctors moved from one circumscription to another, continuity was lost, and progress was no longer observable: the new doctor started from scratch and produced the same negative reports, lacking a longer- or medium-term perspective. Reality as seen by a young graduate of the medical school may often appear much more negative than that of a senior doctor who grew old in his post in the same circumscription. And yet, they observed the same reality. Doctors themselves had a sense of the faultlines and hidden traps in what were supposed to be "scientific" documents. In 1910, doctor Radu Chernbach from the communal hospital in Huşi went as far as to demolish the credibility of this type of scientific literature, which, he wrote, encouraged the

> [...] idea in our country that all our peasants are ridden with pellagra, tumors, syphilis and neurological disorders; one after another, doctors kept producing official statistics collected at the village fête showing that all those seen there suffered from pellagra, TB, syphilis, or granular conjunctivitis. It looked as though they were vying with each other in showing the greatest number of sick, infirm and degenerate people, and the public watched this macabre sport with smiling contempt for the competing authors of that turgid prose which even reached the pages of *Monitorul Oficial*. Today, we still encounter echoes and atavistic legacies of that literature of disasters, but they are rare, and the official statistics presented by these improvised med-

ical scientists are of a falseness to despair of. Every [case of] gastritis, every stomach upset, every feverish labial herpes was palustral, every solar erythema was pellagric, every conjunctivitis was granular. This means that the statistics were inflated with thousands of cases of pellagra, paludism, and granular conjunctivitis. Nowadays, in certain regions, there is a race to have as many cases of syphilis registered as possible, which means that every genital ulcer, every periostitis and osteitis, every cardiac lesion etc. is caused by syphilis. And the obligatory, fashionable treatment for all these is an intramuscular injection with mercury."[67]

From the heights of the medical science of 1910, doctor Chernbach could easily afford to criticize his peers who, three decades earlier, saw in each ailment the illnesses that were "fashionable" in their time. But he forgets that, between 1880 and 1901, medicine had been revolutionized. As far as today's historian is concerned, it matters little whether doctor Chernbach was right or not. What is more important is that, after 1880, the specter of pellagra, bandied about by the medical corps, did indeed haunt the country's rural areas. As we shall see later, pellagra became a real national health threat. This serves as a reminder that the public health reports did not simply record the "reality in the field" but also society's imagined or projected fears, which were as important as factual "reality."

---

67  Chernbach, *Câteva scurte observații practice asupra serviciului*, 621–22.

2

## Doctors Remember

The reports and other documentation required by the health legislation were not the only texts produced by doctors. At their own initiative, in old age, some doctors chose to put pen to paper and reminisce about the medical practices in their active period or simply about the world in which they lived. Those caught up in the storms of "Big History" tried to make sense of the major events in which they took part by writing down and publishing their memories. Alongside the health reports, memoirs and personal narratives represent another way of looking at past lives and past times by authors who often produced both sets of narratives. The unique value of life narratives for the historian lies in the fact that the information they contain is often not to be found in other sources. They act like a photographic developer, revealing the hidden details in the fabric of Romanian society during this period. I have opted for a "long" nineteenth century perspective, extending to World War I. Most of the texts used in this chapter were published after 1918, but in general they narrate events from the previous decades. I have only used published texts and make no claim of having covered the entire corpus of Romanian medical memoirs, but I believe I have sourced a significant sample of the printed literature.

*"Having reached the twilight of life, I am haunted by memories"*

Even a cursory glance will show that the life narratives of doctors form a very diverse body of literature. Depending on the stated objectives, each doctor structured his writing differently. From the perspective of literary theory, all the texts discussed here are "self-referential writings."[68] Only a few of them can be included in the canon of the autobiography, defined by Philippe Lejeune as "a retrospective prose narrative written by an actual person about his or her own existence, with an emphasis on his or her individual life and in particular on the history of his or her personality."[69] Probably the only truly autobiographical work among those cited is the autobiography of doctor Victor Gomoiu, and some chapters in the recollections of

---

68  For a good introduction to the genres of self-referential literature, see Pop, *Memorie și suferință. Considerații asupra literaturii memorialistice a universului concentraționar comunist*, 33–59.

69  Lejeune, *Le pacte autobiographique*, 14.

doctor Constantin Dumitrescu Severeanu. All the other texts belong to related genres: memoirs and diaries. As our primary interest is not of a literary-theoretical order, I shall refer to this body of texts with the generic terms "memoirs" or "recollections." It is perhaps also worth noting that I shall not look at these narratives from the angle of the relations between "truth and mystification," the perspective used by Ana Selejan in a recent study of journals and memoirs by prominent literary figures of the period 1947 to 1970.[70] From our perspective, all these texts are to some extent a "mystification" of reality, in the sense that they are a reconstruction of the self for the benefit of others. In addition, the period covered by our medical texts (1840–1918) does not appear to be as ideologically "complicated" as the post-World War I period: aside from personal animosities, undeniably strong in some authors, the most pervasive influence on the doctors' texts is the nationalism that permeates their views of their professional status and practice.

But before attempting to identify the specific historical value of these sources, let's look at *the ways in which these texts are structured* and the *motivations* behind their writing. In other words, why and how did doctors write memoirs, and what were their sources?

Generally speaking, we can divide the literature into two main categories: biographical memoirs, in which the emphasis is on the author's own life story, and historical memoirs, which look at historical context and circumstance, and, if written in the nineteenth century, at processes of nation-building. In the latter category, the author is no longer the main character; he is a witness of Big History, especially in moments of crisis or tragedy. In 1926, doctor Vasile Bianu published two extensive volumes entitled *Însemnări din Războiul României Mari* (Notes on the war for Greater Romania), in which he wrote: "These *Notes* will help our valued readers form a fairly precise idea of the course of the War for Greater Romania. My most perfect reward will be if the reader derives from them moments of contentment and spiritual elevation."[71] It is obvious that the aim of the *Notes* is to transmit a message infused with ethical and national values through the narrative of the national epic of the Great War, in which the author, modestly, participated. At the other end of the spectrum, writing about the War of Indepen-

70   Selejan, *Adevăr și mistificare în jurnale și memorii apărute după 1989.*
71   Bianu, *Însemnari din războiul României Mari* I, 10.

dence (1877), doctor Gheorghe Sabin confessed ingenuously: "It had never crossed my mind to put pen to paper and write my impressions of the little over ten months I spent under the Flag during the War of Independence."[72] But his objective was as noble as that of doctor Bianu, and revenues from the sale of his memoirs were earmarked for the erection of a monument at Râmnicu Vâlcea[73] to commemorate the local soldiers who fell in Bulgaria during the war. Perhaps the best example of this type of historical memoir is doctor Nicolae Krețulescu's volume *Amintiri istorice* (Historical recollections). Doctor Krețulescu, who, quite surprisingly, explained that he had written the text "to please my friends,"[74] ended up writing a comprehensive history of the nineteenth century, in which he embedded many details of an autobiographical nature. Krețulescu, who was a major political figure in his time, wrote in order to place himself in the line of European politicians who had played an active role in history and wrote about it: "[I]n other countries [...] few are those—by this I mean men who played a political role in their country—who failed to maintain the useful tradition of keeping records of the events and circumstances of their lifetime, and of publishing them while they lived or leaving them within their families."[75] The War of Independence turned out to be a compelling historical milestone that deeply engaged the minds of doctors. Some, like Zaharia Petrescu,[76] kept daily logs of their participation in the campaign. Others, such as the afore-mentioned doctor Sabin and doctor Ludovic Fialla,[77] returned to it decades later and published their memoirs of the events.

Romania's participation in the second Balkan War, too, was covered in doctors' memoirs. Doctor Neculai Burghele, for example, treated with a sense of humor the Bulgarian campaign of 1913, which ended with many fatalities caused by cholera.[78] In contrast, doctor Dimitrie Gerota had a totally different perspective on the same 1913 campaign, a perspective that undoubtedly derived from the author's highly rebellious temperament.[79]

72   Sabin, *Amintiri din războiul Independenței*, ix.
73   Capital city of the county of Vâlcea in southern Romania.
74   Kretzulescu, *Amintiri istorice*, 5.
75   Ibid.
76   Albulescu and Brătescu, *Însemnările unui medic din Războiul pentru Independență. Jurnalul de campanie al lui Zaharia Petrescu.*
77   Fialla, *Reminiscențe din resbelul româno-ruso-turc.*
78   Burghele, *Amintiri din timpul războiului român-bulgar.*
79   Gerota, *Impresiuni și aprecieri din timpul acțiunei militare în Bulgaria.*

The narrative produced by doctor Panaite Zosin occupies a special place in the memoir canon: his text is first and foremost a manual of life teachings for his son and for young people in general. It was, in fact, a confession written in old age about the failure of a life, because doctor Zosin considered himself defeated. Expelled from high school for his socialist activism, arrested "several times"[80] as a student because of his political sympathies, he was tainted by the stigma of these episodes for the rest of his life. His youthful socialist activism became a serious handicap in his career, and it was only after the age of forty that he "chanced upon a full-time paid post."[81] His text is perhaps the most lucid exposition of the avatars of the political in a doctor's career.

Doctor Ştefan Episcopescu appears to be yet another of life's vanquished. He wrote his "secret memoirs" sometime between 1847 and 1850. The text, which remained unpublished until 1981, is likewise highly moralizing in tone. Whereas doctor Zosin's life was marred by the negative outcomes of his youthful political orientation, the misfortune in doctor Episcopescu's life had more prosaic causes: an uninspired marital choice. Towards the end of his life, doctor Episcopescu decided to leave behind for posterity a written account of the "little drama" of his unhappy marriage. He was obviously keen to preserve for eternity his own version of his noble intentions and his lifelong, ultimately failed, efforts to save the marriage. His wife, the daughter of the *medelnicer*[82] Matei Ciupelniceanu, never wrote her memoirs, so her verdict on her marriage to doctor Episcopescu remains unknown. What we do know, however, is that, as she lay dying, eighteen years after the divorce, she did not call on her former spouse, a doctor, to be "in attendance"[83] at her deathbed. From our perspective, the troubles of doctor Episcopescu's marriage have to take second place to other facts in his life: for example, his statement that, upon his return from studies in Vienna in 1805, as a young doctor, he managed to amass a fairly significant fortune simply from his medical practice: "Every day I could afford to get two pairs of carriage horses and a riding horse, had an income of twenty-three golden

---

80   Zosin *Calea unei vieţi*, 17.
81   Ibid., 18
82   Second-rank dignitary at the court of Romania's ruling princes from the early modern period to the mid-nineteenth century. [Translator's note]
83   Gheorghiu, "'Memoria de taină' a lui Şt. V. Episcopescu," 311.

ducats and enjoyed a brilliant train of life."[84] By 1847, when he was writing, those happy youthful days must have seemed very remote. The doctor's rationale for writing is also worth noting. He earned an entire chapter in Constanţa Vintilă-Ghiţulescu's book *Evgheniţi, ciocoi, mojici*[85] due to his memoir, which he wrote and published for very mundane reasons: "Seeing that my income had diminished, and being burdened with children and added expenses, I used what was left of my rest time after the daily rounds and filled [...] a few sheets."[86] These "sheets" turned him into one of the best-known doctors of the first half of the nineteenth century. We should not be fooled by such modesty: doctor Episcopescu was very much aware of the power of the written and printed word, and this earns his text an inclusion in our body of memoirs written by doctors.

Returning to our analysis, it is worth remembering that, at the time of publication, most of the doctors who wrote historical memoirs were more than just doctors, having become involved in politics at some stage in their careers. On the cover of his *Însemnări* [Notes], doctor Bianu is introduced not only as "Army Reserve Colonel and Doctor and former chief medic of' the I.C. Brătianu Hospital in Buzău," but also, significantly, as 'Senator for Huedin." Doctor Sabin is simply presented as the "prefect of Vâlcea County." In 1892, when he published his memoirs of the War of Independence, the old doctor Fialla used the title page to showcase a lifetime of achievements and honors as "[s]enior professor of anatomy and chief surgeon of the civilian hospitals of Bucharest. Former chief surgeon of Red Cross mobile hospitals in Turnu-Măgurele in the year of the war. Awarded medals for active combat in the War for Romanian Independence. Officer of the Star of Romania. Commander of several orders, etc., etc." This shows to what extent published historical memoirs were a way of legitimizing their authors' social prestige. At the same time, we should not underestimate the powerful patriotic and national sentiment, which might sound old-fashioned today, but was felt to inform the actions and writings of historical agents in the nineteenth century. The legitimizing function of memoirs was not something that only individuals harnessed to boost their status. The state, too, used the publication of such *testimonials* to buttress its own national ideology and

---

84  Ibid., 307.
85  Vintilă-Ghiţulescu, *Evgheniţi, ciocoi, mojici*, 273–96.
86  Gheorghiu, "'Memoria de taină,'" 309.

sense of historical mission. For example, the memoirs of doctor Fialla were re-issued in a special edition in 1906,[87] while Zaharia Petrescu's campaign diary was re-issued for the centenary of the war of independence in 1977 as a "tribute to the Romanian regimental medics who, in the war of 1877–1878, made admirable efforts to safeguard health, offer comfort and save the lives of our brave soldiers."[88]

At the opposite end of the spectrum are autobiographical memoirs, which foreground the authors' lives against the backdrop of the period's social and historical context. The best example of this type of life narrative is that of doctor Vasile Gomoiu, published in a six-volume edition in 2006.[89] It is unfortunate that the editors offered no information about the manuscripts they used for this edition of a text that is otherwise full of fascinating detail. This category also includes memoirs by the doctor Constantin Dumitrescu Severeanu, another narrative with the pervasive moralizing ethos of a conduct manual for the young: "Later, the idea occurred to me that perhaps it would not be such a bad thing to add a narrative of the small events which marked my life from tender childhood to venerable old age, if this would be of benefit to some of the children who read this and, taking me as an example, strove to do similar things, and even endeavored to do better. Should any of them find anything bad here, let them not do like me, but take only the good things and derive some profit from them, like I did: I learned from others how to avoid bad deeds and how to strive to do good."[90] Doctor Ioan Bordea reminisces nostalgically about his years as a young village doctor: "Having reached the twilight of life, I am haunted by memories of my years as a rural doctor, and a mysterious power seems to urge me to write about those times, so that I might revisit the idealism and continuous, selfless toil by which I tried to serve and enlighten my people."[91]

Thus, writing your memoirs—and not only in doctor Bordea's case—means revisiting the past and at the same time putting before others a sense of mission and meaning to your life. Consequently, no memoir or life narrative is innocent: it is in fact a tool for constructing identity and manipulating posterity. The texts vary widely in terms of ingredients and dosage for the

87 Fialla, *Reminiscențe din resbelul româno-ruso-turc anul 1877.*
88 Ibid., 3.
89 Gomoiu, *Viața mea (memorii).*
90 Severeanu, *Din amintirile mele* I, 9.
91 Bordea, *Zile trăite*, 3.

type of identity built with an eye to eternity. Some authors see themselves as the forgers of modern Romania, others as eyewitnesses and minor contributors to Big History, and yet others present themselves as average "men amongst men." But they all wish to legitimize social status, or a way of acting and, ultimately, living.

It is now time to look at the record-keeping habits of the memoirists. In the late nineteenth century, Nicolae Kreţulescu deplored the Romanians' lack of a tradition of diary-keeping: "[V]ery few people in our country, I think, have had or have the habit of noting down—if not daily, at least occasionally—facts and events as they unfold,"[92] adding that he was one of these few. However, there is evidence that shows that some of the memoirs we are looking at were based on at least partial jottings committed to paper as the events were in progress. Here is doctor Sabin, for example, in his narrative of the War of Independence, explaining that he wrote down "what happened around me, what I saw and felt, with the help of an old notebook which went with me everywhere during the war and which I subsequently preserved like a holy relic at the bottom of an old chest. I cannot recall why I started writing in it, but I did note down almost day by day facts and events of some importance, as well as minute details which later slipped my mind entirely."[93] Doctor Severeanu wrote in the same vein: "[A]t the time when I entered the Medical School at Mihai Vodă under its director, Doctor Carol Davila, I happened upon an old ledger which someone had abandoned in a corner and, out of instinct, without anyone to tell me so, I took it and started writing in it every day, more or less in earnest. I wrote about students' pranks, about things overheard as we were marched off to the front under the command of some under-officer, or about hilarious incidents at lectures. I kept many notes from that time, which I am now entering in *My Recollections.*"[94] However, doctor Bianu's *Însemnări* were, to a greater extent than similar works by his peers, written on the basis of daily notations, entered under their respective dates even in the final text: "[T]hese day-by-day *Notes* cover things seen, heard, read about and extracted from newspapers and journals during the holy war for the union of our nation [in Romanian: *războiul sfânt de întregire a neamului*], alongside the author's own comments

---

92  Kretzulescu *Amintiri istorice,* 3.
93  Sabin, *Amintiri din războiul Independenţei,* xi–xii.
94  Severeanu, *Din amintirile mele* I, 9.

on his feelings and states of mind."[95] Like doctor Bianu, doctor Neculai Burghele chose to write down daily entries in his account of the sixty-day campaign in Bulgaria in 1913.[96]

Keeping a diary was perhaps more widespread than doctor Nicolae Krețulescu presumed. But, whether written from daily notes or not, doctors' memoirs are based largely on *memory* and claim to recount events which were *seen*, *heard* or *read-about* by the authors. In addition, doctor Bianu embedded in his narrative first-hand oral and written accounts of the fighting on the Romanian front in Moldova (1917) by participants, at the time wounded and placed under the doctor's care in military hospitals.

### "Doctor, scratch me"

Let's now return to the proposed object of our research, which is the use of medical memoirs as sources for the study of medicine in the nineteenth century. In their life narratives, doctors address many topics of interest to the historian. A major such topic is the status of the doctor—the district doctor in particular, who was constantly on the move to the villages in his circumscription. This is how doctor Ioan Bordea recalls his weekly routine as a junior country doctor: "I would start on Monday morning very early and return Saturday evening, with my body broken by all the journeying along very bad roads and my heart burdened with the endless pain, needs and injustices which I saw only too well, but for which most of the time I could offer no remedy apart from a kind word."[97] The countless—and largely ineffectual—inspections district doctors had to carry out and, more generally, the precariousness of their position, stand out as a major grievance in several other sources. Apart from the difficulties inherent in their lowly position in the hierarchy of the health system, district doctors were also often harassed by the local notables. Doctor Bordea enjoyed the support of a well-connected local landowner with "much influence at the Ministry of the Interior,"[98] but others often risked losing their jobs "because the doctor, being paid by the county, could lose his job even when he was supported by

---

95  Bianu, *Însemnari din războiul României Mari* I, 10.
96  Burghele, *Amintiri din timpul războiului român-bulgar*.
97  Bordea, *Zile trăite*, 6.
98  Ibid., 16.

the General Directorate of the health system, who had appointed him; the prefect, who allocated local budgets and had administrative powers, could abolish the circumscription of a so-called troublesome doctor, thereby abolishing his post. Two or three months later, he reinstated the circumscription and requested the appointment of another doctor. In effect, the district doctor was powerless, while the prefect could do as he pleased."[99] In addition, district doctors often declared themselves powerless in the face of the period's major health challenges in the rural world, especially when confronted with epidemics. Doctor Bordea's entire life was marred by his sense of powerlessness as he took part in a rural drama in which the savior character, the doctor, was unable to do much, apart from offering advice and suggesting primitive means of disinfection with lye and lime, methods which were hardly adequate.[100] The junior district doctor's sense of powerlessness and frustration is more than palpable in Bordea's memoirs.

Higher up in the hierarchy of the health system we find the junior doctor Victor Gomoiu, as an intern at Professor Gheorghe Stoicescu's clinic at Colţea Hospital in Bucharest. He had his fair share of professional surprises, but he managed to see them off successfully, judging from an episode he recalled. He wrote:

It was in early May of this year, 1908, that Professor Stoicescu called me to his office at the hospital, asking me to do him a favor and visit the village of Vişina to look after a good friend of his, Mr. Bălescu, who had had an accident. The patient was going to pay well—twenty *lei*[101] per day—and the Professor asked me "to stay with him until he was fully recovered." During this period, I was going to be relieved of my hospital duties on order of the chief himself. My chief's request was compelling, and the patient's pay was attractive. I alighted from the train at the destination, and from there the "boyar's"[102] carriage conveyed me to his "court." [...] As the recovery process evolved quite rapidly, the boyar started receiving the visits of the villagers. One Sunday afternoon, as I was reading in the garden, a man came to tell me that the "boyar wanted to see me." As I entered the room, which was full of villagers,

99   Ibid., 15.
100  Ibid., 21–22.
101  Sg. *leu*, pl. *lei* = national currency in the Kingdom of Romania.
102  Boyar is the term used to designate the Romanian old-regime noble elites.

the "boyar" uncovered his voluminous belly and ordered: "Doctor, scratch me." He wished to show to all those assembled—people whom he normally ordered about—that he even had a "doctor" there, ready to do his bidding. Faced with such insolence, I stopped on the threshold and, turning towards the corridor, I called out to his wife: "Lady, come and scratch your swine." You should have seen the faces of the boyar and his visitors. I went out and sought the boyar's son, asking for a carriage to take me to the station. In vain did the boyar try to apologize for his rudeness. Without even waiting for the fee which was due to me, I chose to return to Bucharest.[103]

The liberal professions, including medicine, did not carry significant social prestige in mid-nineteenth century Romania. Nicolae Krețulescu's memoirs make this abundantly clear. This is what he has to say about his return from Paris, armed with his new degree from the School of Medicine:

A few days after my arrival in Bucharest, I went to pay my respects to Prince Alexandru Ghica,[104] who had known me prior to my departure for Paris, before he became ruling prince. Prince Ghica received me most affably, and the first question he asked amiably was "what had been my reason for studying medicine, an occupation for which I was not suited, for I was better off following in the footsteps of my parents and grandparents," to which I replied that the old days were long gone and it was time for us to join the ranks of civilized nations, and that my aim in studying medicine was to raise the status of the liberal professions, held in such contempt in our country, and show that being a doctor, a pharmacist, an engineer or an artist should not only be deemed suitable for foreigners.[105]

We may presume that Prince Ghica was not particularly impressed with the answer. Bucharest society in general was quite bemused by the professional choice of young Krețulescu, the son of a high-ranking boyar: "[O]ne evening, some time after my arrival in Bucharest, I went over to present my medical doctor's diploma to the medical commission; the members of the commission took it in turns to consider the document with attention and

---

103 Gomoiu, *Viața mea*, vol. 1, 235–36.
104 Ruling prince of Wallachia between 1834 and 1842.
105 Kretzulescu, *Amintiri istorice*, 56–57.

intense curiosity. Like everybody else in Bucharest, they wondered why the son of a grand boyar—the term used at the time—should abandon his position in society and go make a doctor of himself."[106]

The fact that scions of the top echelons of the native nobility should embrace liberal professions was met everywhere—in the capital city of Bucharest and the provinces alike, and by everybody, from the ruling prince to the corner shop retailer—with amazement and even consternation. In this process, young men such as Krețulescu abandoned the best and most sought-after positions in the period's social hierarchy in favor of socially less prestigious, but modern, roles.[107] Not many people were prepared to accept the change in ethos. Krețulescu was not the only one to opt for this change, as he himself wrote in his memoir:

> Alexandru Golescu-Arăpilă, who had returned to his native country with a civil engineering degree from the École Centrale in Paris, had just been appointed to oversee the building of a carriageway from Ploiești to Câmpina. Around July 1844, wishing for a change of scene, I obtained a leave and left Bucharest to join him as he travelled to his new project. We hired a carriage by the day; as we arrived at an inn near Băicoi, the coachman asked to rest his horses, so we stopped in the shade of the carriage to have our lunch. At the same time, two merchants travelling like us towards Câmpina and resting on the inn's shaded veranda, were looking us up and down and commented: "Look and behold what became of the sons of boyars, there's a Golescu who is now a road surveyor and a Krețulescu who works as a doctor." We overheard their conversation, barely able to contain our amusement.[108]

The choice of a medical career by the son of a high-ranking boyar in the mid-nineteenth century was largely regarded as incompatible with the family's social prestige, but it became an emblem of a rapid upward mobility for the son of a country priest in Mehedinți County at the start of the following century. It is also true that, between 1840 and 1900, the social prestige of the doctor and of medicine as a science had increased apace with processes of

---

106 Ibid., 58.
107 On the adoption of liberal professions by the sons of the native nobility, one can consult with profit the beautifully written sub-chapter "Boier fără slujbă, doctor fără voie" [Boyar without a function, doctor against one's will] in the afore-cited study by Vintilă-Ghițulescu, *Evgheniți, ciocoi, mojici*, 89–96.
108 Kretzulescu, *Amintiri istorice*, 58–59.

modernization in Romania. By the early twentieth century, in cities at least, the doctor had become an admired professional whose services were much in demand. This change in perspective is best illustrated by the testimony of another celebrated author of memoirs. Constantin Bacalbaşa, a journalist and politician, but not a doctor, describes the arrival in Bucharest, in 1906, of doctor Norden, who had been called to consult King Carol I. The German doctor found himself overwhelmed by demands: "Half of the residents of the capital city sought an appointment. The German scholar had to turn away hundreds of people for lack of enough time."[109] While the circumstances surrounding the episode are exceptional, the anecdote itself is significant.

Another domain of medicine well documented in memoirs is surgery. As is well known, before the introduction of aseptic techniques, surgical procedures posed huge risks to patients, and this is the reason why in 1840 few doctors took up surgery as a specialism, as doctor Kreţulescu explains: "At that time in Bucharest, surgery was in the same state as today in the East; the idea of surgery as a science did not exist; surgical instruments were mere ornaments on display in hospital cabinets; they languished there, unused, until they rusted away."[110] Little by little, in the decades that followed, the instruments gradually made their way out of the cabinets and were put to use, with various degrees of success, as described by doctor Constantin Dumitrescu Severeanu: "I witnessed another operation. It was a firefighter who fell as he rushed to a fire and had his hand crushed by the fire cistern that rolled over him. As no military surgeons were available, Davila asked for the kind services of Turnescu and Patzelt. They opined that they had to amputate the hand above the wound. Gangrene set in; they cut even further, the gangrene extended and, eventually, the patient died.")[111] A banal blood transfusion, performed before blood groups and transfusion techniques had been established, ended tragically, even though it was performed as a last-minute attempt at saving a life by a celebrated practitioner, doctor Carol Davila: "[O]ne of the operations which caused a sensation at Mihai-Vodă Hospital in 1857 was a blood transfusion. A soldier admitted to hospital had lost a lot of blood and Davila decided to introduce blood from another person; he asked those present, and a medical assistant offered to be a donor. A venesection was per-

109 Bacalbaşa, Bucurescii de altădată, 175.
110 Kretzulescu, Amintiri istorice, 60.
111 Severeanu, Din amintirile mele I, 136.

formed; Davila filled a tin syringe and introduced the blood into the patient's forearm. The man who received the blood died a few hours later, and the donor himself died a few days later, having been infected with erysipelas."[112]

As seen, the risks of surgical procedures remained significant as long as no Listerian aseptic techniques were used. Doctor Severeanu, one of the pioneers who introduced aseptic techniques in Romania,[113] remembered the times, towards the end of the nineteenth century, when "doctors did not wash before operating. I saw the famous *Pean*[114] performing surgery in his tailcoat because, he said, it was cleaner than his day-to-day jacket."[115]

But in this domain, as in others, modernization led to progress: the application of aseptic principles turned the surgeon into the *Master Wizard* of early twentieth-century medicine. The examples I am about to give are not from the better-documented successes of hospital surgery, but, again, from surgical practice outside the hospital, an aspect which is still under-researched. In 1902, following his participation in one such procedure as a medical student, Victor Gomoiu earned his first "client fee." He writes:

> Mr. Gerota had started using me as an assistant in some of the operations. One day (in June 1902) he even called me to his house to "help him with an operation." My God, the excitement of it! To avoid any error of the type I sometimes committed in hospital (as he had an operating room at his home), I washed my hands and, after preparing everything himself, he passed me the handle of the Maisonneuve urethrotome, which he had inserted into the patient's urethra, took the knife and performed the internal urethrotomy. When it was over, and the patient had left, Mr. Gerota gave me a rouble (a five-*lei* coin). I was so shocked, I did not wish to take it, but as my chief insisted, I left with the money he had forced into my fist. This was the first client fee I had ever earned.[116]

A few years later, the same Victor Gomoiu became a kind of assistant at operations performed "in the city" by a famous surgeon of the time:

---

112 Severeanu, *Din amintirile mele I*, 135–36.
113 Jianu and Bercuş, *Constantin Severeanu. Epoca şi opera*, 195.
114 Pean [sic] refers to Jules-Émile Péan (1830–1898), one of the most celebrated French surgeons of the nineteenth century.
115 Severeanu, *Din amintirile mele I*, 136.
116 Gomoiu, *Viaţa mea*, vol. 1, 107.

Thoma Ionescu performed surgery in the city (in the patient's house) and I helped him transport the entire equipment of his surgical theatre. We used two carriages to carry the operating table, basins, boxes with sterile gowns and instruments, bandages, brushes, soap, etc.; as the diagnosis was never precise, I had to foresee all the possibilities, especially with regards to the instruments. For all this he had some special suitcases ready. We loaded everything into them at the hospital, and we unpacked them at the patient's house, where we assembled an operating theatre of some sorts. During the procedure, I handed him everything that he needed and then we put [the suitcases] back in the carriers to return them to the hospital.[117]

This was no easy task for the assistant, but it shows how widespread the practice of "at home" surgery was in this period. The young Gomoiu's experience illustrates not only the way in which surgery was practiced in the city at the time, but also the type of work that went into the apprenticeship of a future great surgeon in early twentieth-century Romania.

Occasionally, the doctors' memoirs include references to the "competition": these were the empirical healers operating in cities and villages, the only ones available prior to the introduction of a national system staffed by trained doctors. Doctor Severeanu, the son of a peasant, remembers using the services of one such healer in his childhood: "I was in a fight once, and my opponent pushed me against a wooden fence, so that the bone in my arm came off the shoulder joint; it was put back together by a master peasant skilled in such things. [...] I suffered from fever and jaundice, of which I was cured by a man who made an incision at the base of my nose. The old man said he had performed the cutting *with a silver coin*, because the iron coins were rusty and caused bad bruises. I also had an eye condition (catarrhal conjunctivitis) of which I was cured by an old peasant who scratched the conjunctivitis away with a sharp wheat bristle."[118] He also remembers another famous peasant oculist active around 1860, who "was a master in cataract removal using a needle (a darning needle) and people used to flock to be treated."[119]

---

117 Ibid., 142.
118 Severeanu, *Din amintirile mele I*, 23.
119 Severeanu, *Din amintirile mele II*, 138.

We cannot conclude this section without a reference to doctor Dimitrie Gerota's recollections of the Bulgarian campaign of 1913. The text was written in the heat of the events, with the obvious aim of analyzing the shortcomings of the army health and sanitary services in wartime. His narrative includes proposals for improvements in the Romanian army's health services and, as such, it also acts as an original type of memorandum addressed to the health authorities. This is not the place to address the disastrous organization of the army's medical services in the 1913 campaign. From our perspective, it is much more rewarding to look at doctor Gerota's observations about the attitudes of army personnel towards the peasants in the supply columns *en route*. The son of a priest from Craiova,[120] doctor Gerota was deeply touched by the lives of these people. "I have made enquiries," he wrote, "and became firmly convinced that, although the groups of 400–500 carriers had to be led by an officer who was supposed to look after their welfare and that of their cattle, ultimately on these marches it was not rank that provided protection, but God. Dressed only in shirts, rained upon, tired, unwashed, covered in dust, going without water and food, these were martyrs whose plight touched me profoundly, for I became convinced that their deprivations were worse than those of the troops!"[121] The exceptional conditions of the war campaign foregrounded their inferior social status: nobody listened to their grievances; they were used and abused without scruple and without the least consideration for their person or their belongings. Being a peasant recruit in the 1913 campaign meant being in hell.

Memoir literature turns out to be an important, even indispensable, source for the historian of medicine and the medical profession in the nineteenth century. This is because, as they wrote down their memoirs, often in old age, doctors opened up their hearts and captured details of the past that other sources had hardly addressed, if at all. Memoirs often mention marginal practices, such as "in the city" surgery, practices seen as incompatible with the period's medical theories and as such often passed over in silence. Another example of such rare glimpses into social history is the great number of empirical healers, with or without specialized skills, pullulating in Romania's towns and villages prior to 1900. A detail such as this, so viv-

---

120 Atanasiu, "Activitatea științifică și socială a lui Dimitrie Gerota," 415.
121 Gerota, *Impresiuni și aprecieri din timpul acțiunei militare în Bulgaria,* 12.

idly captured by doctor Severeanu in his memoirs, as we have seen, is rarely given center-stage prominence in other historical sources.

This survey of the published body of doctors' memoirs addressed a limited number of themes relating to the social history of nineteenth-century medicine in Romania. There are many others awaiting the attention of scholars intending to probe still uncharted depths in the lives and practices of doctors in the recent past: they could, after all, be our great-grandfathers.

*****

Summing up Part One of this study, I must highlight the fact that public health reports and the doctors' memoirs are very different historical texts: the former are administrative documents issued in compliance with the health legislation, while the latter are writings initiated by individual authors and bear the imprint of their subjectivity. From the perspective of today's historian, the data to be found in the two categories of texts are complementary, and this twin gaze is greatly beneficial to the historiography. The health reports yield abundant information, ranging from near-photographic images of Romania's cities, towns and villages in the later nineteenth century to data on the socio-professional status of doctors and their relations with the medical authorities and the wider population. In fact, the entire medical corps was involved in collecting field data on the rural population's health and lifestyles for what ultimately amounted to a huge ethnographical project. This was the case because the health reports covered wide-ranging aspects of the peasants' lifestyle, from dress, personal hygiene and the architecture of rural dwellings to the topography of the household, food and eating habits. Towns and cities were also covered in the reports: the critical descriptions of urban public spaces in the reports of the Higher Medical Council make memorable reading. Equally memorable are the graphic reports on public hospitals and other institutions, which the venerable members of this medical body were required to inspect regularly.

With the literature of the health reports, the historian is taken by the hand and led along the perennially sludgy roads and across the equally sodden courtyards, which lacked shelter for the cattle. He or she is also helped to visualize the tiny room where all the members of large families lived on top of each other in the winter, in a foul atmosphere which the period's doctors—and even more so today's historians—found repulsive. The journey continues through the pungent smells of urban markets sweltering in the heat of summer, or through the "mephitic" gases of the badly built and badly maintained latrines in provincial hospitals, which were often little more than adapted residential buildings and monasteries. A journey of this kind is a descent into hell, and it must have felt very much like one for the affluent, educated urbanites of the time: a descent into the hell of modern Romania. "But how modern was 'modern Romania'?" the authors of the reports seem to wonder.

The other genre considered here, the memoir literature by doctors, focuses more on the individual and his place, role and fate in the medical profession. The memoirs are essential sources for the history of this professional group. Like the health reports, they have the merit of providing an upward perspective from ground level by doctors in rural practices and urban hospitals, all of whom were individuals directly involved in the health system of modernizing Romania. The memoirs describe their careers and those of their peers, who were often also their competitors. We see, for instance, doctor Vasile Gomoiu, in the early years of his career, being used, with minimal rewards, by the renowned surgeon Thoma Ionescu, in the hope of later professional "endorsement," which never came. Eventually, the young Gomoiu rebelled, but his rebellion forever closed the door on a much-desired academic career. Doctor Gomoiu's memoirs have an exceptional documentary value in the honesty with which they depict the struggles and frustrations of a junior medic (born in a rural family) in pre-World War I Bucharest. The picture they present is a bleak one: a world of moral decay, "arranged" exams and contests, favoritism, nepotism, an academic environment devoid of ethical values, all of which, experienced and observed by an insider, must have been a huge disappointment.

# PART TWO

# MEDICAL DISCOURSE
# ON THE PEASANT AND THE VILLAGE

## 1

### "THICK LAYERS OF FILTH COVER THEIR SKIN": ON THE HYGIENE OF BODIES AND CLOTHES

Despite the huge volume of Romanian texts on the peasant and the rural world, the medical discourse on these subjects can be sub-divided into a relatively small number of themes. All doctors who authored these texts addressed approximately the same topics: hygiene of the body and clothes, hygiene of the home and the household, eating habits and alcoholism, the specific illnesses of the rural population, and, finally, racial degeneration. These topics are discussed in Part Two of this book, starting with the hygiene of the body and clothes.

When I began this research, I was surprised by the representations of the peasant and the rural world offered by the medical literature of the second half of the nineteenth century: a world of poverty and pain, in short, a vision of social hell. But the ambient culture in which I grew up and was educated fostered an image of the rural world that was situated almost at the opposite pole: a rural idyll populated by peasants in clean, festive dress, a world with "millennia-old traditions," a positive, quintessential emblem of the Romanian and of Romanianism. I was not aware then that this positive image was a creation of the nineteenth century and that, gradually, the emphasis shifted from negative to positive elements to the extent that, in the latter half of the twentieth century, the positive representation became the dominant one. Today I know that both representations were manipulated by hegemonic culture to achieve alternative and competing views of the peasant and the rural. I concluded that the true peasant of the nineteenth century is to be found halfway between the doctors' image of the savage rustic on the one hand, and of the bearer of true identity values created by folklorists and ethnographers on the other. I shall now investigate the medical discourse on practices of the hygiene of body and clothes among peasants in the last decades of the nineteenth century.

### The Peasant, A Being Wretched in His Body …

The descriptions doctors give of the hygiene of their rural co-nationals are in general extremely negative. Personal hygiene is no exception. However, one cannot overlook the fact that, quantitatively speaking, body hygiene remained a marginal theme in the medical discourse. Doctors normally turned the spotlight on themes that they considered more important, such as the hygiene of the dwelling, eating habits, and the effects of alcoholism.

In a late nineteenth-century doctoral dissertation, the young doctor Constantin Popescu observed: "Women and men alike never have full-immersion baths, and men only wash their hair in exceptional circumstances [...] It is easy to imagine the state of the peasant's skin. A thick layer of filth covers it, and those who have ever spent time amongst peasants know full well the characteristic odor exhaled by their dirty skin and clothes."[1] Here is a voice that firmly claims that peasants never had baths! In other words, according to these sources, the levels of personal hygiene were abysmal. Doctors generally equated the absence of soap from rural households with the peasants' lack of personal hygiene. In this logic, the peasants did not use soap; therefore they did not wash themselves. While it may not be easy to prove or disprove the historical accuracy of this logic, we do have evidence that soap was already routinely used in elite households in the eighteenth century.[2]

Contemporary observers singled out a characteristic foul odor as the best indicator of a deficient personal hygiene. Allegations that peasants smelled were made by many doctors in the period, but perhaps not with the same scientific precision and feeling for colorful adjectives as those dis-

---

1 Popescu, *Contribuțiune la studiul stării higienice și sanitare*, 21.
2 Vintilă-Ghițulescu, "'Primeneli și sulimanuri': despre igienă și modernitate," 207.

played by Nicolae Manolescu. Manolescu, who started out as a district doctor in Buzău County, wrote that, as he walked along the potholed roads of his circumscription to perform the endless inspections in villages and hamlets required by law, he often gained knowledge of his catchment area based on "olfactory" impressions:

> Many times, as I went from one village to another, I was accompanied by a junior village hall official (in Romanian: *vătăşel*). We were on foot, and the wind blew from his side towards me. The air around my young clerk was so foul that, as it drifted towards me, a miasmatic-empyreumatic-alcoholic stench forced me to change places with him. His clothes were impregnated with the miasma of domestic combustion and his pulmonary exhalations reeked of methylic products. The miasmatic infection came from a lack of general body hygiene, and the empyreumatic whiff was the result of long-term exposure to the burning stove in the home. This composite noxious atmosphere of the peasants' dwellings, especially in winter, is difficult to describe, but suffice it to say that upon entering those homes, I would have preferred to be devoid of the sense of smell or of the ability to breathe.[3]

Doctor Manolescu speaks from his own experience. But the spotlight on smells as social markers was a relatively recent development. In a classic study,[4] Alain Corbin claims that an interest in social smells was a major turning point in olfactory history in the nineteenth century. Referring to France, he wrote about the "stench of the poor," a topic, as we have seen, that our doctors appear to never tire of. Here is a description very similar to doctor Manolescu's, although it was written three decades earlier in France: "On entering this house," noted doctor Joire in 1851, "I was struck by the foul-smelling odor breathed there. This odor was literally stifling and unbearable and seemed like the smell of the most fetid dung; it was particularly strong around the patient's bed, and was also spread through the whole apartment, despite the outside air that came in through the half-open door. I could not remove from my nose and mouth the handkerchief with which

---

3    Manolescu, "Aparatul de încălzit camerele ţărăneşti în plaiul Buzău," 553.

4    Corbin, *Le miasme et la jonquille. L'odorat et l'imaginaire social, XVIIIe–XIXe siècles*, 167. The study was published in English translation as *The Foul and the Fragrant: odor and the French social imagination*, Berg Publishers, 1986.

I protected myself the whole time I stayed with this woman. Yet neither the inhabitants of the house nor the invalid seemed to notice the inconvenience of the miasma."[5]

Returning to Romania, let us look at the first-hand account by a doctor from a rural hospital in Gorj County, who evaluated his patients' personal hygiene in the following terms:

When admitted to hospital, our patients are in a wretched state of filth. [...] It is an acknowledged fact that the Romanian, from the day he is born and until the day he dies, does not look after the cleanliness of his skin; if he is lucky enough to be recruited into the regular army, then willy-nilly he will sometimes cleanse his filthy body. But when he enters the hospital, the patient is in a lamentable state. [...] I do not refer simply to those parts of the body that are more exposed and in contact to exterior objects, parts such as the face, hands and feet, but especially to those areas of the body such as the armpits, the groin, the perineal area and the genital organs, where secretions are more abundant. These areas in our patients' bodies are in an unspeakable state of dirt and are sources of terrible infections.[6]

Another observer, doctor Gheorghe Crăiniceanu, had a marginally less catastrophic perspective on the personal hygiene of the peasants who, he noted, had at least occasional partial ablutions. And, because this relatively positive discourse is quite rare, it is worth quoting: "The peasant is generally cleaner than is often recognized, apart from those situations when he is unwillingly exposed to dirt when he threshes grain or labors on muddy fields and roads; otherwise, he would not put a morsel in his mouth in the morning without first washing his face and hands and without crossing himself. [...] Sometimes, for example when inspecting new recruits, one encounters the odd case of extreme bodily filth, but such cases are usually to be found among individuals who are utterly destitute. Women take greater care of their bodies, as indicated by the fact that they are more likely to wash their feet."[7] Such positive evaluations are not typical. In fact, most doctors described the personal hygiene of peasants in the same somber tones, empha-

---

5   Corbin, *The Foul and the Fragrant*, 150.
6   Bianu, "Spitalul rural Horezu," 278.
7   Crăiniceanu, *Igiena țăranului roman*, 174.

sizing the lack of full-immersion baths, and only superficial and partial ablutions, amounting to an almost total neglect of the body.

Perhaps more important than *what* was written about the peasant is *the manner* in which it was written. Quite often the authors did not maintain the kind of neutral tone achieved by doctor Crăiniceanu quoted above, instead preferring the use of irony and mockery. Doctor I. C. Drăgescu excelled in the use of such devices, as when he wrote: "[T]here are people who run from water and who only ever bathed once in their lifetime: at their christening. The peasant will only take a bath when he accidentally falls into water. For this reason, those regions of the body that sweat most profusely are the most malodorous. Some peasants only wash once a week, on a Sunday, and even then, only splash a little water on their face and hands."[8] But doctors made no references to instances of involuntary "bathing" when peasants were surprised by rain as they labored in the fields. This is simply because such an example would have suggested the idea that, in fact, the peasant worked hard,[9] which would have created a shift in the generally negative register of the discourse. Some doctors who wrote about the peasants did so with hilarity and barely concealed contempt. Here, for example, is the young doctor Constantin Popescu describing the parasites on the peasants' bodies and clothes: "The parasites are habitual guests in the peasants' clothes and hair, so much so that it is generally considered as a moment of great tenderness when a young man places his head in his sweetheart's lap for her to pick the lice and nits and kill them. And all this is done in public. In fact, in the countryside everybody searches in everybody else's hair: parents do it for children, children do it for the parents, and the old folk sit in a corner hunting for bugs in clothes and hats."[10]

To recapitulate, the doctors' verdict on the bodily hygiene of rural residents can be summed up as follows: peasants never had full-immersion baths; in the summer, some of the adults, but especially the children[11] bathed in rivers, but never used soap; in sum, bodily hygiene was essentially limited to partial ablutions.

---

8   Drăgescu, *Igiena poporană*, 44–45.
9   On the stereotype of the "lazy peasant," see Bărbulescu and Popovici, *Modernizarea lumii rurale*, 105–70.
10   Popescu, *Contribuțiune la studiul stării higienice și sanitare*, 21.
11   Crăiniceanu, *Igiena țăranului roman*, 175–76.

Hygiene of the hair is a special sub-chapter in the story of rural hygiene. If the general hygiene of the peasant left much to be desired, it would seem illogical for things to be different for hair. Doctors identified the same issues in this area or rural hygiene: "[F]ew are the peasants who wash their hair more than once a week; most of them do so on the eve of major holidays. They rarely pass a comb through their hair, sometimes not even once a week. Children have their hair washed and combed more often, mainly because they are more prone than the adults to have lice."[12] For aesthetic reasons, women used various ointments for their hair, as described by doctor Manolescu: "To give some luster to their hair, some rub oil, butter, or pork fat onto it. They use basil to impart a fragrance to these oily products."[13]

The medical discourse on bodily hygiene among the peasant population is two-tiered: on the one hand, there is a descriptive discourse wherein doctors claim to be describing a factual situation; on the other, there is a normative discourse outlining the period's standards in hygiene and sanitation, standards which by and large remained an unattained ideal in the rural world. The normative discourse features prominently in school textbooks. In one such text, doctor Eugen Rizu urged schoolchildren: "[E]very morning, we have to wash our hands, cheeks, ears, neck and chest with cold water and soap. [...] Twice a week, we have to wash our feet and our hair. [...] At least once every two weeks we have to wash our entire body."[14] Once more, it was doctor Manolescu who offered the most emphatic normative discourse:

The peasant would be able to take a step forward in terms of his personal hygiene if he paid some attention to the natural covering of his head. Such attention takes only a little willingness and mainly consists in: combing the hair every morning; cutting and trimming the hair and the beard at least every two to three weeks; shaving the beard every Saturday evening, or even better, every Sunday morning, and washing the face and the neck every morning. Such hygienic care would arouse an agreeable feeling in the brain of anyone undergoing it, a feeling which would cause his face and eyes to shine with a cheerfulness and alertness which an unwashed and ungroomed man could never display. It would also encourage a desire to think beautiful

---

12  Manolescu, *Igiena țăranului*, 88.
13  Ibid., 201.
14  Rizu, *Schiță de igienă și medicină populară*, 108–9.

thoughts and endeavor things worthy of a real man. Such measures would also have a hygienic role in exterminating the microbes and parasites that lurk between the hairs and could, if left, penetrate the skin and even inside the organism, where they could cause various illnesses. It is from the hairy regions of the body that the minute, disease-carrying creatures can spread from adult to adult, and from parent to child.[15]

What is of great interest in this text is not so much the content of the hygienic norms it prescribes, but the emphasis on the social and moral values of these norms. As Georges Vigarello observed, talking about the "popular" virtues of water in modern France, hygienic norms become part of a broader social pedagogy.[16] The social implications of hygiene became more complex in the nineteenth century. Returning to our text, it is obvious that, apart from pointing to the social and moral dimensions of hygienic norms, the author also wished to reveal the new dangers to the body in the post-Pasteur era: the threat of lurking "microbes and parasites" required more advanced practices of personal cleanliness.[17] The new developments featuring in the above-cited text were so entrenched in Western medicine that a well-known historian of nineteenth-century medicine in France felt entitled to suggest the use of the term *moral medicine*.[18] What this means in practice is that prescribing norms of personal hygiene to the popular classes was implicitly a form of moral education and an essential component in the civilizing processes to which these classes were subjected.

And now we must ask the question which will have occurred to any reader who has attentively followed the argument so far: how and how often did Romanian peasants cleanse their bodies in the latter half of the nineteenth century? And the answer is: it is impossible to know, given the lack of credible sociological surveys from the period itself. But this does not mean that we should not at least advance an intuition as a plausible working hypothesis. Our guide on this journey has been the medical discourse about the peasant, a type of discourse which is rife with traps, lies, and, as Ionela Băluță has observed, is situated at the junction of the scientific and the po-

---

15  Manolescu, *Igiena țăranului*, 88–89.
16  Vigarello, "Igiena corpului și modelarea formelor," 349.
17  Ibid., 352.
18  Faure, *Les Français et leur médecine au XIXe siècle*, 124–25.

litical. The interpretation of this type of discourse is undermined by two major characteristics: its repetitiveness and its positioning on the border-line between science and ideology.[19] While claiming objective and scientific respectability, the medical discourse is in fact deeply ideological, as we know today.

Another method of analyzing the content of the medical discourse in Romania is by comparing it to what is known about nineteenth-century cultures of hygiene in historiographies that are far richer in primary sources as well as in secondary studies on public hygiene. In other words, should we doubt the claims of Romanian doctors, we can try to see what was happening elsewhere, for instance in France, which was a template for modernization in Romania. Surely, "our" standards of personal hygiene could not have been higher than "theirs."

Regarding full-immersion baths, we know from Georges Vigarello that in the West in the early nineteenth century, this was a therapeutic rather than a purely hygienic practice, and was recommended by doctors with some caution. The period's established rules of hygiene required only partial ablutions. Towards the mid-nineteenth century there was a major shift in conceptions of personal hygiene, which resulted from new discoveries in chemistry. According to the new, energetic view of the human body, the skin as an organ became a portal that ensured exchanges of corporal bodies with the environment. It was at this moment that the much-feared complete bath started to be recommended. This remained the privilege of the elites until it began spreading out more democratically to become the "popular" bathing of the last decades of the nineteenth century. The post-Pasteur era saw the emergence of new, and ominous, views of the relationship between the body and its environment, views that led to the adoption of the stricter norms of personal hygiene familiar to us today.[20] Romanian doctors insistently deplored the infrequency of the submersion bath, which had become the norm by the late nineteenth century, and complained about the malodorous peasants. They mention the practice of partial ablutions of hands, face, and feet. Yet, in approximately the same period, their French peers described the hygiene of their rural co-nationals in equally negative terms: in 1886, "the

---

19 Băluță, *La bourgeoise respectable. Réflexion sur la construction d'une nouvelle identité féminine dans la seconde moitié du XIXe siècle roumain*, 127–28.

20 All references in this paragraph are to Vigarello, "Igiena corpului," 337–53.

peasant of Morvan washes his face a little when shaving, but the rest of his body has not seen a drop of water since he was born."[21] Even later, in 1890, doctor Francus was revolted by the low levels of hygiene among the peasants of Forez and Vivarais: "Everybody knows that our peasants take less care of themselves than the Swiss and English do of their animals."[22] These descriptions echoed each other, often using identical imagery. The French and Romanian peasants, and doubtlessly others, too, lived in what has been termed the "age of scarce water" well into the late nineteenth century. They attached a very different meaning to practices of personal hygiene, associating the cleanliness of their bodies and their habitat with the requirements of a spiritual time and space. Cleanliness was something one observed in preparation for sacred occasions and festivals rather than simply for modern hygienic purposes.[23] In other words, peasants only washed on a Saturday to be clean for the Sunday service. Doctor Doctorul N. Takeanu, the chief medical officer of Covurlui County in 1887, recalls that, although the peasants in his area were far from clean, there had been a time when the weekly bath was habitual: "*Baths* and personal cleanliness, which used to be one of the major qualities of our village housewives, have disappeared from common usage in these localities; nowadays, lacking rivers in which they could bathe in the summer and having lapsed from the salutary habit of the weekly bath, I have met persons who cannot recall whether they ever washed their body in their entire life."[24] But, in the last decades of the nineteenth century, the weekly submersion bath remained a hoped-for acquired habit not just in villages, but to a great extent in urban areas, too. As late as 1907, the regimental doctor M. D. Călinescu concluded that "to a large extent, county capitals lack communal bathing establishments; in other towns, if such establishments exist, they are very rudimentary."[25] However, the last three decades of the nineteenth century saw the emergence, admittedly on a small scale, of an interest in personal hygiene. Some doctors, such as for example doc-

---

21  Goubert, *La conquête de l'eau. L'avènement de la santé à l'âge industriel*, 225–26.

22  Weber, *La fin des terroirs. La modernisation de la France rurale (1870–1914)*, 223. For the English-language excerpt, see Eugen Weber, *Peasants into Frenchmen: The Modernization of Rural France 1870–1914* (Stanford: Stanford University Press, 2006), 149.

23  For more on this topic, see Bărbulescu, *Imaginarul corpului uman. Între cultura țărănească și cultura savantă (secolele XIX–XX)*, 232–33.

24  Takeanu, "Raport general asupra serviciului sanitar din județul Covurlui," 2401. Italics in the original. [Translator's note].

25  Călinescu, "Propunere de a se prevedea băi pe lângă toate," 206.

tor Romniceanu in 1871[26] and doctor C. I. Istrati in 1879, popularized the new French practices of bodily hygiene.[27] We must note, however, that what was under discussion in this period was not so much the practice of personal hygiene, as the infrastructure this required. In the 1880s, Romania was still in the age of the urban communal bath, which was still only available to those who paid an entrance fee. Doctors attempted to popularize the health benefits of the communal baths as a priority, but they also wanted to find ways whereby the communal bath could be transformed into what later became public baths open to the wider population. In Romania, public baths were a creation of the first decade of the twentieth century. It was in this period that the first plans and projects for their implementation were laid out. The beginnings were modest, but the sheer existence of such baths was an advantage, even though the public baths were not always adapted to meet local needs. Thus, in the village of Moara Domnească, we are informed with some sadness by doctor B. Drăgoşescu that "the building of the public bath was transformed into the headquarters of the village hall, and in another village into a school [...]; other public baths are almost completely abandoned, some operating in the summer, and even then only occasionally, such as, for example, the bath in the village of Poenarii-Vulpeşti (Ilfov County), Damieneşti (Roman County) and others."[28] However, one should not imagine that everywhere in rural areas the public baths either did not fully operate or were deflected from their intended role. The fact that they were recorded, and that written evidence was made available to future historians, suggests that such cases were the exception rather than the rule.

Gradually, and slowly, especially from the first decade of the twentieth century onwards, the state began to intervene in support of creating the infrastructure required by modern practices of personal hygiene. This was not solely the case in the urban environment, where progress was fairly easy to measure. We refer here chiefly to the public baths built on some of the Crown Domains and some that were attached to rural hospitals and medical practices. These were the early foci from which the taste for and discipline of personal hygiene were supposed to spread gradually among the rural masses.

26 Romniceanu, "Despre băi," 189–91.
27 Istrati, "Despre locuinţa ţeranului," 106–16.
28 Drăgoşescu, "Băile populare," 401–2.

Nowadays, readers of the gloomy medical discourse on the peasant and the rural world in the late nineteenth century are likely to be struck by the otherness of the representations offered by these texts. Indeed, the keywords here are otherness and exoticism. Today, it is not possible to make the kind of appraisals of the rural world based on claims that doctors could confidently make in the late nineteenth century. Why is this the case? Because practices of personal hygiene among peasants have changed to such an extent that assertions such as those made in the nineteenth century can no longer be made? Whoever has grown up and lived in contemporary Romania's rural areas knows only too well that in terms of personal hygiene the only noticeable progress is the generalization of the weekly bath.[29] Even after the 2002 census, rural dwellings equipped with bathrooms and sanitary conveniences remained an ideal rather than a reality in Romania: the census found that only 13.4 per cent of rural dwellings had a bathroom (compared to 83.2 per cent in urban areas), 15.1 per cent had running water, and 12.9 per cent had a sewer system (compared to 85.6 per cent of urban houses).[30] Without such amenities, modern personal hygiene is not possible. The fact that only 15 kilometers from Cluj-Napoca there is a village which has no running water or a sewage disposal system is a sober reminder of the slow pace of change. To my knowledge, only three houses in the village have fully-equipped bathrooms with toilets.[31] The nineteenth century is our next-door neighbor!

### ... And Wretched in His Clothes

The information from historical sources is no better when it comes to the hygiene of clothes among Romanian peasants. If doctors are right in claiming that the peasant does not wash himself and leaves his body in a state of perpetual filth, it is hardly surprising that he will not wash his clothes. Body and clothing are in such intimate contact that they will contaminate each

---

29 Weekly bath in this context should not be understood to be the same as in urban areas: for adults, it consisted mainly of partial ablutions, which covered more extended regions of the body, such as the hands, feet, chest, and armpits. The full immersion bath was not possible as long as a body-sized tub was not available.

30 *Recensământul 2002: Principalii indicatori pe județe și categorii de localități. Rezultate preliminare* [Census of 2002: Key indicators by county and categories of locality. Preliminary results], 82. The document is available at: http://www.recensamant.ro [last accessed: October 12, 2011].

31 This represents less than 1 per cent of the dwellings in the village.

other: the peasant is perceived as wretched in his skin and in his clothes. The head of the medical services in Tecuci County even claimed that "they never wash their whites, their shirts or their trousers,"[32] which seems doubtful. The medical representations of the peasant's rudimentary hygienic habits place him socially, and morally, on the bottom rung of the social ladder. This reinforces a claim I have made earlier, namely, that imposing hygienic norms in the peasant world is a significant part of a broader pedagogic programme. Doctors associated sanitary practices, and cleanliness in general, with intelligence levels and higher moral values. To these were added, in the post-Pasteur era, the fight against microbes. Doctor Manolescu in fact fuses all these representations into one highly educational narrative when he writes about the "freshening" (in Romanian: *primenirea*) of the peasant's shirt: "[T]he peasant never changes his shirt, he wears it night and day during the week [...] This is a very bad habit because, in the course of six days, even though the peasant will have his body ventilated during his labors, his shirt will be nevertheless infiltrated by the many products secreted and excreted by the skin. To these unwholesome products, we may add a multitude of microbes of all sorts [...]. In this way, a soiled shirt will have a general languishing effect on the body, causing a loss of energy which any sentient human will feel, as well as hosting foci of infection-carrying microbes; conversely, a clean shirt will stimulate the skin in a pleasant manner and the reflection of this stimulation in the organism is a pleasant movement, which cannot fail to awaken an alertness even in the most benighted of men."[33] It is to be presumed that, even if changed weekly, doctor Manolescu's moral shirt will be washed prior to use.

When they wrote about peasant dress, doctors consistently selected several micro-themes that they developed again and again. Ostensibly, they described the peasant's dress to pass judgment from a hygienic angle. But, because at times they went into great detail in terms of fabric, style, and even accessories, in doing so they turned into ethnographers. The classic writings by the doctors Nicolae Manolescu and Gheorghe Crăiniceanu from 1895, for example, are outstanding sources for the ethnographer wishing to contextualize his or her findings historically. I shall return to this, but what in-

---

32  Crăiniceanu, *Igiena țăranului român*, 153.
33  Manolescu, *Igiena țăranului*, 172–73.

terests me here primarily is finding the doctors' criteria for evaluating and assessing the peasants' clothes.

One frequently made comment concerns the poor adaptation of dress to environment, season, and climate. In their great indolence, doctors believed, peasants did not cover themselves adequately to keep the cold out in winter, but wore excessive layers in the summer. Doctor Mihail Mingarelli, for example, wrote about the peasants of Mehedinți County that they would let their children go about "with uncovered heads and bare feet, and wearing just one shirt, as I myself saw them in courtyards and in the streets in this current year when thermometers indicated minus 26 degrees Celsius."[34] One would hope that such instances were exceptional, but they were probably quite common: doctor Gheorghe Crăiniceanu, for example, was indignant when he saw "unmarried lasses" who, to prove their robustness, would step out without shoes, even in winter.[35] Earlier records mention children walking around with bare feet in the snow, or, less dramatically perhaps, children who could not attend school for lack of footwear, by that time considered by many to be indispensable articles of clothing.[36] Doctors noted that the peasants would wear the same "defective" hat in summer and winter: "The hat, of a defective shape which was inappropriate for the cold season, became an instrument of torture in the summer heat."[37] The peasant lacked common sense when it came to dress, doctors concluded, and was not mindful of the traditional cautionary saying, "riding a sledge in the summer and a horse-drawn carriage in winter." Specific traditional items of clothing were singled out for universal condemnation in the medical literature. Doctor Nicolae Manolescu knew well that "the white pantaloon, the șalvar, and the woollen baggy trousers" (in Romanian: "nădragul, șalvarul și poturul") had originated as Eastern imports and, in time, had lost much of their initial "heaviness and ungainliness." Nevertheless, he condemned these items of dress in the name of practical modernity, but also on aesthetic grounds: "These are impractical clothes: looser than they should be, heavier than necessary for the greatest part of the year, outside of the summer months, and more richly adorned with braiding than is required by good taste."[38] It is

---

34 Mingareli, "Raport general asupra serviciului sanitar," 2521.
35 Crăiniceanu, *Igiena țăranului român*, 120.
36 Vintilă-Ghițulescu, "'Primeneli și sulimanuri,'" 204.
37 Manolescu, *Igiena țăranului*, 91.
38 Ibid., 189.

quite clear that doctor Manolescu disapproved of *şalvars*, which by 1895 had become far too "Oriental" in the new European kingdom by the Danube. Instead, he recommended the trousers, a "rational" article of dress, which ensured an adequate balance between cost (the amount of fabric used), functionality (by allowing freedom of movement), and aesthetic values (they "do not require accessories").[39] Doctors were true Europeans when it came to the cut and style of garments, Europeans from a small nation searching for its place in the continent's new industrial order. On the other hand, they were also protectionists, and as often as they had a chance to they deplored the decline of the home textile industry and the purchase of foreign merchandise "from the market." Their main target of their attack was the replacement of hemp as a prime raw material with cotton, a choice which some considered a "national loss."[40] Furthermore, some considered the abandonment of the rural textile industry a major mistake. Fabrics, often the "product of foreign manufacturing," were now purchased directly at the market, noted the chief medical officer of Tecuci County ruefully.[41] Those were the early stages in the modernization of rural dress codes, which de facto meant the abandonment of traditional peasant styles and of the home textile production. The process was to take a long time and was not completed until some time during the first decade after World War II.

The peasant sandal (in Romanian: *opinca*, a variety of buskin) was a key sartorial element of the peasant's identity. The doctors who addressed the ways in which people dressed in rural areas discussed these items at length. Was this leather sandal—usually worn over a type of fabric legging—hygienic as footwear? What were the pros and cons of this type of footwear? These were some of the issues discussed by doctors. But, as these sandals were an emblem of identity, placed halfway between archaism and modernity, they were treated with a degree of respect. In other words, while they were not considered very hygienic, they were not dismissed on all fronts. Firstly, the fact that these sandals were a native, traditional style of footwear worked in their favor. In addition, they were practical, "easy to put on and take off, and with a good fit on the leg, light and warm."[42] It would ap-

---

39  Ibid., 190–01.
40  Ibid., 79–80.
41  Crăiniceanu, *Igiena ţăranului român*, 153
42  Manolescu, *Igiena ţăranului*, 243.

pear that the peasant sandals were ideal footwear. However, they were not robust enough and hardly practical in "rainy weather." Nevertheless, it was the only type of footwear that most peasants could afford. The peasant sandals remained in use well into the next century. In the late 1990s, as I conducted field work at Raşca in Cluj County, I found specimens of "rubber peasant sandals," the last variant of this type of footwear before its demise: they were made of pieces of discarded car tires and were in use sporadically until as late as the 1980s. Once the sandal finally disappeared and the consumption of wheat flour became generalized, two key elements of the peasant identity were lost: the peasant could no longer be called derisively either "sandal-shod rustic" (in Romanian: *opincar*) or "eater of polenta" (in Romanian: *mămăligar*). It was the end of a historical cycle.

2

## "THE MAJORITY LIVE IN WORSE CONDITIONS THAN THE ZULUS": DOMESTIC SPACE AND HEALTH

### *The Underground Hovel: The Scourge of the Rural Habitat*

In the 1820s, in a classic book, Dinicu Golescu launched the catastrophic representation of the rural habitat that became one of the key tropes in nineteenth-century Romanian literature. Golescu's village has "no church, no houses, no fences around the yard, no cart, no oxen, no cattle, no sheep, no poultry, no granary for winter provisions, in short, nothing; there are only some chambers under the ground, which they call hovels [in Romanian: *bordeie*]; upon entering these, the only thing to see is a hole in the ground, big enough for a man with his wife and children to crouch in front of the hearth, and up and above it, a basket made of twigs daubed with dung [...]. Anyone entering these hovels will be hard put to find any object of value, either the clothes on their backs or any other things around the home; even the pot for making the corn gruel [in Romanian: *mămăliga*] is owned together by five or six associates."[43] But the hovel as an emblem of poverty had previously been the discovery of foreign travellers in the region. Here, for example, is the Austrian consul Ignaz Raicevich's description of the villages in the plains of Wallachia in the 1780s: "The villages of the lowlands are inhabited by poor people; they all have an air of misery and desolation about them. These dwellings, or rather burrows, are dug into the ground and are called *bordeie*. From afar, one can only see the smoke rising from chimneys, but as one approaches, one sees roofs above small earth domes; they are made of wooden sticks and mud, so the grass grows on them."[44] Western travellers were perpetually bemused by these villages of the plains, composed mainly of hovels: for them, these places were the embodiment of unmitigated negative otherness. Dinicu Golescu, who travelled westward, gained new insights into the lives of peasants on his estates in Muşcel, and more generally into his native country, from the opposite perspective of what to him was the utmost positive otherness of Western Europe.

---

43 Golescu, *Însemnare a călătoriei mele Constantin Radovici din Goleşti făcută în anul 1824, 1825 şi 1826*, 76–77.
44 Raicevich, *Voyage en Valachie et en Moldavie*, 126.

In addition, these early medical testimonies about the rural habitat also emerged in Wallachia, a few years after Dinicu Golescu's work. Doctor Constantin Caracaş included what to our knowledge is the earliest description of peasant homes in a medical monograph published in 1830. His representations do not differ very much from those of consul Raicevich and boyar Golescu:

> [T]he dwellings comprise one small, modest room and have a porch made of weaved sticks daubed with cow dung both inside and outside, and covered with bulrushes or corn cobs. Many live in hovels, which are dwellings dug into the ground; fences for safety or trees planted for their benefits to health, beauty or rest are rare; instead most houses are surrounded by mounds of cattle dung and other refuse. And if their habitations are like this, the sheds meant for cattle are even worse; most of these are made of wooden trellis, or there are none at all, which leaves the animals exposed to winds and rain, standing forlorn in the midst of mud-choked courtyards and often deprived of the necessary fodder in winter.[45]

In this short text, doctor Caracaş surveys the key topoi of the medical discourse on the peasant home. Everything is listed, from the modest size, the unhygienic building materials (such as the mix of clay and cow dung), to the ever-present mounds of cattle excrement, the muddy, neglected yards, and the absence of shelters for the cattle. In the second half of the nineteenth century, doctors built their texts around these symbolic images, continuing an already existing tradition of negative representations of the peasant dwelling. They were not the only ones to critique and propose solutions for improvement. Mihail Kogălniceanu, author and politician, writing in the mid-1840s, and the writer Costache Negruzzi, in the 1850s, both addressed these topics in the periodicals of the time.[46] What the health professionals contributed to the debate was the transfer of pre-existing representations from the realm of lay wisdom to the rarefied spheres of science. In the early 1880s, doctor C. I. Istrati declared emphatically that he studied the "lack

---

45  Samarian, *O veche monografie sanitară a Munteniei*, 124–25.
46  I am grateful to Constanța Vintilă-Ghițulescu for bringing to my attention the two texts dedicated to rural peasant homes by Kogălniceanu and Negruzzi. She herself draws on these sources in her study *Evgheniți, ciocoi, mojici*, 311–14.

of hygiene among the inhabitants of our rural areas" from the perspective of the "man of science."[47] But his findings only confirmed what had been known for over a century before doctors paid any attention, namely that the peasants lived in unhygienic, unhealthy conditions. Istrati, too, primarily blamed the dwellings, and especially the underground hovels, of rural, lowland regions. He, too, indulges in detailed descriptions of such homes and emphasizes the wide areas of their spread:

> There are entire counties, particularly in Vlaşca, Teleorman, parts of Dolj and in Gorj as a whole, where houses consist of holes, hovels dug in the ground. Those with greater skills dig holes with a depth of one to two meters into which they throw straw and corn cobs, which are then set alight if the weather continues dry for a few days. The heat generated by these combusting substances helps dry the walls and reduces the water content of the clay that generally forms the country's alluvial geological foundation. In the last stages, superimposed layers of wood, corn hobs and straw are added on top, often also covered with earth, until a degree of depth and inclination is achieved which is believed to be enough for meteoric water to flow out rather than in. Often, there are no windows at all. In such cases, light penetrates through the chimney of the hearth or, in summer, through the window. If windows are provided, they are placed on one side of the house between the criss-crossing barns which form the roof, next to the door or the door itself, which is a mere opening at the top of a flight of clay stairs, serves as window. In general, these houses have a single, large room, with a floor in the shape of a parallelogram; sometimes there is a smaller room next to it, and most often, there is a niche in a corner, a sort of small, dark grotto which serves as a pantry for a bagful of corn and other provisions.[48]

It is quite obvious that doctor Istrati uses a language rich in scientific terms to reformulate a description of the peasant home that essentially does not differ from those of his predecessors. It is enough to remind ourselves of the even more eloquent scientific style used by doctor Nicolae Manolescu to describe the body odor of his junior clerk at the time when he was district

---

47  Istrati, *O pagină din istoria contimpurană a României din punctul de videre medical, economic şi national*, 320.
48  Ibid., 322–23.

practitioner. The aim of this terminology, as mentioned before, was to turn a non-specialist text into a scientific one through a shift from simple narrative to analysis. Both doctor Istrati and doctor Manolescu claim that, rather than simply describing a rural environment, they are in fact engaged in a scientific project.

If we compare the descriptions of rural habitats from the late eighteenth and early nineteenth centuries, such as, for example, those written by consul Raicevich and boyar Golescu, with the medical texts, they appear as mirror images: they all tell tales of miserable hovels and abject poverty. And yet, these two very similar series of texts are interpreted in very different ways, mainly because the social and intellectual contexts in which these texts were produced are different. Dinicu Golescu and most of the foreign travellers who left such narratives embedded their observations about rural habitats within the broader context of the merciless exploitation of the peasants by the land-owning boyars and the revenue collectors. Golescu's text expresses pain as well as a Christian, enlightened compassion for the unjust fate of these "creatures of God."[49] But the doctors of the latter half of the nineteenth century were no longer imbued with a Christian ethos; they were the products of a triumphant, secular, Western education that emphasized progress and science. For them, these "creatures of God" were mere primitives whom they felt entitled to treat with derision and a barely concealed contempt. Doctor Istrati's peasants lived in houses "which were almost invariably insalubrious and primitive, and in conditions which suggest that little progress has been made since prehistoric times."[50] This was an elegantly euphemistic way of saying that the peasants still lived in the prehistoric past where their hovels belonged. A few pages later, the same author confidently states that the majority of rural inhabitants "live in worse conditions than the Zulus."[51] It became obvious that a Europeanized Romania, as imagined by doctor Gheorghe Crăiniceanu in a study that won the Romanian Academy Award in 1895, had to tackle the problem of hovels. These blots on the new Romania's European CV had to "disappear."[52]

---

49 Golescu, Însemnare, 77.
50 Istrati, O pagină din istoria contimpurană a României din punctul de videre medical, economic și național, 321–22.
51 Ibid., 329.
52 Crăiniceanu, Igiena țăranului român, 103.

However, the hovel as a type of rural dwelling stubbornly resisted all suggestions of change by the top echelons of the medical profession and all attempts at administrative reform by the health authorities of the late nineteenth century. In 1894, "Regulamentul pentru alinierea satelor și pentru construcția locuințelor țărănești" (Regulations for the alignment of village streets and the construction of peasant dwellings) stipulated in article 22 that "all hovels had to be dismantled and replaced with dwellings built according to the guidelines contained in [the] present regulations" within five years.[53] Those who did not comply would "be prosecuted in accordance with the provisions of the preceding article, and their hovels will be dismantled."[54] In other words, Romania had to enter the new century free of the stigma of the peasant underground dwellings. We do not know whether individuals who continued building hovels after 1894 or failed to dismantle existing ones by 1899 were ever taken to court.[55] The suspicion that in fact article 22 was never enforced are confirmed by doctor Petre Cazacu, who, in 1906, wrote that the article had no legal consequences "at any time and in any place in our country."[56]

What we know is that in fact the hovels endured, and that much ink continued being spilled over them in medical writings. The conditions of rural dwellings engaged the minds of known medical figures of the Romanian Kingdom, but because this became such a fashionable topic, even medical graduates believed that including the description of a hovel in their doctoral dissertations was mandatory. Constantin Popescu was one of these junior doctors. Here is his description:

> None but those who ever entered such a *bordei* know how much squalor hides behind these figures [i.e. the statistics on the construction of residential buildings – *author's note*]. From the mouth of the hovel one goes down a series of steps dug into the ground, then upon opening a door one enters a tiny room no deeper than one and a half meters from the surface. This serves both as kitchen and as pantry, and the only source of light is the chimney or

---

53 "Regulament pentru alinierea satelor și pentru construirea locuințelor țărănești," in *Buletinul Direcțiunei Generale a Serviciului Sanitar,* year VI, 1894, no. 12, 187.

54 Ibid.

55 For a more detailed discussion of the enforcement of the regulations for the alignment of village streets and the construction of peasant dwellings, see Bărbulescu and Popovici, *Modernizarea lumii rurale,* 56–60.

56 Cazacu, "Locuințele sătenilor," 544.

the door, if it is kept open. The wooden roof has an outward cover of straw, bulrushes or corn cobs. These are plastered or whitewashed on the inside, where they form the ceiling of the hovel. The source of light is a small sheet of dirty glass of around 30 square centimeters, which opens right at ground level. There is a niche stove which is heated from the hearth, the beds are made of planks and do not exceed 20 cubic meters in volume. The underground part of the dwelling goes down to 1.50 meters and rises above ground up to around 2 meters or a little higher. This is *the only* room, and in it live and sleep on top of each other the man, wife, their lads and unmarried lasses, the younger children, the odd goose or a hen with its chicks, a lamb, calf or newborn piglets. As the ventilation is reduced and the room badly lit, the air is always foul, and especially the children look very pale. Some hovels are better than others, but this description fits the most common type.[57]

Doctor Popescu's not-so-good-yet-not-so-bad average hovel is representative of the known descriptions of this "scourge" of the rural habitat.

But let's depart from the evolutionary paradigm of progress chosen by our doctors, most of whom placed the hovel at the bottom of human habitations, somewhere between prehistoric cave dwellings and inhabited tree hollows.[58] First of all, we should perhaps try to establish how widespread this type of habitation actually was in the nineteenth century. The earliest statistical data on the human habitations of Muntenia[59] are to be found in the 1859 census. This census has the advantage that it presents separate figures for rural and urban hovels, although not, unfortunately, for other types of buildings. It shows that at the time, Muntenia had 1,213,950 residential buildings (a cumulative figure for residential buildings and outbuildings, both in rural and urban areas), 3,297 hovels in towns, and 84,998 hovels in villages,[60] a total of a little over 88,000 hovels. However, although their spread was wide, they were more numerous in the counties of Dolj, Mehedinți, Romanați, Olt, and Teleorman, Romania's south-western areas, which in total had 65,369 rural hovels, a percentage of 76.9 in the region.

---

57    Popescu, *Contribuțiune la studiul stării higienice și sanitare*, 11–12.
58    See the entry "Locuința" [The dwelling], in Bianu, *Doctorul de casă sau dicționarul sănătății*, 429.
59    Muntenia was the Romanian-language designation for Romania's southern province, also referred to in many documents as "Wallachia" (in Romanian: *Valahia*).
60    Marțian, "Recensiunea din 1860," 128–33.

Both partial and general data are available for the next decades, but they are not as reliable as the census. However, drawing on figures forwarded by county doctors, a series of *Reports on Public Health in the Kingdom* [*Rapoartele asupra stării sanitare a Regatului*] published aggregate data on the numbers of hovels on Romanian territory. In 1892, when he became head of the Health Services, doctor Iacob Felix counted "a relatively large number of hovels, 56,000 approximately.[61] By 1897, when he published his last report as director of the services, the Kingdom allegedly had only 46,915 hovels left,[62] 10,000 less than five years earlier! If true, this was an impressive achievement of his tenure in office, but we do know that the figures sent by the county medical officers were far from exact. Unfortunately, the population census of 1899, widely considered as Romania's first modern census, did not collect data on dwellings. Six years later, the country was preparing to celebrate the "ruby" jubilee of Carol I's reign with a General Exhibition to be held in Bucharest between September 24 and 27, 1906. In the run-up to this event, G. D. Scraba initiated a social survey of the "condition of the peasant" on the basis of a questionnaire, which also addressed the issue of rural dwellings. In his analysis of the census of 1912, although he rated the data collected by Scraba as "approximate,"[63] Leonida Colescu still thought they were sufficiently accurate to be used for comparison. This is how we will use them here. One characteristic of Scraba's data was the grouping of hovels by ethnicity of the residents. More specifically, he considered dwellings occupied by ethnic Romanians and Gypsies separately, presumably in order to highlight his view that hovels were not the typical habitat of the Romanian population. Obviously, the number of houses (i.e. overground dwellings) inhabited by Gypsies was not recorded. Consequently, in what follows we shall ignore Scraba's arbitrary classification. Nationally, but only for the rural areas, the census recorded 42,907 hovels and 1,109,905 overground dwellings.[64] In other words, in 1905, hovels accounted for only 3.72 per cent of the total of rural dwellings, which suggests that this type of habitation was already marginal numerically across the entire country. But, as we know from earlier data, almost half of the total number of hovels was recorded in Oltenia, with Moldavia and

61  Felix, *Raport general despre igiena publică și despre serviciul sanitar ale Regatului României pe anul 1892*, 90.
62  Felix, *Raport general asupra igienei publice și asupra serviciului sanitar al Regatului României pe anii 1896 și 1897*, 284.
63  Colescu, *Statistica clădirilor și locuințelor din România*, 43.
64  Scraba, *Starea socială a săteanului după ancheta privitoare anului 1905*, 19.

Muntenia sharing the rest almost equally. The counties which in 1859 topped the list for the number of hovels on their territory remained the same in 1905. Thus, Romanați remained by far the county where the hovel predominated: 11,529, more than a quarter of the county's rural dwellings, were hovels. The figure stands close to the total number recorded for the entire territory of Moldavia: 11,660.[65] The county of Dolj comes second, with Teleorman in third place. Even though between 1859 and 1905 the number of hovels decreased by 67 per cent,[66] in the traditional areas of the country's south-east the hovel remained a fairly widespread habitat. With respect to the census of 1912, Leonida Colescu joined the doctors in deploring the fact that "the *bordeie* continued to be in use as human habitation in Romania, in some places in fairly great numbers."[67] In actual fact, every year the numbers continued to decline to the point that by 1912 only 30,672 underground huts were still in use in both rural and urban areas across the entire Kingdom.[68] Yet, even though "in towns hovels have become a rarity,"[69] in the county of Romanați the number of hovels remained high, even in urban areas: in Caracal, for example, the number of hovels amounted to a quarter of the total number of buildings, while in Corabia this was 9 per cent![70] The census of 1912 was a truly modern census in terms of the details it collected, such as the number of rooms per house, the building materials used for walls and roofs, etc. Hovels, however, even though varied in structure—a variety Colescu himself also noted—were regarded as nothing more than primitive dwellings harking back to ancient times. Their—hopefully declining—numbers were recorded, but the statistics remained opaque: no further details were noted and consequently we know very little about them.

There were doctors, however, including some important figures of the profession, for whom the *bordei* was not necessarily the least hygienic type of human habitation. A hovel made of well-fired clay, doctor Istrati wrote, was hygienically superior to overground houses made of wattle and daub.[71] Doctor Felix compiled a classification of the ethnic groups in modern Ro-

---

65  Ibid., 18–19.
66  The number of hovels went down from 84,998 in 1859 to 28,524 in 1905.
67  Colescu, *Statistica clădirilor și locuințelor din România*, 20.
68  Ibid., 18.
69  Ibid., 21.
70  Ibid.
71  Istrati, *O pagină din istoria contimpurană a României din punctul de videre medical, economic și național,* 326–27.

mania based on the lack of hygiene in their homes: Romanian peasants secured an honorable third place. At the top of the league of unhealthy homes were those belonging to two ethnic groups from the region of Dobrudja, the Lipovans[72] and the Tatars, whose hovels and clay houses were deemed by the doctor to be "the dirtiest" and least hygienic. These were followed by the homes of Jews in Moldavia's small market towns, which he described as "sordid little shacks, lacking in air and light."[73] Interestingly, doctor Felix makes no mention of the Gypsies and their hovels. Doctor Manolescu, however, places the Gypsies' hovels in a separate category as "the most primitive of dwellings,"[74] home to the most primitive of the country's inhabitants. Doctor Manolescu held a view of the Gypsies that was shared by the entire nation: "There are only a few Gypsies who possess a tiny amount of the physical and moral assets of the civilized human."[75]

Nobody in modern Romania appeared to understand the real reasons why peasants continued to live in hovels. This was largely because nobody, before Gheorghe Focşa in the mid-twentieth century, was curious enough to gain insight into what the residents themselves thought about living in this type of home. And yet, the fairly diverse techniques used in the building of hovels, and their spread in specific regions, were signs that should have given the Romanian elites a pause for thought. As early as 1868, Ion Ionescu de la Brad observed—with reference to two specific districts in the low-lying areas of the country of Mehedinţi—that "the hovels, built under the ground and lined with bricks, were better, more hygienic, and more comfortable than the houses proper."[76] Of course, Ionescu was not a doctor, but an agronomist, "inspector-general for agriculture," and a man with little time for the period's elite-driven stereotypes, such as representations of the peasant as lazy, which he rejected vehemently: "[L]azy, the man who works to feed and make all the others rich? What a blasphemy!"[77] But Iacob Felix belonged to the medical profession, and was the Director-General of the Kingdom's Public Health Service. It was in this exalted capacity that he wrote about hovels in the coun-

---

72  The Lipovans were Old Believers of Russian ethnic origin.
73  Felix, *Raport general asupra igienei publice şi asupra serviciului sanitar al Regatului României pe anii 1896 şi 1897*, 285.
74  Manolescu, *Igiena ţăranului*, 47.
75  Ibid., 48.
76  Ionescu, *Agricultura română din judeţul Mehedinţi*, 151.
77  Ibid., 204.

ties of Olt, Teleorman, and Romanați as being "dry, comfortable," and, in his view, "healthier" than "some of the smaller houses made of wattle and daub, with low ceilings, and small windows which could not open."[78] Clearly, this shows that, gradually, members of the central administration became aware of something that Leonida Colescu, "Director-General of the Office for Statistics," was not shy to claim in 1912, when he said that the hovels were not always "mere holes dug into the ground."[79] In some areas, they could be, he wrote, as extensive and well-equipped as overground dwellings, and "made of good-quality materials such as clay or brick, with a rise above ground level and with roofs made of clay tiles, bulrushes, planks, straw, conifer bark, or wattle and daub. 'Superior' hovels such as these could be seen mainly in Oltenia, and to a lesser extent in Moldavia."[80] Such observations suggest that the hovel as a residential structure differed considerably from the dramatically simplified images doctors kept offering, even though they were in a privileged position to observe the reality in the field.

One has to look at twentieth-century sources for more merciful and nuanced representations of this type of habitat, but these did not come from the medical profession. Both immediately before and after World War I, the hovel as a typical dwelling of the rural habitat became the focus of attention for the new school of geography-anthropology. Constantin S. Nicolăescu-Plopșor, for example, claimed that, originally, the hovels of Oltenia were the direct product of specific features of the regional steppe environment, such as the lack of available wood.[81] He noted that contemporaneous hovels, for example some hovels in Romanați, which used wood profusely, no longer offered the possibility of understanding the "direct influence of the geographic environment on the human environment, which could no longer be observed."[82] Geographers, like doctors, believed that, in its original form, the hovel was a primitive, basic structure, which copied animals' dens. In the eyes of these modern observers, the hovel remained trapped in an enduring vision of a primitive underground dwelling, a negative view that eventually led to its demise.

---

78  Felix, *Raport general asupra igienei publice și asupra serviciului sanitar al Regatului României pe anii 1896 și 1897*, 284.
79  Colescu, *Statistica clădirilor și locuințelor din România*, 20.
80  Ibid.
81  Nicolăescu-Plopșor, "Bordeiul în Oltenia," 129–32.
82  Ibid., 129–30.

In the mid-twentieth century, under Romania's new People's Democracy, the ethnographer Gheorghe Focşa conducted important fieldwork in the region of Oltenia, which led to a new interpretation of the thorny issue of the hovel. Because he conducted his research within the paradigm of the peasant as the bearer of the national identity, Focşa was primarily interested in the "decorative elements" of the hovel's architecture, but he also collected other invaluable data on those hovels still available for observation in the field. He classified the hovels of northern Oltenia as "primitive," contrasting them to the more "evolved" type of southern Oltenia, which corresponded to Colescu's "superior" hovels. Some of these, for example in the district of Caracal, could comprise as many as six rooms. In 1949, at the time this research was conducted, there were still peasants from the plains who remembered the building of the first overground houses in their villages. In Grozăveşti, the first such dwelling was erected in 1884; in other localities, this happened even later, such as in Amăreştii de Jos, in 1905, and in Castranova, in 1909.[83] This time we have an opportunity to learn from the peasants themselves why they chose to build and live in hovels. The reasons they offered were of the most prosaic and practical kind: they kept "warm in the winter and cool in the summer."[84] Unfortunately, the researcher did not dwell on these issues, but the peasants' answers show, predictably, that they did not perceive the hovel as a symbol of poverty and ignorance. The simple explanation was that, as practical people, they adapted their home to the local economic resources and climate. Gheorghe Focşa's study is a comprehensive survey of the richness and variety of hovel architecture in Oltenia. It is also a salutary reminder that our suspicions of the medical literature are well-founded: rather than being serious studies of the rural habitat, the medical sources turn out to be collections of stereotypes of the peasant world, at least until the early twentieth century.

## Overground Homes: Clay, Dung, and Straw

But the range of peasant dwellings does not end with the hovel. The hovel is simply an exemplary case that encapsulates all the "hygienic ills" of the rural

---

83  Focşa, *Elemente decorative la bordeiele din sudul regiunii Craiova*, 10.
84  Ibid., 5.

habitations, often described using stereotypical images ranging from "veritable animal lairs"[85] to tomb-shaped dwellings presaging the residents' premature death. But the doctors tell us that overground houses were not much better. Often, the criteria used in the classification of rural dwellings are the materials available for the construction of walls and roofs in the geographic areas considered. Houses in the plains were built of clay and covered with straw or bulrushes, whereas in the mountainous areas the main materials were wood and clapboard. Doctors who chose to describe rural dwellings often gave information on building techniques collected with an ethnographic attention to detail. Doctor Manolescu noted that in low-lying areas, where wood was scarce and expensive, but sometimes also in hilly or mountainous regions, the most popular construction technique for walls was based on "wooden strips daubed with clay."[86] The frame structure was made of wood, and the walls consisted of a lattice of twigs daubed with a layer or two of clay mixed with chaff or small pieces of brick. The wall was finished off with "a mixture of watered-down mulch [...], cattle dung and wheat or maize chaff."[87] Another technique was "rammed earth building,"[88] which consisted of compacting (ramming) a moistened paste of "clay and sand between formwork planks, which are gradually raised as the wall is erected."[89] Burning straw was placed in the middle of the room to dry and harden the walls.[90] Doctor Manolescu saw rammed earth houses in the counties of Teleorman and Romanați,[91] while doctor Istrati was aware that the technique was "practiced" in Dolj.[92] As for the timber-frame houses, they were built using a straightforward technique for fitting and joining wooden beams together and daubing them with clay, so we shall not dwell on them here.

In the last three decades of the nineteenth century, the medical corps started showing an interest in issues of health and hygiene in rural areas, including the hygiene of homes. Interest in the latter was expressed in two *Regulations on the Alignment of Village Streets and the Construction of Peasant Dwellings* (1888 and 1894), and in the multi-volume study *Igiena țăranului*

---

85   Baer, *Considerațiuni generale asupra locuințelor rurale în România,* 8.
86   Manolescu, *Igiena țăranului,* 21.
87   Ibid., 22.
88   Ibid., 23.
89   Istrati, *O pagină din istoria contimpurană a României,* 324.
90   Manolescu, *Igiena țăranului,* 23.
91   Ibid.
92   Istrati, *O pagină din istoria contimpurană a României,* 324.

*român* (The hygiene of the Romanian peasant), published by the Romanian Academy in 1895. After 1900, social research and action entered a new phase: the descriptive information collected previously was complemented with statistical data, which greatly enriched the picture of the rural homes previously put together by researchers. Two milestones marked social research in the post-1900 period. The first occurred in 1906, when doctor Petre Cazacu published the outcomes of his surveys of peasant habitats.[93] The second was the census of 1912, which offered the first general and comprehensive image of modern Romania's human habitats. These two sources complement each other very satisfyingly. Doctor Cazacu's results came from his survey of all of Romania's 32 counties and covered 28,509 homes in 164 localities. District doctors served as ad-hoc pollsters. This survey, as well as the census six years later, lists a novelty among the construction techniques traditionally used in rural areas before 1900: houses made of unfired mud bricks (in Romanian: *chirpici*). This must have been an upgraded version of similar, earlier techniques and imitated buildings made with fired bricks.

Table 1: Types of rural dwellings by construction materials and techniques

| Building materials | Bricks | Stone | Wood | Adobe[94] | Wattle and daub | Mud bricks |
|---|---|---|---|---|---|---|
| 1906[95] | 7.74% | 0.44% | 21.29% | 22.1% | 37.26% | 5.63% |
| 1912[96] | 8.9% | 0% | 36% | 13.3% | 38.6% | 1.7% |

Fortunately, today's historians and ethnographers can use Leonida Colescu's study of the data collected in the 1912 census, the most comprehensive survey of modern Romania's rural habitat. His study reveals a fairly wide range of regional variations in building techniques, depending on the available materials and the levels of economic development in the regions.

93 This research, conducted to mark King Carol I's jubilee, complemented already published work coordinated by G. D. Scraba.

94 In Leonida Colescu's description, "adobe houses were made of moistened clay which was compacted with a mallet into a thick paste." Colescu, *Statistica clădirilor și locuințelor din România întocmită pe baza recensământului general al populațiunii din 19 decembrie 1912/1 ianuarie 1913*, 28.

95 Petre Cazacu, "Locuințele sătenilor" [Peasant dwellings], in *Viața românească*, year I (1906), vol. III, no. 10, 543. Compared to the 1912 census, this study has separate categories for hovels (2.23 per cent), and houses made of "straw and mud" (in Romanian: *ceamur*) (3.26 per cent), which I have not included in Table 1.

96 Colescu, *Statistica clădirilor*, 28.

But even as early as 1895, doctor Manolescu had noted correctly that most houses in rural areas (38.6 per cent) were made of wattle and daub, followed by wood (36 per cent), and adobe (13.3 per cent). In 1912, the majority (87.9 per cent) of houses in rural Romania were built using these materials and techniques. Brick, used in 8.9 per cent of houses, was in fourth place, a suggestion that the pace of modernization in this area was still slow. As already mentioned, there were county-by-county variations, and regional particularities at province level. For example, in Muntenia, "house frames" were built predominantly with wattle and daub (62.6 per cent), wood (24.7 per cent), and brick (10.8 per cent). Oltenia was the kingdom of wood (72.7 per cent), but brick came close with 15.5 per cent (the highest provincial percentage), followed by wattle and daub (10.1 per cent). In Dobrudja, mud brick houses were in the majority (41.1 per cent), followed by adobe (20 per cent), and wattle and daub (14.1 per cent). Finally, in Moldavia, the percentages were relatively more even, with the top three positions taken by adobe (35.2 per cent), closely followed by wood (30.4 per cent), and wattle and daub (30.2 per cent). However, one administrative unit down, at county level, the percentages of building materials often form spectacular mosaics: in the county of Constanța, for instance, no less than 41.1 per cent of rural houses made of stone. The county of Romanați offered an interesting contrast, with 37.3 per cent rural brick houses, but also 6,957 hovels,[97] the highest percentage of underground homes in Romania at the time. Fălciu County provided an intriguing contrast, too, with 92.8 per cent of the houses made of adobe brick.[98] The broad cross-province patterns conceal many diverse regional patterns. Unfortunately, our picture is not complete, as we lack data for districts and villages.

In conclusion, using the statistical data at his disposal, Leonida Colescu guides us on a journey into a rural world he considers backward and primitive, a world where often peasants built their homes using materials readily available in their environment and a range of traditional building techniques. Nevertheless, the resulting picture is one of a multiform and complex rural habitat.

---

97  Colescu, *Statistica clădirilor și locuințelor din România*, 18.
98  Ibid., 27.

## The "Hygienic Ills" of Rural Dwellings

By and large, doctors deemed rural dwellings to be unhygienic. The above-cited descriptions offer clues, but what exactly were the specifics of the criticism against this type of human habitation? Firstly, the dimensions of these homes were found to be inadequate. They were modest dwellings, much too small in terms of surface and cubic volume for the number of individuals living in them. These overcrowded residential spaces became the very emblem of poverty, squalor, and deprivation. Here is a description of a typical peasant dwelling of the last decade of the nineteenth century, by doctor Manolescu, who knew the rural environment well: "The peasant's home comprises a maximum of two habitable rooms, with a porch in the middle and a small storage room called a cellar, where he keeps various items of food: sacksful of cornmeal, flour, seeds, etc. [...]. Of the two habitable rooms, in fact only one is in use, the other serving as a spare room. The young wife and nubile maiden keep their dowry assets in this room, which is also used for entertaining friends and guests."[99] This was the classic structure of the average peasant home and the manner in which the rural population used their residential space. Not only were the homes diminutive, but the defective hygiene was worsened by the peasants' "bad habits." The homes and their residents were both evaluated and judged. Typical for the rural world, the way in which the entire family huddled together in one room around the hearth and the open fire was judged as one of the scourges of the rural habitat, the behavioral equivalent of the hovel. Not all the rural homes were as spacious as that described by doctor Manolescu. Many lacked the second room, the "reception room." There were still many of these homes left in 1905, when doctor Petre Cazacu surveyed 9,907 dwellings comprising "one room and a hall (porch)," which amounted to 34.75 per cent of the total number.[100] Alongside these, there were the many homes that did not even have a porch, comprising only one room. These amounted to 3.77 per cent.[101] The dwellings with "two rooms and a hall," as described by doctor Manolescu a decade earlier, represented 50.38 per cent[102] of the total num-

99  Manolescu, *Igiena țăranului*, 36–37.
100 Cazacu, "Locuințele sătenilor," 549.
101 Ibid., 548.
102 Ibid., 549.

ber of rural dwellings. It is Leonida Colescu again who, in 1912, produced the most comprehensive picture of the ways in which rural dwellings were compartmentalized. He did so starting from a very precise definition of his terms. For the first time, we come across a more rigorous definition of what a "room" meant: "A room is any partition in the house, separated from other rooms by walls rising to the ceiling, which is large enough for an adult-sized bed."[103] This definition, I believe, partly explains the discrepancies between the data collected in 1905 and in 1912. It is worth recalling that for the first two decades of the twentieth century, three different and more or less detailed surveys of rural dwellings are available. For 1905, there is the ambitious survey coordinated by G. D. Scraba with data collected by village mayors and head teachers,[104] and the less extensive one produced by doctor Petre Cazacu from data sent by district medical officers.[105] The third survey is the census of 1912. Unfortunately, the methodologies differ and as such the data cannot easily be compared. However, as shown in Table 2, the 1912 census and Scraba's survey are comparable in terms of the categories used, and both consider overground houses separately from hovels.

Table 2: A statistic of rural dwellings by number of rooms in 1905
(G. D. Scraba) and in 1912

| | 1 room | 2 rooms | 3 rooms | 4–5 rooms (1912) | Over 5 rooms (1912) |
|---|---|---|---|---|---|
| | | | | More than 3 rooms 1905 | |
| 1912[106] | 20.2% | 45.4% | 21% | 10.9% | 2.5% |
| 1905 (Scraba)[107] | 27.5% | 52.6% | 15.2% | 4.7% | |

Nevertheless, the results are divergent, with wide differences in percentages in all the categories. It is quite obvious that the short period that elapsed between the two surveys cannot in itself explain these differences.

---

103 Colescu, *Statistica clădirilor și locuințelor din România*, 41.

104 Scraba, *Starea socială a săteanului după ancheta privitoare anului 1905*, 5.

105 Cazacu, "Locuințele sătenilor," 541.

106 Colescu, *Statistica clădirilor*, 44.

107 Scraba, *Starea socială a săteanului după ancheta privitoare anului 1905, îndeplinită cu ocaziunea Expozițiunii generale române din 1906 de către Secțiunea de economie socială*, 18.

It is hard to believe that between 1905 and 1912, the rural dwellings with three rooms increased from 4.7 per cent to 13.4 per cent. Although the two surveys were similar in their statistical objectives and national coverage, the lack of professionalism in the way in which they were conducted is apparent in the less than reliable results.

Table 3: A statistic of rural dwellings by number of rooms in 1905
(P. Cazacu)[108]

| One room | One room and hall (porch) | Two rooms and hall (porch) | Several rooms |
|----------|---------------------------|----------------------------|---------------|
| 3.8% | 34.8% | 50.4% | 11% |

Even a quick comparison of Tables 2 and 3 reveals that doctor Cazacau's data also differ quite significantly from Leonida Colescu's. They seem to be surveying different rural environments. This is further evidence of the ease with which improvised "surveying" and impressionistic polling can distort the reality in the field. It was this lack of reliable statistical data that was to encourage the myths of degeneration projected onto modernizing Romanian society. In what follows, I shall only use data from the 1912 census, which were undoubtedly the only accurate ones.

The overall picture of the rural environment on the eve of World War I is hardly flattering for the young Romanian state: in 1912, the huge nationwide percentage of one-room dwellings—20.2 per cent—concealed wide regional disparities, ranging from 32.4 per cent in Moldavia to only 9.4 per cent in Oltenia.[109] In all provinces of the Kingdom, however, the dwellings with one or two rooms—those which hygienists deemed to be the least healthy—formed the majority by far, as the figures show: in Moldavia, they amounted to 71.4 per cent of rural dwellings, in Muntenia to 61 per cent, in Oltenia to 68.9 per cent, and in Dobrudja to 54.1 per cent.[110] Taking into account the later observations of doctors and ethnographers, who agreed that in dwellings of up to three rooms the entire family in fact used only one

---

108 Doctor Petre Cazacu's study, and therefore Table 3, too, both include hovels. Cazacu, "Locuințele sătenilor," 548–49.
109 Colescu, Statistica clădirilor și locuințelor din România, 44.
110 Ibid.

room, you can conclude that in 1912, this was the case for 76.5 per cent of rural homes. This confirms the picture of overcrowded rural housing doctors deplored with a mix of compassion and revulsion. Besides the hovels, which, according to the taxonomy favored by the period's intellectual elites, were not even deemed fit for humans, the greatest concern—at least for Leonida Colescu—was Moldavia's huge percentage of one-room homes. This should have been a general cause for concern, not simply for Colescu: "The statistics reflect a worrying situation which should attract the attention of all our leaders. For isn't there a link between this unfortunate layout of Moldavia's dwellings and demographic events peculiar to this region, such as an excessive death rate, even in normal years, combined with a decreasing birth rate?"[111] For Colescu, as well as for many doctors, the state of the peasant dwellings was a clear symptom of a social malady that had a direct impact on natality and mortality.

Overcrowding caused many of the "hygienic ills" of rural dwellings, such as when an ailing occupant needed to be isolated: as soon as one member of the family fell ill with a contagious disease, "almost all the others succumbed to it,"[112] doctor Istrati believed, in agreement with the entire rural medical corps. Some doctors commented on the negative impact of overcrowding not only on the physical, but also on the moral well-being of occupants forced to live in the same room:

In this one room, the mother gives birth in painful convulsions; a sick child dies in agony, as his siblings, older and younger, look on, terrified witnesses to these great crises. These terrible images will forever leave an imprint on their imaginations; all the children, from an early age and even later, as grownups, sleep huddled together on top of the stove; cases of incestuous rape are not unheard of. In that one conjugal room, children grow up quickly as their eager curiosity is subjected to temptation by their parents' example. All this has a powerful influence on their still immature imagination. Almost every day, we can see a nomadic population of girls leaving their family homes, migrating to the cities, where they start their careers as servant maids, only to graduate to drunkenness and prostitution. They end up having their fate

---

111 Ibid., 45.
112 Istrati, *O pagină din istoria contimpurană a României*, 335.

decided by hospitals and courts of law. Those who return home, do so with an acquired propensity for vice and promiscuity.[113]

These are terrifying images of moral decay among the rural population, the origins of which are firmly located by doctors in the rural environment. Around approximately the same time, another doctor spoke about the "affective faculties" of his rural patients in these terms: "No sense of shame, a proclivity to bestial amorous relations [...], and vices such as: drunkenness, sloth, stealing, lying and, in women especially, a love of luxury."[114] We are not far here from doctor Antoniu's images.

Doctors made long lists of other factors undermining the hygiene of peasant housing, which they kept reiterating in their writings. Firstly, there were the diminutive windows, covered with the only translucent materials available to the peasant: the bladder of the pig slaughtered for Christmas, or a piece of greased paper. These perpetually closed windows hardly permitted any ventilation. Next in line for criticism was the heating system, often used for cooking as well. Often, this was an open fire with a funnel that sucked in the smoke and expelled it no further than the attic. It was a defective system doctors never ceased criticizing for "charging the atmosphere with products which are harmful to life."[115] As early as 1870, doctor Felix knew from hygiene treatises that people themselves contributed to the excessive dampness of the rooms and that this was not without health consequences: "In these cramped, badly ventilated and overcrowded houses, the walls drip with vapors from kitchens, laundries, and other sources of household fluid waste. The effects of fermentation of this waste cause many conditions, most importantly generalized scrofula and scrofulous conjunctivitis."[116] Peasant homes also suffered from defective foundations and badly built walls. This was especially the case in dwellings made of "compacted earth," a building technique doctor Istrati knew was "practiced" in Dolj County. These houses, he wrote, "had so much moisture that many, especially on the walls facing the north and the north-east, were covered by luxuriant vegetation"[117] and as such were highly unhygienic.

---

113 Antoniu, *Cercetări asupra stărei țăranului român*, 13.
114 Ștefănescu, "Raport asupra mișcării bolnavilor în Spitalul rural Horezu în cursul anului 1886," 379.
115 Manolescu, *Igiena țăranului*, 56.
116 Felix, *Tractat de hygiena publică și poliția sanitară*, 360.
117 Istrati, *O pagină din istoria contimpurană a României*, 327.

Before we conclude this discussion of peasant dwellings, it is worth remembering that their occupants were not just humans, but also frequently animals, as many doctors reported. Doctor Manolescu devoted a special sub-chapter to the "animals that can be seen in the home of the peasant."[118] I know as much from memories of my rural childhood in an Oltenian village during the 1970s and 1980s. We are not talking about continuous human-animal cohabitation, but about humans and animals occasionally and exceptionally sharing the same domestic space. Quite often, in the cold days at the end of winter, peasants would take in the newborn lamb or the hen with her chicks. But doctors often claimed that the peasant lived with animals in the house, or that he loved animals more than his family members, implying that peasants were closer to animality than to humanity. Such claims illustrate the period's deep-seated social divide between the judging intellectual and the peasant who is being judged.

In conclusion, doctors' descriptions of rural homes in Romania in the nineteenth century until the eve of World War I create an image of miserable dwellings, built of readily available materials—clay, wood, straw, fodder, and cow manure—overcrowded, unheated, and badly ventilated. As we have seen, this type of accommodation had disastrous consequences for both the physical and the moral well-being of the occupants. Then, as now, the abode was deemed to be an image of its occupant and owner. In the eyes of the doctors who sat in judgment of the rural dwellings, these homes conveyed that the peasant was primitive, ignorant, immoral, and degenerate both physically and morally. Quite often, these wretched creatures—especially those living in hovels—seemed to belong to a species which stood apart from the observers. The tragedy of modern Romania's elites was that they had to save this peasant mass from poverty, illness, and death, because in numbers, origin, and manpower this multitude represented the real nation. However, the intellectual elites wanted to mold the emerging nation not in the image of this multitude, but in their own image: a modern, highly educated, Europeanized, and prosperous nation.

Stepping out of the peasant's house, you encountered a courtyard very much like the interior of the house itself. This is how the chief medical officer of Gorj County described a rural courtyard in 1886:

118 Manolescu, *Igiena țăranului,* 70–72.

[T]he yards of the rural inhabitants are major foci of infection. In any one village, you will be hard put to find a single house with a clean yard; in the others, you will have to walk with your boots on, as there are no paths to the entrance door. Cattle manure, urine, and meteoric waters create a slush that never dries up, not even in summer. Even the cattle, tired of standing in the mud, seek refuge by clambering onto the porch. Residents carry the mud into the house on their boots or buskins [*opinci*], thus creating foci of illness indoors.[119]

The typical imagery of rural courtyards is replete with the ubiquitous mud and the mountains of manure rising up to the eaves of the cattle sheds, wherever these existed. Another widespread stereotype about rural households was the lack of outbuildings to shelter cattle against the elements. As early as 1887, some county doctors, for example in Dolj, reported to "Mister Director General" that the inhabitants in their regions had "started the building of cattle sheds," even though the majority still "kept the cattle outdoors, without any shelter, even in rough weather."[120] This situation was not specific to Oltenia: the medical discourse abounded in such descriptions for the entire country throughout the nineteenth century. Yet, browsing this huge documentary mass for more balanced testimonies to counterbalance widespread and presumably widely accepted stereotypes is not easy. Doctor Manolescu, the son of a peasant from the Buzău region,[121] is one of the few to offer a less judgmental view on rural hygiene. In the previous chapter, he observed that the personal hygiene of peasants was better than was usually assumed. In the same study, of 1895, he paints rural courtyards in less somber hues than most of his peers. He noticed items and features many observers did not see or chose to ignore: "Sheds for cattle and horses, enclosures for sheep and goats, pens for poultry and pigs, barns and haylofts; in vine-growing areas, stills for making plum brandy and *raki*, lodges for carts, ploughs and vineyard utensils, etc."[122] Only the more impoverished households in both mountainous and low-lying areas, which did not have laboring cattle, lacked the necessary outbuildings. Undoubtedly, doctors manipulated the ratio of particular versus general data, because the census of 1912

119 Augustin, "Raport general asupra serviciului sanitar," 3602.
120 Chintescu. "Raport general asupra serviciului sanitar din județul Dolj," 2404.
121 Cealic, "Nicolae Manolescu," 451.
122 Manolescu, *Igiena țăranului*, 16.

still yielded a significant percentage of 23.1 of rural households lacking out-buildings across the entire territory of the Kingdom.[123] In other words, doc-tors who inspected or simply visited Romania's villages in the last decades of the nineteenth century could observe a wide range of peasant households, from prosperous ones—and these were not many—to the basic hovels of areas adjacent to the Danube. The palette they used in their descriptions largely depended on their expectations, their socio-professional back-ground, and not least, the empathy they felt with the peasant environment. To most members of the medical corps, this environment was profoundly alien: they had little understanding for it and, ultimately, they despised it.

The hygiene of the household and of the entire village left as much to be desired as the interiors of the houses. The idyllic village of the romantic writers looked totally different to the doctors: "[O]n a cold and peaceful au-tumn morning, the village could be seen through a dark haze of vapor ema-nating from rubbish heaps, of smoke from the stoves and of (noxious) gases from poodles; there are heaps of rubbish everywhere; the chimneys do not rise high, some of them end in the attic, stopping short of the roof (in moun-tainous areas); and there are fever-inducing poodles everywhere."[124] The de-scriptions of the modernizing doctors have nothing in common with the picturesque narratives of foreign visitors or the bucolic poetry of the roman-tics. For them, a backward rural society stood in the way of the European-izing drive in the reform program they had in mind for Romania. It was like this then, as it is now.

On work deservers further attention here. It is the study of doctor Istrati, *Despre locuința țăranului* [On the peasant's dwelling], originally submitted as a competition piece for a post at the chair of hygiene at the "Mihai Bravu" Gymnasium in Bucharest in September 1879.[125] It was immediately re-pub-lished in a scientific journal with high impact among medical circles in Bu-charest, *Jurnalul Societății Sciințelor medicale din București* (The journal of the Society of Medical Sciences in Bucharest), in the November 1 issue of the same year,[126] and serialized only a few days later in two issues of the Na-tional Liberal Party daily, *Românul* (The Romanian).[127] The following year,

---

123 Colescu, *Statistica clădirilor și locuințelor din România,* 32.
124 Manolescu, *Apărătorul sănătăței cuprinzător,* 54.
125 Jianu and Vasiliu, *Dr. C.I. Istrati,* 56.
126 Istrati, "Despre locuința țeranului," 293–301
127 Istrati, "Despre locuința țăranului." *Românul,* year XXIII, 1016–17, 1020–21

an "extended" version of this study became a chapter[128] in a volume that established doctor Istrati as one of the best observers of modern Romania's medical and social realities: *O pagină din istoria contimpurană a României din punctul de vedere medical, economic și național* (A page from the contemporary history of modern Romania, seen from a medical, economic, and national standpoint). This work became a classic and remained a much-cited study on the topic until World War I. It is noteworthy that in September 1879, doctor Istrati turned twenty-nine, having obtained his doctoral title in June 1877.[129] Only two years after completing his postgraduate medical studies, the young doctor thus became the much-talked-about author of a "hit" medical volume. Born in Moldavia in a modestly upwardly mobile family of land-owning free peasants (in Romanian: *răzeși*), he spent the first twelve years of his life in the village Rotopănești, not far from the town of Fălticeni, where his father was the administrator of a cousin's landed estate.[130] His school records suggest that he was a highly academic urbanite, rather than a keen student of the rural world. He was educated at a public school and the private Meltzer boarding school, both in Roman, before being admitted by competition as an intern student at the Academia Mihăileană[131] in Iași (1864).[132] In 1869, he left Iași to become one of the last students at doctor Carol Davila's National School of Medicine before it closed, and he completed his medical studies at Bucharest University.[133] Looking at this summary biography, one may wonder what entitled doctor Istrati to write in such stridently negative terms about Romania's rural environment in 1879. What we know about him suggests that his knowledge of this environment was not deep. And yet, this young, well-educated, up-and-coming doctor, familiar with the latest breakthroughs of the French school of hygiene studies, from which he cited copiously, chose in 1880 to publish an ambitious overview of the major social issues engaging the minds of Romania's elite medical professionals. It was obviously a successful strategy: the study rapidly became a classic and the young doctor became a medical celebrity overnight.

128 Istrati, *O pagină din istoria contimpurană a României*, 320–41.
129 Jianu and Vasiliu, *Dr. C.I. Istrati*, 49.
130 Ibid., 14.
131 Academia Mihăileană was an institution of higher learning founded by Moldavia's ruling prince Mihail Sturdza in 1835.
132 Jianu and Vasiliu, *Dr. C.I. Istrati*, 16–19.
133 Ibid., 20–23.

The next milestone in the history of the Romanian medical discourse about the rural world was the publication of two studies, both entitled *Igiena țăranului român* (The hygiene of the Romanian peasant), by the Romanian Academy, in 1895, following a contest. The two Academy Award-winning studies, written by doctors Gheorghe Crăiniceanu and Nicolae Manolescu, comprised detailed chapters on the hygiene of peasant dwellings, on which I draw in the present study. In the short period in which he was district doctor in his native Buzău County, doctor Manolescu published several well-received articles on rural hygiene and health care provision in the specialist periodical *Jurnalul Societății Sciințelor medicale din București*. Like doctor Istrati's work, one of doctor Manolescu's studies was then reprised by the newspaper of the National Liberal Party, a periodical that constantly devoted pages to works of social medicine and hygiene. Doctor Manolescu was undoubtedly much more cognizant of the rural world than doctor Crăiniceanu, but the latter had a comprehensive knowledge of Romanian medical literature.

One decade later, in 1906, as the country celebrated King Carol I's ruby jubilee, the Romanian General Exhibition's Section X (hygiene, public assistance, social economics) was devoted to the hygiene of the rural world, with a significant focus on the hygiene of the peasant dwellings. This was the topic of the volume published on this occasion by the "organizing secretary" of the section, G. D. Scraba,[134] and of the congress linked to the same event. At this congress, doctor Petre Cazacu presented the outcomes of an extended survey of rural dwellings, to be published later by the prestigious periodical in Iași, *Viața românească*.[135]

The last and most comprehensive stage in the study of rural dwellings was the population census of 1912. It comprised data on most aspects of rural housing, and the historian regrets that such information was not collected earlier, at least starting in 1860. The census amounted to a highly precise and systematic survey, which can help towards the verification of the stereotypes circulated in the medical discourse of the late nineteenth and early twentieth centuries. The historian can only dream of never realized surveys on other aspects of the discourse on rural hygiene.

---

134 Scraba, *Starea socială a săteanului după ancheta privitoare anului 1905*, 17–20.
135 Cazacu, "Locuințele sătenilor," 540–51.

3

## "THE PEASANT'S ONLY FOOD IS MĂMĂLIGA":
## FOOD AND HEALTH

### The Peasant at the Table

Inadequate personal hygiene and dwellings, as well as inconvenient house-hold arrangements, all contributed to outbreaks of illnesses. But nutrition made its own contribution to the poor health of the rural population. Let's first look at the general picture of the dietary habits of the rural population as presented to us by the medical discourse of the late nineteenth and early twentieth centuries. One of the earliest doctors to tackle the subject was Constantin Caracaş. In 1830, he published a monograph in which he sum-marized what were later to become the key medical tropes on nutrition:

[T]he meals of the [...] peasants were simple, modest and random, for they consist mainly of corn mush (in Romanian: *mămăligă*) made of maize flour, which they use as bread, and which on days of fasting they eat only with salt, onion, or garlic. Sometimes they prepare dishes made of various greens, which they cook with a little water and flour, or mushrooms and wild fruit, often gathered some time before and left to dry; more rarely, they cook with beans, pulses, or soured cabbage. They live for two thirds of the year on this sober and meagre nutriment, so that their robust bodies weaken, while those of infants and those of the infirm become prone to gastric illness. The rest of the time—for the three months when they are allowed to break the fast—they eat a little more, adding foods such as fermented milk, hard cheese, eggs and fish, especially salted fish of which they are very fond; very rarely, they have meat, which they cook in a simple manner, with a little water and onions, or which they fry. At table, they only drink water; those who go laboring in the fields or perform other work, partake of a little plum brandy.[136]

More than four decades later, Ion Ionescu de la Brad was appalled when he evaluated the peasant's food in relation to his labor:

---

136 Samarian, *O veche monografie sanitară a Munteniei*, 100.

The Romanian [peasant] fasts for half of the days of the year; and what does he fast on? Boiled vegetables and *mămăligă*: a diet based on vegetables especially designed to deprive the body of its strength and mortify it! Many fellows fast by eating only *mămăligă* with onions or vinegar, or *mujdei*, which is minced garlic dipped in vinegar! Pickled cucumbers and cabbage also play an important role in the food the laborer eats when fasting. But even when he breaks the fast, he still fasts, as fasting is understood in the West, because he eats eggs, milk, and cheese. Our laborer has an egg and makes a meal of it! He only eats meat rarely and when he does, it is lamb in the spring, beef in the fall and pork in winter. Habitually, he will have his meat in the form of *pastrami*, which is meat from which the juices are pressed out and then it is dried.[137]

Twelve years after these lines were written, doctor C. I. Istrati produced a detailed analysis of the peasant's nutrition and reached the same conclusions: many of the medical conditions in the rural world originated in a deficient diet. This is how he summed up his findings:

[A]ll this is proof that, generally, our peasant nourishes himself with indigestible substances which, apart from beans, are not very nutritious; this means that, to sustain himself physiologically, he has to ingest an enormous volume of food with a high content of acrid and irritant spices. The alimentary regime of today, which includes an abuse of greens and of low-quality fruit which are often either unripe or past their prime, results in an unfortunate effect on the peasant's body and mind, as well as on his progeny. This is the cause of the debility, morbidity, and mortality that are now rife among peasants, as well as of their low capacity for work and of their involuntary sloth.[138]

Doctor Istrati's comments have steered us towards the highly sensitive topic of the consequences of this type of nutrition. All the period's doctors, irrespective of their specific focus on one medical aspect or another, look at the peasants' hygiene and at its impact on morbidity and mortality in the rural world, search for the causes of this disastrous situation, and suggest "remedies" for it. One gets the impression that, for doctors, society was nothing

---

137 Ionescu, *Agricultura română din județul Mehedinți*, 203.
138 Istrati, *O pagină din istoria contimpurană a României*, 267–68.

more than a sick body: they studied the symptoms and their social effects, and suggested a treatment. They tried to cure individuals, but also society as a whole—or at least this was the ambitious aim of the hygienist discourse. In 1895, having completed a detailed survey of the nation's alimentary practices, doctor Nicolae Manolescu reached the following, inevitable, conclusion: "The peasant lives on a poor diet, a diet which, today, cannot produce the energy which he needs to go about his daily tasks. It is an inadequate nutrition, not only because for half of the year he is sustained only by foods from the vegetal and mineral kingdoms, but also because of the types of foods he ingests and of the little amount of foods from the animal kingdom allowed him by religion. The lack of proper food is linked to the general causes which prevent the peasant from escaping the poverty trap."[139]

After 1900, nutrition studies gained in scientific credibility: doctors were no longer content to describe the foodstuffs prepared and served on the peasant's table, but, adopting scientific methods, started calculating average rates of annual consumption by type of ingredient, as well as daily rations by category of nutrients. Engaging with the basic chemical principles of alimentation, the doctors adopted radically new formats for their studies, which became researches in culinary chemistry, often based on animal and even human testing, soon to become a legitimate methodology. But their conclusions did not essentially differ from those of their predecessors, as illustrated by the following passage: "[B]y analyzing the alimentary habits of our peasant with regard to total daily consumption, to the daily ratios of nitrates, fats, and hydrocarbonates, and the proportion of vegetal and animal foods, and by comparing these to the values established by *Voit*,[140] we obtain results which by now are familiar and well-established: [the peasant consumes] large amounts of food with a significant lack of animal content, an unbalanced, unhealthy and debilitating vegetarian diet."[141] In a study published in 1907—the year of a major peasant revolt—doctor Nicolae Lupu calculated the daily food consumption of a sample of 150 peasants from Fălciu County and obtained the following results, which support other evidence of the peasants' debilitating diet: "1,000 grams corn flour; 50 grams barley flour; 20 grams wheat in various forms [...]; 40 grams meat;

139 Manolescu, *Igiena țăranului*, 352.
140 Carl von Voit (1831–1908) was a German physiologist and dietician.
141 Urbeanu, *Îmbunătățirea alimentației țăranului român*, 25.

20 grams milk (a spoonful); 5 grams eggs (one egg every ten days) [...]; 115 grams cabbage juice (in Romanian: *curechi*); 800 grams borscht."[142] In terms of "principles of nutrition," this translates as follows, as analyzed by doctor Lupu: "[T]his means that, compared to the daily food rations necessary for sustenance, the diet of the villagers I have observed contains slightly fewer albuminoids than the above-mentioned average, while fats are well below this average (20 grams), and hydrocarbonates are much higher."[143]

The Congress of Social Sciences of 1906 held debates not only on issues relating to rural housing, as exemplified by doctor Petre Cazacu's studies, but also on aspects of the peasants' alimentary practices. Doctor G. Proca, later joined by doctor Gh. T. Kirileanu, conducted the most extensive survey of nutrition in the rural world during the pre-World War I period. The objectives were ambitious: a questionnaire was sent out to 3,480 schoolteachers, but only 439 (12 per cent) of them responded.[144] Even so, the results were significant. But a survey of "peasants' nutrition, assessed in terms of quantity and quality"[145] was not an easy task, and some of the results appear to be somewhat "creative." For example, across a sample of twelve families in Argeş County, the average caloric value calculated for the daily consumption of an adult was between 4,000 and 6,000 calories. In Mehedinţi, in eleven of the twenty families surveyed, the caloric intake of an adult reached 5,480 calories. Similar values were calculated in Olt, Prahova, Neamţ, and other counties. The conclusion was self-evident: "Everywhere, the [caloric] values entered for the actual food intake were generally too high."[146] But there was no way back, and doctor Proca was forced to adjust the figures that seemed in excess and to accept those that appeared in deficit, before, inevitably, reaching a foregone conclusion: "The rural laborer is perpetually exposed to the risk of not having enough to eat; the rural population is threatened with malnutrition from eating insufficient amounts of food not only from one year to the next, but also from one season to the next."[147]

Whether they use the hygienist language of the late nineteenth century,

---

142 A naturally soured juice obtained by fermenting wheat, rye, or beet chaff, and used for preparing a traditional East-European sour soup. Lupu, "Alimentaţia ţăranului," 222.
143 Lupu, "Alimentaţia ţăranului," 223.
144 Proca, Kirileanu, "Cercetări asupra hranei ţăranului," 609.
145 Ibid., 610.
146 Ibid., 612.
147 Ibid., 616.

or the language of the latest, turn-of-the-century breakthroughs in chemistry, doctors represent the peasant's nutrition in the same terms they use to represent the peasant himself: primitive, backward, and uncultured. Following up on doctor Istrati's comments of two decades earlier, doctor Adolf Urbeanu was also appalled by his findings:

> [T]he great majority of humankind has a preponderantly vegetarian diet, dictated by lack of means to purchase the more expensive animal foodstuffs. But not even in the most impoverished European nation do people have a poorer, more badly balanced and monotonous cuisine than that of our own peasantry. It can only be compared to the nutrition of savage populations, who have remained untouched by civilizing influences. I wish to state from the very beginning, and on the basis of data and figures, that I have rarely seen a more irrational, primitive, and insufficient system of nutrition among all the nations whose eating habits have been studied so far.[148]

These examples show that, from 1830 until World War I, doctors used the same terms to describe the Romanian peasant's nutrition, irrespective of whether they wrote within the hygienist paradigm or from the later, more modern perspective of food chemistry. The imagery they deploy is profoundly negative, repetitive, and colored by the stigma of primitivism and low levels of education.

## Mămăligă ... *and Again* Mămăligă

Leaving behind the general studies on rural nutrition, we now proceed, guided by the same doctor-observers, to take a closer look at what the peasant had on his table. Can there be anything unwholesome about a "traditional cuisine" that today still offers the delicacies we savor? Doctors are no ethnographers and, therefore, they do not write from the positive perspective of the peasant as bearer of a native tradition, but from the opposite perspective, i.e. of the primitivist paradigm.

The main criticism that doctors levelled against peasants' nutrition was the fact that it was almost exclusively based on vegetables. The key item in

---

148 Urbeanu, *Îmbunătățirea alimentației țăranului roman*, 26.

the alimentation of the peasantry was corn flour, made into a boiled porridge of varying degrees of thickness.[149] It was a fact noticed not only by doctors, but also by foreign travellers to the Romanian lands and by local observers. From the second half of the eighteenth century onwards, most travellers, those who were in transit as well as those who spent a longer time in the region, noted that the derivatives of maize were a key item in nutrition. The Swiss traveler François Recordon,[150] for example, wrote that "corn is their main food; they use corn flour to prepare a very thick mush, in fact, a kind of bread, which they call *mămăligă* and which is very tasteful when fresh."[151] It was not long before *mămăligă* ceased to be simply a core food item to become a social symbol. The peasant was "often called *mămăligar*," doctor Manolescu observed.[152] Doctor Istrati went even further and commented on the manner in which the elites dissociated themselves socially and symbolically from the masses by banning this food from their tables. "They do so not because they find it unpleasant to taste or indigestible, but simply because this is the food of the people and is not on the menu at the Grand Hotel du Boulevard des Italiens in Paris," Istrati wrote sarcastically.[153] Yet, in the 1890s, in a press overview of the "most pleasing foods," doctors Iacob Felix and Nicolae Kalinderu both listed *mămăliga* among such foods.[154] But one must remember that there were several variants of *mămăligă* and that rustic *mămăligă* was cooked into a thicker mass in rural areas: the peasants could break it, or cut it into slices using a length of "sewing thread."[155] In addition, they also used corn flour to prepare a related food called *mălai*, which was a type of corn bread baked in an oven or in a closed clay pot (cloche). These food items have retained their place in the Romanian "national cuisine": many of those now reading these lines must have dined on *mămăligă* some time over the last months. The bread-like *mălai* can still be purchased, but today mainly as a gastronomic product in the patisseries of Cluj. I can still recall that, as a child in Mehedinți County in the 1970s, I used to watch with excitement as my paternal grandmother (who was born in 1910) baked

---

149 The Romanian *mămăliga* is similar to the Italian *polenta*.

150 François Recordon (1795–1844) lived in Wallachia (Țara Românească) from 1815 to 1821. He published a monograph on Țara Românească, *Lettres sur la Valachie* (Paris: Lecointe et Durey, 1821).

151 Cernovodeanu, *Călători străini despre Țările Române în secolul al XIX-lea*, 669.

152 Manolescu, *Igiena țăranului*, 271.

153 Istrati, *O pagină din istoria contimpurană a României*, 239.

154 Crăiniceanu, *Igiena țăranului roman*, 235.

155 Manolescu, *Igiena țăranului*, 272

*mălai* in her own clay cloche. She also cooked a traditional dish called *zăbic*, which doctor Manolescu encountered in 1895,[156] and which was made by frying pieces of corn bread and eggs in fat. When my grandmother died, an entire world disappeared with her.

By the late nineteenth century, corn was ubiquitous in the peasant's alimentary patterns. Gradually, maize replaced competing cereals: millet, which by 1895 was only still cultivated and consumed in the counties of Ialomița,[157] Romanați, and Brăila;[158] and barley, still consumed by "many peasants in Moldavia," according to doctor Manolescu.[159] It also replaced buckwheat, grown and used in Moldavia and "around Brăila."[160] But maize and corn produce soon came to be overshadowed by suspicions that they caused an illness that spread in the last decades of the nineteenth century: pellagra, which will be discussed later in the book.

The peasants' vegetarianism consisted not only in a diet based almost exclusively on *mămăligă*, but also in the vegetable-based seasoning of this food item. Doctor Manolescu knew of this small range of accompanying and seasoning vegetables and was not very optimistic about their effects on the peasant's health: "Eating *mămăligă* with onions or leeks, or pickles and *mămăligă*, or sauerkraut, garlic porridge, cucumbers, prunes (in Romanian: *chiseliță*), vine leaves, and sour grapes with *mămăligă*, all of which [i.e. these combinations of foods] can be encountered all over the country, means eating according to an impoverished vegetarian system, like any herbivorous creature who eats only crushed, mushy, or boiled vegetables."[161] Seen in this light, the peasant ate more like an herbivorous animal than like a human. If further evidence was needed, the wasting away of the teeth, as doctor G. Z. Petrescu claimed, in humans and cattle alike, was the result of a herbivorous diet.[162]

The most widely consumed vegetables in rural areas, as singled out by doctors, were beans, onions, garlic, cabbage, and cucumbers. Vegetables and herbs such as carrots, parsley, tomatoes, kohlrabi, and even potatoes were quite rare. Romanian peasants came under frequent accusations that they

---

156  Ibid., 274.
157  Ibid., 274.
158  Crăiniceanu, *Igiena țăranului roman*, 246
159  Manolescu, *Igiena țăranului*, 277.
160  Crăiniceanu, *Igiena țăranului roman*, 246
161  Manolescu, *Igiena țăranului*, 306.
162  Petrescu, "Tocirea dinților la om," 87.

did not possess the skills or the willingness to cultivate vegetables and herbs in their gardens. Here is doctor Istrati, complaining ruefully: "There are entire villages in our country in which one can hardly dig out an onion."[163] This was especially the case, he said, in Moldavia. The data collected by doctor Manolescu for Muntenia and Oltenia show that the Romanian peasants of these regions habitually bartered with vegetable-growing Serbian and Bulgarian villagers for garden produce. We have records of individual peasants who engaged in barter: Barbu Ciurcu from the village of Alimăneşti, in the district of Şerbăneşti in Olt County,[164] and Vasile Marin from the village of Coteştii-din-Deal in Dâmboviţa County[165] are only two examples. Theoretically, doctors had to act on the failings they found, rather than simply describe them and make recommendations. I. C. Drăgescu, the chief medical officer of Dolj County, for example, consulted with the county's prefect over plans to encourage and spread "the cultivation of vegetables and the baking of bread among the Romanians."[166] Their project, launched in the spring of 1900, was only partially successful, and doctor Drăgescu complained that "nothing was done about the bakeries, and even today, in all the villages, the Bulgarians go around selling detestable bread."[167] However, in two of the county's districts, the most impoverished ones, the villagers were persuaded to start growing fruit and vegetables, and the Bulgarians were finally driven off the market. Exactly how the peasants in the districts Amaradia and Jiul de Sus could be persuaded to grow vegetables, even if only for their own use, doctor Drăgescu does not say. However, he did identify the individuals who were in a position to solve many of the problems of the rural environment: the deputy prefects who, in the doctor's view, could have emulated the "German praetor" he had personally seen when travelling in Transylvania, using a whip to "chase peasants away from the tavern and on to labor in the fields."[168]

Doctors' representations of the almost exclusively "vegetarian" diet of the peasants was another way of saying that meat was only rarely to be found on their tables, sometimes when it was least needed. The question arises: why should foods of animal origin have been so important in the nutrition

163 Istrati, *O pagină din istoria contimpurană a României*, 228.
164 Manolescu, *Igiena ţăranului*, 337.
165 Ibid., 325.
166 Drăgescu, "Raportul D-lui medic primar al judeţului Dolj," 259.
167 Ibid.
168 Ibid., 260.

of the peasant population? In the period's scientific imaginary, human societies were often compared to animal societies. In addition, social Darwinism, which the educated classes were familiar with, had imposed the idea of a "struggle for existence," which set communities and societies against each other. Within the food chain, herbivores were bound to become a prey to carnivores, a law that applied to nations, too. The epigraph placed by doctor Lupu at the start of his study on the alimentation of the peasant was a telling quote from the study of a French hygienist: "Nations with a nutrition based on vegetables are fated to be conquered, in the same way that the masses of herbivorous animals appear destined to become food for the carnivores."[169] In his study, doctor Lupu in effect attempted to prove his claim that "our peasants have descended the zoological ranks down to the level of herbivores."[170] If this was the case, it was a sad destiny for modern Romania.

Any doctor who acquires notions of food chemistry as part of his studies will know that a body's energy comes largely from nutrients of animal origin to be found in meat, fat, and milk. In the period under consideration, a nutrition based on animal foods was deemed to result in an active lifestyle, while a vegetarian diet suggested stagnation and backwardness. Mechanistic metaphors crept into the medical discourse, for example when doctor Israti compared "the individual and the nation" to a train engine that releases mechanical energy in proportion to the quality of the fuel used. Likewise, the human engine, individual and national, was more likely to function properly if fed high-quality produce.[171] In other words, only a well-fed nation could aspire to a glorious historical destiny. This was not the case with the Romanian nation, doctors thought. If we look at the foods on the peasants' table through the eyes of doctors, we might see that meat was not altogether absent. Peasants were engaged not only in farming, but also in animal husbandry, and some of their cattle were slaughtered for personal consumption. Both meat and bread were not staples, but food items reserved for "special occasions." But not all the animals in the peasant household were raised for their meat. Each culture creates its own alimentary hierarchy, which includes certain species and excludes others. Romanian peasant culture was no exception. In addition, societies have their own hierarchies of meat fit for

169 Lupu, "Alimentația țăranului," 217.
170 Ibid., 231.
171 Istrati, *O pagină din istoria contimpurană a României,* 223–24.

human consumption. In the peasant system, pork is the preferred meat, followed, according to the evidence, by lamb. Pork in winter, and lamb in summer and fall, was the essential pair in the meat consumption of the peasant in the modern age. Doctors offer plenty of evidence. Doctor Manolescu, for example, found that the "villager ate a lot of lamb,"[172] while doctor Crăiniceanu believed that "pork was the preferred meat of the Romanian."[173]

Research conducted in an ethnic Romanian village in Transylvania has shown that the pork-lamb pair retained its relevance for peasant consumption well into the second half of the twentieth century. Recent dramatic changes in contemporary nutrition, which demoted lamb from its top position, has caused discontent among the locals, unable to purchase their preferred choice of meat.[174] Beef was never fully accepted in the food circuit. Even in the second half of the twentieth century, beef occupied an intermediary place between meat fit for human consumption and prohibited meat: veal was "good to eat," meat from cows only in exceptional circumstances, and meat from bulls never. My own findings in the field in the first decade of the twenty-first century entirely confirmed the views expressed one century earlier in the first ethnographic study of nutrition in the rural world: "On occasions, he [the peasant] buys beef or uses some of the meat when a cow needs slaughtering because it is ill or has broken a leg, so that it is not all wasted [...]. It is sinful to eat meat from the bull. Calves are only slaughtered when they are ill, otherwise they are allowed to reach maturity."[175] Things are still the same. But why do peasants avoid beef? When questioned, some peasants from Bucovina revealed the real reasons why beef was not on their menu: "The peasant will not touch beef, there are folk who never put a morsel of beef in their mouth their entire life, and never would, for it is considered sinful to do so. Cattle toil for you and feed you and make you rich, you cannot eat them! In the old days, in Horecea, when they spotted someone eating beef, they said he was an evil heathen. At Mihalcea, they are loath to eat beef, they'd rather be fasting. So it is in Moldavia, where they say: we take their milk, shall we now take their flesh as well?"[176]

172  Manolescu, *Igiena țaranului*, 259.
173  Crăiniceanu, *Igiena țaranului român*, 259.
174  Bărbulescu, *Relația om-animal. Studiu de caz: porcul domestic*, chapter 1, "Porcul și animalele gospodăriei țărănești" [Pigs and other animals of the rural yard].
175  Lupescu, *Din bucătăria țaranului*, 58.
176  Niculiță-Voronca, *Datinele și credințele poporului român adunate și așezate în ordine mitologică*, 236. The

Cattle, therefore, were on the list of prohibited sources of food, at least in the peasant world. Alongside horses, they were in the category of auxiliary, laboring animals and were not supposed to end up on a plate. Starting with the late nineteenth century, we have evidence that firmly supports this. Doctor Manolescu, for example, was convinced that "all over the country, beef is not a habitual food amongst peasants, and many are loath to touch it."[177] Doctor Gheorghe Crăiniceanu assures us that only veal was consumed, and only "in town."[178] In Mehedinți County, the head doctor of the hospital in Strehaia communicated to doctor Manolescu that, in that area, "the peasants shun beef in the same way that Jews shun pork,"[179] and doctor Crăiniceanu found that in hospitals "many villagers refused to eat beef."[180] Again, the most shocking testimony comes from doctor Istrati, who wrote: "[I]n general, our peasants are loath to eat beef, and I have met a great number of them, especially in the southern area of Dolj County, who confessed to me that they would feel defiled eating it, for they had never touched it."[181] The evidence is too numerous to cite, but it all converges towards the same conclusion.

## The Peasant: A Reluctant Vegetarian

As mentioned above, doctors were not content with simply identifying and outlining the "hygienic ills" of peasants' nutrition, but also tried to find their causes. They tried to uncover not only the types of foods that composed the peasant's diet, but also the reason why this diet was the way it was. But, as the medical discourse on nutrition was eminently negative, doctors in fact listed the causes of the disastrous situation they observed in the field. These causes were few, and easy to identify. Poverty was the main cause, followed by "ignorance" and, in third place, a religious tradition—fasting—that peasants strictly observed. In addition to these major causes, doctors identified several secondary causes. One was the disruption of the peasants' already precarious diet during the regular periods of labor on the landown-

first edition of this study was published in 1903.
177 Manolescu, *Igiena țăranului*, 313.
178 Crăiniceanu, *Igiena țăranului român*, 259.
179 Manolescu, *Igiena țăranului*, 327.
180 Crăiniceanu, *Igiena țăranului român*, 257.
181 Istrati, *O pagină din istoria contimpurană a României*, 251.

er's estate, where laborers were offered an even worse fare than the meals they had at home. Another cause was the lack of culinary expertise. Let's consider each of them in turn.

The severe material deprivation of the majority of the rural population was a prime cause of their deficient nutrition. Levels of poverty, wrote doctor Istrati, sometimes drove peasants close to starvation, a situation the elites often chose to ignore:

> The poverty of the peasant's garden is terrible. Go to the countryside, and you will see dozens of houses, belonging to peasants who were allocated land in the reform of 1864, which are squalid and unhealthy, some even lacking a fence; how can these people be expected to have a garden for vegetables and fruit, how can they be expected to have a pig or a cow? In the countryside, poverty reigns supreme, but we are looking away! Penury is causing demoralization, the loss of all desire to live and the destruction of aspirations. The peasant's state of misery is such that he does not know if he has anything left to eat tomorrow![182]

Living from hand to mouth is an apt saying for the kind of existence these peasants led, doctors say. Doctor Istrati's generic poverty is fleshed out and given a human face by the health sub-inspector Charles Laugier, who, in 1905, wrote a report on the outbreak of collective food poisoning in the village of Popești, in Iași County. The protagonists of this episode are members of the Crivei family, around whom doctor Laugier constructs a sort of fairy tale in which the poor, humble hero is destined for a great future: "In the village of Popești, on the eastern edge of the village, there lives in a miserable hut a poor peasant, forty years old, Vasile Crivei by name, with his wife and four children—Maria, aged eight; Sultana, ten; Gheorghe, five; and Dimitrie, two."[183] The Crivei family was so poor that they did not even have a crust of bread between themselves. On the first day of Christmas, the family's reserves of corn were gone, and the doctor's fairy tale does not mention a pig, the traditional pig whose meat ethnographers considered a sign of domestic "plenty" in rural areas. Vasile approached the tavern keeper, who was unable to give him a loan. As for his village neighbors, they were all "as needy

---

182 Istrati, *O pagină din istoria contimpurană a României*, 265.
183 Laugier, "Intoxicație alimentară," 26.

as he was."[184] The situation seemed hopeless. After two days of starvation, the "unfortunate mother" resorted to desperate measures. She took the uninspired decision of turning poultry feed into food for human consumption. She used "husks of barley, oats and corn left behind by the thresher, which she had kept for feeding the poultry."[185] She ground these into a "dirty, blackish, coarse [flour] which she then cooked into *mămăligă*."[186] The entire family became ill and lost consciousness. The tale had a happy ending at the rural hospital at Podu Iloaiei, where the patients were given a powerful laxative and were treated back to health in a few days. The doctor decided to keep them in hospital for one extra day to "give them some proper food."[187] As a researcher in the twenty-first century, the story of the Crivei family brought home to me the extent of poverty and malnutrition among the rural population, of which doctors in previous periods never ceased to complain. The "generic," prototypical peasant so often represented by doctors in fact concealed a multitude of individuals and situations, and I am concerned here with the unique experiences of these living men and women. These were the people who, on Christmas day, could only put leftover corn mush on the table. This happened somewhere in Moldavia in 1905, the same Moldavia that, as the 1912 records show, had the highest number of monocellular homes in the country. Poverty reached terrifying levels, at least for a large section of the rural population, terrifying enough to trigger the major jacquerie of 1907.

"Ignorance" came second after poverty, and was not necessarily related to it. Peasants represented a section of the population characterized by low levels of education, ignorance, and superstition, according to the doctors, who vied with each other in such negative representations of the peasants' mental universe. Large sections of the intellectual elites in the late nineteenth century—bar some conservatives—agreed that the modernization of the rural world was a two-tiered process: one key project was to ensure the economic sustainability of the peasant household by allocating land, while the second was changing the peasants' mentalities through education. In other words, the solution to the "rural question" could be neatly summed up as land and

184 Ibid.
185 Ibid., 27.
186 Ibid.
187 Ibid.

schooling. Each of these projects had its heroes: land distribution had the ruling prince Alexandru Ioan Cuza[188] at its center, while Spiru Haret[189] made "enlightenment" through schooling his lifetime's mission. In the last decades of the nineteenth century and until World War I, most of the country's intellectual elites believed that one of the most damaging difficulties faced by the peasantry was a lack of education. Education was regarded as a sort of panacea, a remedy for all the "hygienic ills" affecting the rural population.

Returning to the issue of nutrition, the evidence shows that ignorance affected the culinary know-how of wealthier peasants, too, and that their alimentary habits did not differ radically from those of their poorer peers. Poor or wealthy, the peasants had an inadequate diet. Poor peasants could hardly put food on the table, while wealthier peasants did not know what to put on the table. The peasants were simply not aware of the nutritional value of the various foodstuffs available to them, according to doctor Lupu. When they swapped food, they often did so on the basis of (scientifically) very unsound decisions, such as giving away eggs in exchange for salted fish. "In the spring of 1904, I was treating patients with measles in the village of Nereju-Nefliu, Ilfov County," wrote doctor Lupu.

At one of the houses, I saw five little children, each cautiously dunking a piece of *mămăligă* in a bowl where a tiny salted fish swam in brine. It was a meat day. I asked the children's mother what she gave for the fish. Nine eggs, doctor, she answered (nine eggs have a content of 96.47 grams albuminoids and 45.50 grams fat, whereas the tiny fish, which did not weigh more than 100 grams, had only 18.90 grams of albuminoids and 16.81 of fat). When I asked why she would not give them the eggs instead, she answered: You see, they can all dunk in that pot and eat, but they couldn't do that with boiled eggs. And it looked as though she was right. But when I countered by saying that with a little drop of hot fat she could have fried a big dish of scrambled eggs, which would have fed twice that number of children, she simply shrugged, upon which I said: this is where ignorance leads. But I could not blame her.[190]

---

188 Alexandru Ioan Cuza (1859–1866), the first ruling prince after the unification of Țara Românească and Moldavia in 1859. The first land reform was initiated under his reign in 1864.
189 Spiru Haret (1851–1912), Liberal politician and major education reformer in nineteenth-century Romania.
190 Lupu, "Alimentația țăranului," 232.

It is quite clear that this description is meant to suggest an encounter between science (the doctor) and ignorance (the village woman). Doctors collected a wide range of data that suggested that peasants had no idea of the nutritional value of foodstuffs, and were thus unable to manage in a rational manner their meagre alimentary and financial resources. Doctors found, for example, that the meat peasants preferred to purchase was often pastrami (dried, salted meat) or salted fish. Both these products, doctors believed, lost a large percentage of their nutritional values through processing. Doctor Felix calculated in 1862 that pastrami, although three times "more condensed than fresh meat," was also three times more expensive. In addition, he knew from his own experience that the pastrami available in the shops was not a hygienic product:

One day in September 1860, as I visited one village after another during an epidemic of relapsing fever, I bought some pastrami to allay my hunger, for lack of something more delicate; a piece of that pastrami was lost in my travelling bag. In late September, as I did not have any pressing matters to attend to, I set out my "devoted brass companion," the microscope, on the table. I chose that wandering piece of pastrami as a random object of my observations that day. And what did I see? Entire forests of microscopic vegetation; a large part of the pastrami consists of such moldy parasites. It was the first time I observed pastrami under the microscope. I was appalled to realize the colossal self-deceit of pastrami eaters who introduce those non-nutritional substances into their bodies. That vegetation is not directly poisonous, but it is harmful because it diminishes the amount of nutritional content ingested by the body. In October 1860, I analyzed 28 different varieties of pastrami and found 19 of them to be full of those molds.[191]

The pastrami also caused alarm for doctor Gheorghe Crăiniceanu, who found out that "as they were washed in the river Ialomița, the pieces of meat destined to become pastrami were treated worse than sheep hide tossed about in sand and mud."[192] Doctor Crăiniceanu also observed that "fish has already gone bad by the time it reaches the shops."[193] With the last com-

191 Felix, "Despre nutrimentul țăranilor," 365.
192 Crăiniceanu, Igiena țăranului român, 260.
193 Ibid., 255.

ment, we have reached the sensitive domain of food safety, which the modern Romanian state has constantly attempted to regulate, and, implicitly, to control: the earliest general regulations governing the "production" and retail of food and beverages came into force in 1895.[194]

Finally, the last of the most important causes of the Romanian peasant's vegetarianism was religious fasting. All the members of the medical corps who treated nutrition in their writings vituperated against it, often in very aggressive terms. A short survey of the vocabulary used to criticize fasting is revealing: "the most immoral derangement of the human mind"[195]; "the wretched custom of the fast"[196]; "a genuine calamity"[197]; "to approve of fasting [...] would be a crime against the nation, to be condemned both by science and by morality"[198]; and "a true crime against humanity, one which affects our very development as a nation."[199] The examples could continue. All doctors tried to spread the message that fasting led to an unbalanced diet among the peasant population by criticizing the feature they thought was most harmful: vegetarianism. But there were other factors. Firstly, the doctors said, the periods of fasting were far too frequent and long: there was the Nativity fast, Lent, the Saint Peter and Virgin Mary fast, as well as every Wednesday and Friday, and in some cases even every Monday. All this added up to lengthy periods when the consumption of animal produce was prohibited. According to Ion Ionescu de la Brad, these periods amounted to almost half of the year,[200] while doctor Istrati calculated 185 fasting days,[201] and doctor Manolescu 189 fasting days, more than half of the year.[202] For his part, in 1901 doctor Urbeanu calculated no less than 194 fast days, which included the Wednesdays and Fridays. But when Mondays were also included, the number of fast days could reach staggering figures of up to 225 per year.[203] Between 1868 and 1901, the number of fast days appears to have mysteri-

194 See "Regulament asupra privegherii sanitare a fabricațiunii alimentelor şi băuturilor şi a comerțului cu alimente şi băuturi (art. 154, 155, 156 and 157 din legea sanitară)" [Sanitary regulations for the manufacturing of and trade in foodstuffs and beverages], in *Legislația sanitară*, eds. Şuta, et al, 507–38.
195 Felix, "Despre nutrimentul țăranilor," 365.
196 Istrati, *O pagină din istoria contimpurană a României*, 269.
197 Istrati, "Postul la români," 315.
198 Istrati, *O pagină din istoria contimpurană a României*, 277.
199 Mendonini, *Contribuțiuni la demografia României*, 12.
200 Ionescu, *Agricultura română din județul Mehedinți*, 203
201 Istrati, *O pagină din istoria contimpurană a României*, 259.
202 Manolescu, *Igiena țăranului*, 311.
203 Urbeanu, *Îmbunătățirea alimentației țăranului român*, 25.

ously increased. As if the large number of fast days was not enough, some of the fast periods, for example Lent, occurred at a sensitive time in the farming calendar: late winter and early spring, with the capricious weather of March and April, just as the agricultural season was about to start. Doctor Istrati believed that nothing could be more counter-productive than the timing, duration, and strict nature of this fast. This is his reasoning: "[A]s, weakened by winter, he is about to start arduous labor which lasts seven or eight months, he should seek to sustain his body with the alimentary equivalent of the rich hay and barley he gives to his horse; instead, he subjects himself to a diet of straw, of unwholesome substances, for seven weeks!"[204] The calendar of fast and meat days did not correspond to the peasant's real alimentary needs: in periods of demanding work he observed the fast, but enjoyed a richer diet of animal foods when labor tapered off. It all culminated in the period after Christmas, when he enjoyed the richest diet of the year, although he hardly did any work.

Peasants strictly observed the fasts, doctors found. Adding to their apocalyptic picture of nutrition in the rural world were claims that even children were subjected to fasting from an early age, but this was often as much hearsay as the result of direct observation. Doctor Istrati, for example, knew of this from doctor Sabin, who found out that "the inhabitants of the villages Gheboaia and Finta were very strict in their observance of fasts. I found men and women who told me that they would rather see their infants die than damn their souls by giving them milk or eggs during fast days."[205] However, his own experience at the children's hospital in Bucharest convinced doctor Istrati that such incidents occurred. And, if his testimony is not enough, here is doctor I. S. Mendonini, who wrote: "During the free consultations offered at the Brâncovenesc Hospital, I personally saw peasant women whose milk had dried up because of their inadequate nutrition and who came in with sick infants. Ninety per cent of those conditions affected the digestive system and were caused by the fasting imposed on those wretched creatures. The majority of those marasmatic children succumbed to these maladies."[206] Doctor Urbeanu vehemently deplored the fate of peasant children, whom he considered to be victims of the fasts and of the general alimentary depriva-

204 Istrati, *O pagină din istoria contimpurană a României*, 277–78.
205 Ibid., 282.
206 Mendonini, *Contribuțiuni la demografia României*, 13.

tions in the rural world: "I confess that I find it painful to expand any further on this theme by presenting the figures which sum up the misery endured by these peasant children, these innocent beings awaiting the liberation of merciful death. Even death has more compassion than church dogmas, than our laws, than the love of the powerful for the humble slave."[207] That Lent had an impact on mortality can easily be demonstrated with doctor Lupu's statistics for 1870–1897, which show that every year mortality rates peaked in the month of March.[208] Doctor Lupu was convinced that this trend was caused by fasting.

In the above, I have outlined the three causal clusters for the "hygienic ills" of peasant nutrition. Poverty meant that the peasant was unable to purchase foodstuffs of animal origin, thus keeping him on the borderline of alimentary deprivation. Ignorance rendered him unable to improve his diet even when this would have been possible. And finally, the religious prescriptions on fasting condemned him to a strictly vegetarian diet for more than half the year. These three interlocking causes kept the peasant trapped in a vicious circle of adverse circumstances: poverty fed ignorance, and ignorance encouraged an unquestioning observance of traditions. It was a circle of circumstances difficult to break away from.

However, as mentioned earlier, the defective diet of the Romanian peasant had secondary causes as well. Doctors made references to the food allocated to laborers by landowners and leaseholders in the farming season. The food normally available to the peasant was nutritionally inadequate, but the rations offered by the landowners were even worse. It would appear that all the low-quality grain and food leftovers in the landowner's or leaseholder's pantry ended up invariably on the peasant's table during the summer agricultural season. Doctor Lupu saw such scenes with his own eyes.

As I later went to another village—with yet another Jewish leaseholder— [...] I saw a wagon carrying a huge boulder of hardened *mămăligă* and a barrel of cucumbers pickled in brine; this was the food allocation for the field laborers on a long summer's fast-free day! The lad leading the oxen told me in secrecy, "Mister, you come in the evening to see for yourself, for in the eve-

207 Urbeanu, *Îmbunătățirea alimentației țăranului român*, 36–37.
208 Lupu, "Alimentația țăranului," 233.

ning he gives us *mămăligă* which is bitter like bile and black like the earth, of the sort he would be ashamed to give us in full light of day!" But what brought tears to my eyes was a little old woman running behind the wagon holding a small bowl in her hands; I stopped her and asked: what have you got in that bowl, auntie? "A bit of milk, my son, with millet gruel," she said, "to take to my lass working the machine[209] (?) at the boyar's, because she cannot just eat the sour broth from that barrel!"[210]

It must have been a pitiful sight, indeed.

In 1895, doctor Manolescu was more critical of the landowners and their leaseholders. He, too, recalled from his own experience

[...] the spreads laid out for the laborers at harvest time, where each was given a lump of *mămăligă* (of which there was plenty), a piece of cheese which could not have weighed more than 50 grams, and a small onion. The cheese was exceptionally hard and salty, which—the leaseholder claimed— was *better value*, as the peasants ate little and *there was more of it to go round*. There was no mention of borscht with sweet meat in it. Only the more magnanimous of landowners had sour borscht with blue bream (*zope*) made for his laborers. But even then, the portion of fish in the soup was smaller than it would have been if fried, because it was deemed that the liquid made up for it.[211]

By then, the health authorities had started to take such descriptions seriously and attempted to monitor the quality of the food distributed to farm laborers. Special attention was paid to the quality of the corn flour used in the preparation of the daily *mămăligă*. In 1889, doctor Polizu sent a circular to the prefects and the county chief medical officers, instructing them to send "administrative agents" to oversee the food given by owners and lessees to the peasants laboring on their fields. The aim, he explained, was to avoid a repeat of an incident in Tecuci County, where analyses had shown "a reduction of 48.50 per cent in the nutritional values" of the corn flour used for the laborers' food. In the doctor's view, this was bound to contribute to

---

209 This refers to a thresher machine.
210 Lupu, "Alimentația țăranului," 226.
211 Manolescu, *Igiena țăranului*, 308–9.

the "physiological misery" of the "village inhabitants."[212] The perpetual confrontation over these issues between county administration, landowners, and estate leaseholders does not appear to have borne fruit in any noticeable way.

As an ultimate cause of the peasants' poor nutrition, doctors identified their lack of culinary know-how. The overall lack of knowledge about the nutritional content of foodstuffs acquired a new dimension in this period: a lack of cooking skills. In simple terms, peasant women did not know how to cook, as doctor Istrati wrote in his characteristically emphatic style: "As regards the culinary art, most women in the countryside have forgotten all knowledge of it, as they have forgotten everything about growing vegetables in their gardens, or about weaving yarns, bedspreads and men's trousers, etc."[213] The use of the phrase "forgotten how to cook" implies that in the old days they used to know, and that the knowledge had been lost in the meantime. But we see that doctor Istrati includes the loss of cooking skills among other lost female traditions of the countryside, such as maintaining a kitchen garden, spinning, and weaving fabrics and carpets.

According to doctor Istrati, the loss of rural domestic crafts and traditions was one of the superficial signs of modernization and a sign of the decline of the rural world. In this view, in 1880, the archaic village was an ideal template, about to be dislodged by triumphant capitalism. Doctor Istrati was not the only member of his profession to comment on this trend. Doctor Crăiniceanu had his own, slightly more positive take on the loss of traditional skills. He wrote that whereas "Romanian women in most regions have been accused of being unable to cook," he knew in fact "from personal experience, that Romanian women in many villages cooked marvelous food."[214] It would appear, however, that the individual experience of witnesses was not enough to counterbalance the accusations levelled against peasant women. Doctor Crăiniceanu's comparatively positive observations could not by themselves influence the promoters of the hygienist discourse, who believed that the peasants' traditional ways of preparing food were unhygienic and based on culinary ignorance.

---

212 Polyzu, "Circulara D-lui Ministru de Interne," 305.
213 Istrati, *O pagină din istoria contimpurană a României*, 233.
214 Crăiniceanu, *Igiena țăranului român*, 230.

This brings us to the issue of bread and bread making, more precisely to the absence of bread from the peasants' diet. Paradoxically, doctors did not always interpret this absence negatively, given their claims that the peasant woman did not have the skills to prepare it. The village was not the place where one could find high-quality bread, as doctor Istrati noted: "[N]owadays it is rare to find bread at all in the countryside [...], but what is sad is that one can rarely find well-made bread."[215] In general, the preparation and consumption of unleavened bread (in Romanian: *lipie*, a type of flat bread) was met with criticism. Doctor Manolescu claimed that most often the core of this bread was not properly baked.[216] Doctor Istrati commented that making unleavened bread in a baking cloche was the "most primitive way of manufacturing bread."[217]

The author of the present study wishes to add his own testimony regarding the consumption of unleavened bread, the *lipie*. In my own childhood, in the 1970s and 1980s, I had the occasion to eat both the flat bread baked on the hob, first on one side, then on the other, as well as the bread baked in the old, "primitive" cloches. The latter was baked on vine leaves and glazed with a mix of egg and tomato juice and in my memory it did not have much to do with the doctors' descriptions from the late nineteenth century. The unleavened bread made by my grandmother in her own baking cloche was one of my childhood's treats, which I am not likely to sample any time soon. I am persuaded that my perception is not colored by the well-known psychological reflex, which makes us idealize childhood and the magic of the early days. Purely and simply, a bakery product of that quality is no longer to be found on the Romanian bread market.

## Mămăligă, *Sloth, Illness and Death*

Having surveyed the causes of the deficient nutrition of the rural population, I will now follow the doctors' lead and look at its consequences. As seen above, a largely vegetable-based, poor nutrition had important physiological—and ultimately also social—outcomes. Firstly, malnourishment, which was typical of the peasant's alimentation, largely explains what many

215 Istrati, *O pagină din istoria contimpurană a României*, 235.
216 Manolescu, *Igiena țăranului*, 275
217 Istrati, *O pagină din istoria contimpurană a României*, 236.

observers thought was a character failure of the peasant: sloth.[218] Many doctors provided explanations for this. Doctor Felix, for example, in his early days as chief medical officer of Muşcel County, came across an example he believed was convincing: "In the summer of 1860, after a bad harvest, the peasants from several villages in the district of Podgoria (Muşcel County) were left without reserves of corn. Around that time, Mr Nicolae C., who had a built a villa in the area, was looking for laborers, but found none, although he had promised a good pay. The peasants of Leurdeni refused to work, even though hardly any work was available for them. And why was that? It was because the lack of nutrients in their food had rendered them lazy by diminishing the energy they needed to break out of this abnormal situation."[219] Four decades later, doctor Lupu became aware, alongside the country's entire intellectual elite, that malnutrition and its pathological outcomes had "significantly impaired the quantity and quality of labor nationwide. This was a major fact observed by all those who live in the countryside."[220] However, what triggered doctor Lupu's indignation was, as he wrote, the fact that "the higher strata of our society have found no better explanation for the diminution of labor than the so-called *laziness of the peasant*. I am revolted, but cannot find the right words against the inventors of such an explanation, so I will answer them using the words of one of these peasants: '[L]azy, sir, you're saying lazy? But who ploughs the fields, who mows the cereals, passing each grain through their fingers, who paces up and down a thousand times, laboring on these lands which stretch as far as the eyes can see? It is us, not their Lordships!'"[221]

The chief pathological outcomes of malnutrition were the high rates of morbidity and mortality in rural areas, followed by what doctor Lupu called "the premature ageing" of the population, which he describes in the following terms: "At the age of thirty, women look like and have the energy of fifty-year-old women; the men are gaunt, with sallow, ridged and earthen complexions. Those who have depicted ruddy-faced, muscular Romanian lads in our present times have done a disservice to the nation. The majority are in fact very weak and doctors' statistics are there to prove it. The prog-

218 On this topic, see Bărbulescu and Popovici, *Modernizarea lumii rurale*, 105–70.
219 Felix, "Despre nutrimentul ţăranilor," 365.
220 Lupu, "Alimentaţia ţăranului," 227.
221 Ibid., 227.

eny issued from such debilitated bodies are equally enfeebled and this explains the high mortality and low resistance to illness among both adults and children."[222] Consequently, the poor nutrition of the peasants imperiled not only the country's present, but also its future. In 1880, Doctor Istrati held similar beliefs: "If we have malnourished bodies, we stand fewer chances of having children, especially *viable, strong* children."[223] But, while both authors agreed on the outcomes of the peasants' malnutrition, the ensuing dangers facing the nation were different in 1880 and 1906. Depending on their personal perspective, doctors emphasized different aspects of the two periods' social anxieties. Doctor Istrati, writing during the heated debate generated by the modification of article 7 of the 1866 constitution, feared that "the country's future is in danger; and, if that is the case, all our self-imposed sacrifices will only help another nation rise above our defunct one, a nation that will—solely and certainly—benefit from our modest economies and improvements."[224] His target here were the Jews, in a work that teems with antisemitic feeling. Doctor Lupu, who published in the flagship journal of the "Poporanist" movement,[225] *Viața românească* [Romanian life], was more empathetic about the social aspects of the situation. He condemned the country's elites *en bloc*: the "higher strata" had no social utility whatsoever and "contributed nothing to the life and strength of the nation."[226] His well-aimed arrows targeted the Conservative Party when he wrote that "Mr Marghiloman's fine equine specimens"[227] had a better diet than modern Romania's peasant millions. But, beyond a more emphatic social critique, doctor Lupu's observations were also meant to point to the fact that the peasants' malnutrition diminished Romania's chances of "using the mental and physical vigor of its population to gain its rightful place among the civilized nations of Europe."[228] Romania thus found itself at a disadvantage in the competition with other European nations. To compound this negative

---

222 Ibid.

223 Istrati, *O pagină din istoria contimpurană a României,* 269.

224 Ibid.

225 *Poporanism* was a Romanian ideological current that extolled tradition and viewed the peasantry as the embodiment of national identity. It emerged after 1890 in intellectual circles, which included the lawyer and journalist Constantin Stere and the journal *Viața Românească* in Iași.

226 Lupu, "Alimentația țaranului," 227.

227 Alexandru Marghiloman (1854–1925), Conservative politician with a passion for breeding horses. Lupu, "Alimentația țaranului," 231.

228 Ibid., 228.

situation, whereas generally across Europe the consumption of animal produce rose constantly throughout the nineteenth century, the opposite trend
was the case in rural Romania in the last four decades of the century.

### The Good Times of Yesteryear

If such representations of the peasants' alimentation are accurate, it is also
true that doctors were convinced that these developments were fairly recent. Some believed that the peasants' diet had been better. Writing about
bread consumption, doctor Istrati stated rather abruptly that "in the old
days, the Romanian peasant nourished himself solely on bread."[229] But what
did he mean by "in the old days"? He does not say, but the next sentence
takes us into a fairly remote past and a fairly different type of peasant, more
of a "warrior" type: "The Romanian soldier is described as carrying a loaf
of white bread attached to his horse saddle."[230] He does not elaborate. More
than two and a half decades later, doctor Lupu admitted that he did not have
any sources describing the diet of the peasant in the past. However, he too
was convinced that it was much better compared to the food available in
his own period. He argued that it was a matter of logic and common sense
to presume that "in the past, our bravery and fortitude could not be the result of such a diet," by which he meant the deficient diet common in his own
time.[231] Prince Stephen the Great's warriors in the fifteenth century were
unlike the peasants of the late nineteenth century, but the food range available to them was different, too, the argument ran:

> [T]he warriors of the Great Stephen stepped out on the hard and perilous
> road to war armed not only with their spiked maces and their sharp swords.
> They carried with them satchels with small loaves made of wheat and rich
> cheese from their mountain sheep. The milk and cheese of those pastoral
> times have ensured our endurance among nations and our freedom. The
> *mămăligă* and onion of our times of "improved agriculture" and modern
> "labor organization" will lead to our demise and to the subjugation of our

---

229 Istrati, *O pagină din istoria contimpurană a României*, 234.
230 Ibid., 235.
231 Lupu, "Alimentația țăranului," 228.

nation by foreigners, or by our guests within, whom we welcomed as brothers but who have turned into our oppressors![232]

A passage such as this corresponds with the writings of the historian Nicolae Iorga occasioned by the anniversary of the death of the great Romanian military prince four hundred years earlier.[233] The contrast between a glorious princely past and a grim capitalist present is cast here in medical terms.

In 1906, both doctor Lupu and doctor Urbeanu used the available statistical data to support their view that in the last four decades of the nineteenth century the peasants' diet had worsened. Doctor Lupu cited data published in the first issue of the periodical *Viața românească*, which showed that, between 1876 and 1903, the annual domestic consumption of corn decreased from 230 kilograms to 146 kilograms *per capita*,[234] a dramatic decline. Starting from the same statistics but using more sophisticated analytical tools, doctor Urbeanu also found a decline in the average food consumption of the peasant between 1860 and 1900. For corn, despite concurrent rises in production, exports, and population, the average for the period under consideration remained largely the same: 675 grams per inhabitant per day, which is not much. Significant additional drops, however, were found in the rations of foodstuffs that had traditionally been less available to peasants: milk, cheese, pork, and lamb. Even though doctor Urbeanu's overall picture seems to be a little more balanced than similar accounts by his peers, his conclusions are equally terrifying:

The Romanian villager has not evolved towards better eating habits and a more substantial diet; on the contrary, he has had to adapt to a poorer nutrition, which is now inferior in terms of quantity and quality to everything he has known in the past. As a result, he faces declining health and chronic hunger. [...] The alimentary balance sheet of the Romanian peasantry after the last forty years is in huge deficit, as shown in the great number of pellagra sufferers and degenerates.[235]

232 Ibid., 229.
233 See the chapter "O amintire istorică" [A recollection from history], from the volume by Bulei, *Viața în vremea lui Carol I*, 237–41.
234 Lupu, "Alimentația țăranului," 229.
235 Urbeanu, *Hrana săteanului în cei din urmă 40 de ani și îmbunătățirile de adus*, 19.

I wonder, however, how, using the same statistical data and the same computational algorithm, doctor Urbeanu calculated an average of 202 kilograms of corn per capita for the interval 1867–1903,[236] while the author of the statistics in *Viața românească* found a constant decline of the corn rations from 230 kilograms in 1876 to 146 kilograms in 1903.

Against the overwhelmingly alarming tone of the medical discourse on the peasant's nutrition, there were occasional voices of dissent. They were few, and this is precisely why they should be taken seriously. Here is doctor Manolescu again with a summary of information on the peasant's nutrition collected from his peers, his own experience, the declared eating patterns of the peasants themselves, and eyewitness recollections from village school teachers. On the basis of this body of data, doctor Manolescu reached the strange conclusion that "the peasant is now enjoying better food than at any other time in the past, mainly owing to the support he has received from various institutions."[237] It is strange, because it is not supported by any other evidence or claim from his 1895 study. The only other medical professional to corroborate it was doctor Munteanu from the rural hospital in Răducăneni, in Vaslui County, who claimed that during the previous seven or eight years, the "living standards" of the peasant had changed considerably "to the better, a change which I would attribute to a great extent to the solicitude of those in central administration in providing support such as farming credit, the appropriate legislation, and land allocation, for example to young newlyweds and the sale of state lands in small allotments."[238] The seven or eight years referred to here were the years of successive Conservative governments, which had, indeed, sought to improve the situation of the peasantry by adopting supporting legislation.[239] We presume that, at the time, doctor Munteanu positioned himself on the advantageous side of the political barricade. His peers of a more liberal orientation do not seem to have noticed any marked improvements in the condition of the peasant.

One must wait for 1905, and the incisive pen of doctor Radu Chernbah, the head of the communal hospital in Huși, well known for his opposition to

---

236 The average remained more or less constant in the interval considered. Urbeanu, *Hrana săteanului în cei din urmă 40 de ani și îmbunătățirile de adus*, 7.

237 Manolescu, *Igiena țăranului*, 304.

238 Ibid., 345.

239 For the legislation promoted by Conservative governments, see the study by Lungu, *Viața politică în România la sfârșitul secolului al XIX-lea (1888–1899)*, 66–84, 110–38.

the clichés circulated by doctors, to formulate an informed opinion on these trends. With a sweeping gesture, doctor Chernbah brushed aside the entire medical discourse on the peasants' alimentation from doctor Constantin Caracaş's text to his day. "It is wrong to believe," he wrote glibly, "that the diet of our peasants—ranging from the thrifty, hard-working peasants to the elite strata of the peasantry—is indigestible, poor, and insipid. [...] Our villagers partake of very nourishing food. If it were otherwise, how could we explain the exuberant health of their bodies and their capacity for work, joined to the quickness of their minds?"[240] Were these simply assertions based on common sense, or did they reflect the particular circumstances of an individual doctor? It is hard to say. I would incline towards the former, but this may reflect my own particular circumstances. In his campaign to rehabilitate the peasants' nutrition, doctor Chernbah even approved of— *horribile dictu*—fasting! "An erroneous current of thought in public opinion," he wrote, "has led some to condemn fasting. Many of those who, without any calling at all, talk or write about nutrition, commiserate 'tenderly' with the fasting peasant, claiming that this is the cause of his degeneration. This results in a regrettable confusion, because often those who lament most loudly are those who have the least qualification in the matter."[241] Quite obviously, doctor Chernbah had come to this conclusion having read recent scientific research, which had demonstrated that there was no real difference in the assimilation of animal and vegetable albumins. A year later, doctor Lupu had not yet heard of this research.

The fact that the positive appraisals of the peasant's food date from the first decade of the twentieth century may not be an accident. To illustrate the richness and variety of the peasant's diet, doctor Chernbah did not draw on medical sources, but on the series of articles on "rustic cuisine" published by Mihai Lupescu in *Şezătoarea* magazine between 1899 and 1904. These articles were preliminary fragments of the first ethnographic monograph devoted to peasants' nutrition, to be published by the Romanian Academy under the title *Din viața poporului roman*. The manuscript was completed by early 1916,[242] but the onset of war derailed Lupescu's publishing schedule and the work appeared in print almost a century later. However, as already

240 Chernbah, "Alimentația bolnavilor în spitale," 433.
241 Ibid., 434.
242 Lupescu, *Din bucătăria țăranului român*, 14.

mentioned, some of the preliminary material was published in the well-known folklore journal edited by Artur Gorovei in Fălticeni. At first sight, the study of the Moldavian ethnographer is located within the paradigm shared by the majority of the period's medical texts. In 1893, Lupescu himself announced plans for a study of the peasantry, which was to devote separate chapters to the "hygiene of the peasant," footwear, dress, and food.[243] I cannot fail to notice the similarities between Lupescu's project and the classic studies of doctors Manolescu and Crăiniceanu. With the notable exception of a chapter on rural habitation, which is not treated in the volume, all the other themes are there. But, are there any other differences between the ethnographer's study and the medical discourse? What stands out immediately is the neutral tone of the work: there are no accusations here, no subtle ironies. Quite obviously, the author intends to offer a comprehensive picture of everything pertaining to what he calls "rustic cuisine": implements, ingredients, and culinary practices. But far from being simply a collection of "peasant" dishes, the book had a more ambitious scope: it aimed to be an encyclopaedia of folklore traditions and representations of alimentation. Each entry opens with a glossary of peasant terms, continues with an outline of cooking techniques, and concludes with beliefs and imagery linked to the topic under consideration.

In fact, Lupescu's objective was a journey into peasant culture from the perspective of food and culinary practices. The work is embedded in what I earlier described as the "indigenous paradigm," which identifies the peasant as the true bearer of national values. As already mentioned, the medical discourse is generally located within the primitivist paradigm. Even though, superficially, the ethnographic and the medical discourses appear similar, in fact they look at the peasant and his world from radically opposite perspectives. For the ethnographer, the peasant is the bearer of a superior culture, a cultural being *par excellence*, in no way inferior to the observer. Conversely, for the medic, the peasant is a primitive creature in need of guidance—if need be through administrative coercion—towards the light of modernity. And this light did not come from within the rural world itself. For the ethnographer, the peasant is a cultural archetype; for the medic, he is a unit of statistics.

---

243 Ibid., 12.

What is certain is that, from the early nineteenth century, the intellectual elites located themselves within one or the other of the two afore-mentioned paradigms, to build two competing sets of representations of the peasant and the rural world. It would appear that, around the start of the twentieth century, the primitivist paradigm started to recede in favor of the indigenist paradigm, which ultimately pushed positive representations at the forefront of the public discourse on the rural world. It might be worth recalling that in the last two and a half decades before World War I, two important peasantist currents of thought, *sămănătorism* and *poporanism*, asserted themselves in Romanian culture.[244] Such intellectual movements promoted a reappraisal of and return to the moral and aesthetic values of the rural world, all painted in the idealizing palette of the "good old times." These were, indisputably, the times before rising capitalism started changing the face of our economies and societies. The medical professionals felt in tune with the literary discourse of *sămănătorism* and of the intellectual circles around the historian Nicolae Iorga, and many wrote their own works in the spirit of these ideas. For example, in 1914, doctor Neculai Lapteş published a work that was situated halfway between fiction and travel narrative.[245] Standing out among the characters is Father Tudor, a priest from a Moldavian village, who harmoniously combines the patriarchal values of the rural world of old with the Spiru Haret-inspired intellectual values of the author's own time. He was a kind of Popa Zamă[246] *avant la lettre.*

## Our Daily Water

In the hygienist literature, drinking water is a typically urban concern with particular relevance for the city of Bucharest. Much was written about the drinking water of the capital city in the last decades of the nineteenth century until World War I. The abundance of texts reflects the interest of the authorities in this specific aspect of urban hygiene. I will not dwell on this theme here, as it is out of the remit of my research on the rural world. There, until the last decade of the nineteenth century, issues related to the hygiene

---

244 See Ornea, *Sămănătorismul*, and idem, *Poporanismul*.

245 Lapteş, *Din nevoile satelor.*

246 Popa Zamă was a priest in the village Cornova in Bessarabia, made famous by the writings of members of the School of Sociology in interwar Bucharest. See Gusti et al., *Cornova 1931.*

of drinking water remained practically unheard of. In the first *Regulament pentru construirea locuințelor țărănești* (Regulations for the building of rural dwellings), published in 1888, there was only one entry on drinking fountains. Article 11 required the space within a radius of three meters around the fountain to be hygienized with "cobblestones or gravel" and prescribed a height of one meter for the casing liner of the fountain. Nothing further was added on the subject, except an injuction for fountains that did not meet the requirements to be "filled up within a year of the publication of these regulations."[247] I would be curious to know how many fountains were closed in observance of these regulations. Unfortunately, such data are not available, but we can see from the health reports that attempts were made to enforce the rules on the building of wells. The regulations and related punitive measures were maintained in unchanged form in the new legislation of 1894.[248] However, even when non-compliance posed a threat to public health, such legislation proved difficult to enforce in villages, largely because of opposition from the locals, as shown in the following source:

It is difficult to imagine the difficulties we encounter when we try to stop the use of or dismantle infected wells and fountains. Often, we are faced with revolts from locals who do not understand or do not accept our advice. Admittedly, they also often suffer from severe lack of water. In order to demonstrate the risk of contamination, the Health Directorate has ordered for fluorescein to be introduced in all latrines and refuse dumps adjacent to suspected wells in towns and villages. The resulting characteristic coloring of the water should help convince everyone, from the authorities down to the most ignorant of locals.[249]

The issue of fountains and drinking water in the rural environment received greater attention on the three pages devoted to it in the annual report for 1896–1897, which closed with the period when doctor Iacob Felix was at the helm of the Health Services. Here are doctor Felix's comments:

---

247 Şuta et al., *Legislația sanitară*, 296.
248 Ibid., 431.
249 Obregia, *Raport general asupra igienei publice și asupra serviciului sanitar*, vii–viii.

One of the more serious drawbacks is *the lack of clean water*; there are entire villages that do not have the necessary amount of water for domestic use and for the drinking needs of their cattle. In many villages, drinking water is very poor, laden with organic matter and living organisms that cause palludism, enteritis, and dysentery. The wells (fountains) are badly built, inadequately lined, and poorly maintained. There is no protection against seepage of impurities from the surface of the soil. Often, they are surrounded by slurry poodles where cattle have bathed. There are places where wells have depths of only between one to two meters; elsewhere, they are deep enough, but cattle and humans drink from the same bucket. In many places, drinking water comes from holes plugged by tree trunks or bottomless barrels, which collect surface or meteoric water. In many villages, drinking water comes from stagnant ponds, lakes, tanks or small pools infested with domestic effluents and waste from distilleries. Only a small number of villages are lucky enough to be supplied with fresh, abundant water from nearby rivers.[250]

We have every reason to believe that this description is fairly close to reality.

A few years earlier, doctor Manolescu had blamed the peasants' own unhygienic practices for the health hazards of water consumption. He observed, for example, that drinking from the same troughs used by animals was not a problem for the peasant, nor was he troubled by "dirt tracks," areas of mud mixed with corn cobs, such as can still be seen surrounding rural wells. The peasant was thus exposed to illnesses, which, doctor Manolescu commented, he did not associate with the water he drank, because "everybody in the village believes that, when sickness strikes, it is sent by God!"[251]

In 1905, the Health Directorate commissioned a survey of drinking water quality across the nation, "with statistics and a map for the whole of Romania."[252] This, regrettably, remained unpublished, which suggests that the authorities did not think it was an issue worthy of their serious consideration.

It would appear, however, that in the first decade of the twentieth century some progress was made in the domain of drinking water supplies.

---

250 Felix, *Raport general asupra igienei publice și asupra serviciului sanitar al Regatului României pe anii 1896 și 1897,* 281.
251 Manolescu, *Igiena țăranului,* 298–99.
252 Obregia, *Raport general asupra igienei publice și asupra serviciului sanitar,* vii.

These changes were due either to services provided by the state or by private individuals. In 1909, for example, doctor B. Drăgoșescu commented on the hygienic drinking fountains installed in railway stations by the CFR, Romania's national train company, as well as on the "American Northon drinking fountain," which he had seen "on the farm of Major Maca, in Teleorman County, next to Miroși station."[253] He also lists a hygienic drinking well made locally according to a prototype created by doctor Manolescu.

Issues related to the health hazards of drinking water received increased attention as advances in bacteriology showed that water was a medium that carried pathogenic bacteria. But 1903 was still early, as doctor Demostene observed when he wrote that "the morbigenic nature of poor water" did not seem yet to have "attracted the serious attention of the public or incited real interest among the higher social classes."[254] One of those recent advances was the discovery that Eberth's bacillus, which caused typhoid fever, was normally transmitted via drinking water contaminated by patients' excrements.[255] When such an epidemic occurred, waterborne transmission was the first cause to be considered. This was the case in Iași in the summer of 1909, when the health sub-inspector Vladimir Bușilă was sent to the city to investigate an epidemic. Having quickly identified the causes, he then sketched a hideous picture of the city at the end of the first decade of the twentieth century. The most important trigger he identified was "the frightening state of uncleanliness in the city (unimaginable even in the most backward of Asia's towns) and especially the detestable water supply system."[256] The impressions of sub-inspector Bușila are strikingly negative. To him, Iași looked like "a ruin immersed in waste and fecal matter from the midst of which monument after monument rises majestically. The money spent on any one of these would have been enough to build a proper sewage system and cleanse the entire city."[257] He criticized everything. His first target was the combined water supply system, which pumped "drinking water" through defective pipes and "water for general use" from the 2,700 "wells, which are little more than cesspools."[258] This is his nightmarish description:

---

253 Drăgoșescu, "Puțuri igienice," 317–23.
254 Demostene, "Câteva cuvinte asupra apei cea de toate zilele," 667.
255 Bianu, *Doctorul de casă sau dicționarul sănătății*, 726–29.
256 Bușilă, "Epidemia de febră tifoidă din Iași," 409.
257 Ibid., 411.
258 Ibid., 410.

The textile factory near the railway station [...], although it has large available funds and significant revenues, has not arranged for its courtyard to be paved or its dyeing laboratory to have proper flooring, nor does it have a cesspit for the drainage of its waste liquids. These flow across the floor into the heavily potholed yard, emanating a sickening stench which fills the entire factory, in which exhausted children swarm in the dirt. Rivers of filth trickle on across dozens of courtyards all the way to Bahlui. The entire town is crisscrossed in every direction by similar streams of slurry.[259]

He was equally critical of the "barometric company"[260] (a drainage facility), where barrels "were most often emptied down that road [leading out of the city – *author's note*], namely down the main Ion Brătianu Boulevard and onto the outlying suburbs. Formidable swarms of flies are afloat in the heavy, pestilential atmosphere, attacking the traveler and bothering him without respite."[261] A hideous image, no doubt, which, even if not totally accurate, might explain the causes of hecatombs in Iași during the refuge,[262] which occurred only eight years after doctor Bușilă's report.

Issues related to the hygiene of drinking water have been treated here simply because there was no scope for developing them into a distinct chapter of rural hygiene. It was impossible to resist the temptation put forth by doctor Bușilă's report, which steered us away from the countryside towards the urban setting of Moldavia's capital, Iași. Whereas the hygiene of "our daily water"—to use the phrase of doctor Demostene—was not deemed worthy of sustained interest, alcoholism was. It caused quite a furore in the period considered here, inciting much passion among health professionals and in public debate. This is the topic of the next chapter.

---

259 Ibid., 411.

260 The name comes presumably from mechanical pumps equipped with barometers.

261 Bușilă, "Epidemia de febră tifoidă din Iași," 412.

262 During World War I, after the Romanian army's disastrous campaign of 1916, large areas of the country were occupied by German, Austro-Hungarian, and Bulgarian troops. After December 1916, Romania as such consisted only of Moldavia and its capital Iași. Overpopulated with refugees, the city was hit by many epidemics which caused a medical and demographic catastrophe in the winter of 1916 and the spring of 1917.

## 4
## "IS THE ROMANIAN AN ALCOHOLIC?":
## ALCOHOL AND HEALTH

Has alcoholism ever been a social issue in Romania? More importantly, using the terminology of the period under consideration, was the Romanian peasant a drunkard? Over the entire long nineteenth century, doctors—and not only doctors—addressed issues relating to the consumption of alcohol in the rural world. This chapter attempts to retrace the debate on alcoholism as it unfolded.

### The Peasant and His Bottle

Our journey starts around 1830, with the testimony of doctor Constantin Caracaş: "[A]t the table, they only drink water; some partake of a little home-made brandy (in Romanian: ţuică) when they go out to labor in the fields. On Sundays and on other holidays, they all run to the tavern and drink raki and wine until they become intoxicated."[263] Even a cursory look at the text shows that the author locates the peasant population halfway on the scale between moderation and excess in the consumption of alcohol: routinely, all drink only water, in the fields some have a little brandy, but on holidays they all get inebriated. In other words, doctor Caracaş's peasant drinks wine and home-made spirits and, because this is about Muntenia, presumably the latter refers to a liquor made of distilled fruit (in Romanian: tescovină), which they have as they labor in the fields or on religious holidays, of which there were quite a few. The overall picture is one of sobriety, but there are indications that the tavern was quickly establishing itself as a site of dissolution. Almost four decades later, Ion Ionescu de la Brad felt compelled to defend the peasant against accusations of "drunkenness": "[T]he laborer is said to be a heavy drinker. But he only drinks water as a matter of routine, whereas those who spread this calumny drink wine and raki every day!"[264] This was the point in the public debate on drinking patterns when accusations started to pour. References to an era of distilled spirits started making

---

263 Samarian, *O veche monografie sanitară a Munteniei*, 100.
264 Ionescu, *Agricultura română din judeţul Mehedinţi*, 204.

regular appearances in the texts of the intellectual elites around 1850–1855. By 1875, P. S. Aurelian already made a distinction between spirits produced from the distillation of cereals, which were typical for Moldavia, and the homemade fruit spirits of Muntenia. He also wrote about the famous *basamac*, a beverage made with alcohol from distilled cereals, which doctors unanimously vilified as a hazardous poison:

> [A]n industry which has grown in recent times is the manufacture of alcoholic drinks from cereals. The greatest number of stills can be found in the counties across the [river] Milcov; on this side, the manufacturing of liquor made of plums and other fruit still meets the requirements of the population. However, because plum harvests are unpredictable, a new beverage called basamac has started to be sold recently. It is a poisonous mixture of alcohol, water, and who knows what other ingredients.[265]

Even earlier, in 1870, doctor Grigore Romniceanu was aware that fruit *raki* was the specific drink of Muntenia, while in Moldavia locals "consumed grain *raki* exclusively, a drink which was richer in alcohol than in any other part of the country."[266] He, like many others at the time, believed that "drunkenness is one of the greatest weaknesses of our laborers; it can be seen daily from the enormous taxes levied on spirits."[267] The first proponent of the "peasant-as-other" paradigm, doctor A. Sutzu, wrote in 1872 that in Romanian cities and to a lesser extent in the countryside, alcoholism was as widespread as it was in Russia and the Nordic countries.[268] The scientific debate he launched about the links between the spread of alcoholism and the social milieu, both rural and urban, was to be reprised in the early twentieth century.

In 1880, the situation was not yet deemed serious. Doctor Istrati commented that "here, the malaise is not yet very advanced."[269] Elsewhere in his study, he adds darker touches to this rather serene picture, but his comments remain fairly reassuring. Yet, the prospect was far from optimistic, as the number of taverns increased in towns and cities. The capital city, Bucha-

---

265 Aurelian, *Terra nostra*, 185.
266 Romniceanu, "Despre beuturi," 105.
267 Ibid., 106.
268 Sutzu, "Băuturile alcoolice și alcoolismul,"173.
269 Istrati, *O pagină din istoria contimpurană a României*, 293.

rest, was in a leading position. There, "sixty per cent of the new buildings are erected by ordinary innkeepers and owners of confectionery shops. Cafés have multiplied at a scandalous pace, and taverns are one thousand per each school."[270] In fact, according to some of the sources, the entire country was about to be invaded not only by taverns, but also by foreigners:

[B]ecause of the Greeks and the *ţânţari*[271] in Muntenia and the Yids[272] in Moldavia, not one street corner, village road, pathway, junction, or country road has been left to stand free of a tavern. Despite our glorified regulations preventing the Jews from running taverns in the villages, they now reign supreme everywhere. It is quite clear that here *money is power. Money taken by the Jew from the Romanian! For 10 to 15 gold ducats annually, often even less than that, the owners lease the inn on their estate or their village to these criminals, who then inject the blood of the Romanians with their burning, poisoning liquor and suck it out. They take the fruit of their harvests from them, selling them vice and death instead!*[273]

In doctor Istrati's writings, the theme of alcoholism is inextricably linked to the "Jewish question." However, the stereotype of the Jewish innkeeper had not been invented by the doctors, but was part of a widespread discourse[274] the doctors adopted by embedding it into a scientific paradigm. The Romanian state did, indeed, attempt to dislodge the Jewish leaseholders of rural taverns with targeted legislation in 1873,[275] but the degree of success of such measures remains difficult to assess. Doctor Istrati did not seem convinced of the efficacy of administrative coercion. Instead, he noted an increase in the number of taverns in towns, as well as in villages. In Prahova County, for example, he found a village of "*80 families* in which I counted *12 taverns.*"[276] The terrifying nature of such data turned doctor Istrati's study of 1880 into a veritable alarm call about the spread of alcoholism in Roma-

---

270 Ibid., 299.

271 In Romanian, this literally means mosquitoes, designating ethnic Romanians or Bulgarians from Macedonia.

272 Derogatory term designating a Jew, in Romanian "*jidan.*"

273 Istrati, *O pagină din istoria contimpurană a României*, 299–300.

274 See Oişteanu, *Imaginea evreului în cultura română. Studii de imagologie în context est-central european*, 176–95.

275 Iancu, *Evreii din România (1866–1919). De la excludere la emancipare*, 210.

276 Istrati, *O pagină din istoria contimpurană a României*, 314.

nia. The volume became a much read, often cited classic of the hygienist discourse.

In the 1880s, the health reports, as published in *Monitorul Oficial*, helped maintain the public's attention focused on the dangers of alcoholism in the peasant communities, especially in Moldavia. One such example is the report on public health in Covurlui County drawn up by doctor N. Takeanu in 1887. He wrote:

> The alcoholic beverages, which they insatiably partake of, are often of very poor quality (being made of bad, unprocessed grain), and are a poison that is often fatal to our villagers. I have often witnessed their revelries, where I had to watch the sad spectacle of bodies bereft of the vigour, agility, and vivacity these organic excitants are eminently supposed to impart. Instead of seeing well-nourished, vigorous, healthy bodies, we saw mechanical machines, animated for a few minutes by a feeble flicker which could halt their operation at any moment, and often for ever![277]

Doctor Takeanu's generic peasant was a malnourished alcoholic, in imminent danger of degeneracy.

Until 1880, the issue of alcoholism remained under the radar of medical circles in Romania. Interest peaked with doctor Istrati's study, where the problem of alcoholism was intimately linked to the "Jewish question." After this date, for more than fifteen years it disappeared from public debate. In 1894, the deputy for Iași, A. C. Cuza, attempted, and failed, to have Parliament pass a law on the "monopoly on the sale of alcohol." He invoked the growing spread of alcoholism, which he saw as the main cause for the "degeneration of our race" as manifested in the "decline of the ethnic Romanian population and the growing number of aliens."[278] Let's not be deceived by the non-specific language: for Cuza, these "aliens" were predominantly Jews, and the emergence of alcoholism in Romania was inextricably linked to the "Jewish invasion."[279] And while the anti-monopoly legislation was not adopted, the proposal brought alcoholism back to the forefront of public debate, where it remained without interruption until World War I.

---

277 Takeanu, "Raport general asupra serviciului sanitar din județul Covurlui," 2401.
278 Cuza, *Monopolul alcoolului*, iii–iv.
279 Ibid., xii.

1895 was a significant year for the debate on alcoholism: the Romanian Academy published two studies on the Romanian peasant by Nicolae Manolescu and Gheorghe Crăiniceanu. While both authors addressed the issue of alcoholism, they did not treat it as comprehensively as they treated other aspects of rural life, such as, for example, the hygiene of food or the home. This suggests that for both authors, alcoholism and bodily hygiene were not priorities. Could this be an indication that health professionals still did not deem the threat of alcoholism serious enough? It is quite possible, although both doctors were aware of the extent of alcohol consumption among the peasantry. Doctor Manolescu wrote:

> In all regions across the country, the villager consumes vast amounts of raki. [...] The villager consumes plum brandy [in Romanian: *ţuică*] and plum raki, grain raki [in Romanian: *basamac*], raki of grape must [in Romanian: *rachiu de tescovină; boştină; prăştină*]. Transylvanians also drink yeast raki. Muntenians[280] generally prefer plum brandy, Transylvanians drink grape raki, and those from the lowlands grain raki. [...] The villager will drink raki all day long, in the morning and before every meal. When he labours in the fields, for himself or for others, the villager will carry his raki with him and drinks as from a fountain of youth and vigour.[281]

As we have seen, doctor Manolescu's knowledge of the rural world was profound, so these words have the ring of truth. Doctor Crăiniceanu drew amply on the very alarming public health reports published in *Monitorul Oficial* when he wrote that in the southern Argeş county, "the abuse of the available alcoholic beverages among the peasants" was "frightening."[282] He found that in the county of Râmnicu Sărat, "plum brandy was consumed in excess and as a result the rural population decayed both morally and physically. The peasant deems raki to be a panacea which cures almost all ailments; each hour of leisure is spent in a drunken state; enormous amounts of alcohol are offered even to toddlers."[283] The medical corps started bracing itself to meet the growing peril. In 1894, the University of Bucharest an-

---

280 These were the inhabitants of the southern province of Romania, Muntenia.
281 Manolescu, *Igiena ţăranului*, 302.
282 Crăiniceanu, *Igiena ţăranului român*, 285.
283 Ibid.

nounced a contest for the publication of a "scientific-medical" pamphlet entitled *Alcoolismul în România* (Alcoholism in Romania). The winner of the award was the young D. D. Niculescu. His study, published in 1895, was the earliest overview on the topic. In the same year, A. C. Cuza published his proposed bill on the monopoly of alcohol sales and his two parliamentary speeches on the topic. The resulting volume, *Monopolul alcoolului* (The monopoly on alcohol), remained a widely read and much appreciated title until World War I.

1895, therefore, was the moment when the medical discourse made a powerful statement on alcoholism with two major impact studies endorsed by some of the country's key institutions: the Romanian Academy, the University of Bucharest, and Parliament. It was a winning formula. The medical corps started paying attention, and, presumably, so did the intellectual elite. The Romanian Athenaeum in Bucharest hosted public lectures on the topic. In April 1904, doctor Poenaru-Căplescu noted that his was the third lecture on alcoholism to be offered at the Athenaeum before a "well-educated and distinguished audience."[284] The first two had been doctor Al. Obregia's lecture in 1897, and doctor Urechia's lecture in 1901. The first professional association of the Kingdom's doctors, *Asociația Generală a Medicilor din Țară* (The national medical association) was created in 1897. Each year, the Association organized a congress on key themes of social medicine. The theme selected for 1898 was "Paludism," followed by "Pellagra" in 1899, and "Alcoholism" in 1900.[285] At the latter, the key address was given by doctor Ștefan Possa, the author of a voluminous study on alcoholism. This study, published on the pages of the Medical Association's periodicals[286] between 1900 and 1902, as well as in *Antialcoolul* (Anti-alcohol), the review of the Anti-Alcoholic League (Liga Anti-alcoolică) (1900–1901), received highly favorable reviews.

By the end of the twentieth century and the beginning of the twenty-first, most people seemed to agree that alcoholism was spreading in Romania. Medical statistical data on alcohol-related morbidity and mortality were mostly lacking, or very imprecise. Doctor Urechia used the official sta-

---

284 Poenaru-Căplescu, *Alcool și Alcoolism*, 3.
285 "Foreword," in *Buletinul Asociațiunei Generale a Medicilor din Țară*, IV, 1900, nos. 1–2, 4.
286 *Buletinul Asociațiunei Generale a Medicilor din Țară* [Bulletin of the national medical association] was followed by *Buletinul Medical. Organ al Asociațiunei Generale a Medicilor din Țară* [Medical bulletin: A publication of the national medical association].

tistics and determined that the rate of alcohol-induced conditions and death was extremely low: he calculated 304 deaths in 1896 and 411 in 1897.[287] The doctor questioned the accuracy of the officially compiled statistics, which, he commented, might lead one to believe that "there was no alcoholism" [in Romania]. And, as he reviewed the anti-alcoholic campaigns publicized by the Anti-Alcoholic League, he asked with rhetorical humor: "If there is nothing to combat, why should one have an anti-alcoholic league, why so many anti-alcoholic conferences, speeches, theatrical shows, banquets, and other similar weapons?"[288] The doctor was aware that these statistics were inaccurate: the data did not reflect the actual alcohol-related "deaths in the villages, because the cause of death was not recorded; the number of deaths in cities was also incorrect, because often the records listed the affected organs, but did not specify the cause of the lesions. Our public health statistics fail to document alcoholism in our country adequately."[289] Doctor I. Ştefănescu, too, was aware that the spread of alcoholism in Romania could not be assessed accurately on the basis of the official statistics on morbidity and mortality.[290] So were doctors Ştefan Possa[291] and Iacob Felix.[292] However, at his own hospital—the "Paşcanu" in Iaşi—doctor Possa tried to do what the official statistics had failed to do. Between January 19, 1898 and April 1, 1900, he entered in a special register all the patients whom he suspected of being alcoholics. There were some interesting results: of the 2,387 patients who checked in during the above-mentioned interval, doctor Possa identified 281 as alcoholics. This represented 11.8 per cent of the total.[293] But, fortunately, he did not stop with the register. He drew up a questionnaire about alcoholism and its consequences among the rural population. It was distributed to rural schoolteachers via the school inspectors and examiners in ten Moldavian counties.[294] He received responses from 452 schoolteachers, who sent in data for 601 villages.[295] This survey of alcoholism in Romania is the only one of its kind, as far as we know, and as such I shall dwell on

287 Urechia, "Cercetări asupra alcoolizmului în România," 190.
288 Ibid.
289 Ibid.
290 Ştefănescu, "Vindecarea beţiei ca remediu contra alcoolismului," 376–77.
291 Possa, "Alcoolismul," 57–58.
292 Felix, "Alcoolismul poporaţiunei rurale în comparaţiune cu alcoolismul poporaţiunei urbane," 1.
293 Possa, "Alcoolismul înaintea Congresului Asociaţiei Medicilor" II, 107.
294 The data were collected in 1899.
295 Possa, "Alcoolismul înaintea Congresului Asociaţiei Medicilor" II, 104–5.

it at some length. The design of the questionnaire highlights the social categories doctor Possa probed to determine the consequences of alcoholism: the subjects' material status, civil status, birth rate, the physical and mental health of offspring, and the number of antisocial incidents in which the subjects were involved. The survey also took into consideration the hereditary transmission of alcoholism. The numbers of persons identified as alcoholics differed from one county to another: from a minimum of 13 per cent in Fălciu to a maximum of 35 per cent in Neamț, averaging 24.2 per cent across the ten counties. Doctor Possa then collated the responses with the data he had collected in his hospital, and applied the results for Moldavia to the entire country. This allowed him to conclude that "between 20 and 30 per cent of the country's population are alcoholics"[296] But, alongside the alcoholics, there were other types of drinkers in Moldavia's villages: there were "moderates" and even "abstinents." The latter, it is true, were not numerous. In villages like Fălciu and Tutova, they were conspicuously absent. The data on civil status show that unmarried alcoholics were much more likely to live with common-law spouses than unmarried moderate drinkers. Let's take the county of Roman as an example: only 2 per cent of the moderate drinkers co-habited as opposed to a staggering 15 per cent of alcoholics. In Fălciu, things were even worse: 1.49 per cent of moderates and 21 per cent of alcoholics lived with common-law spouses. Doctor Possa's data suggest that a considerable number of alcoholic peasants failed to regularize their matrimonial status. In other words, they chose to live in sin. With respect to material status, it was listed as "good," "mediocre," or "bad." As was to be expected, percentages were calculated only for the latter, showing that alcoholics were generally poorer than moderate drinkers. Across all of Moldavia's ten counties, the number of poor moderate drinkers was smaller compared to alcoholics. For example, in Suceava, 35 per cent of alcoholics lived in poverty, compared to 5.30 per cent of moderates. In Tecuci Country, more than half (56 per cent) of alcoholics lived in dire poverty, compared to 15 per cent of moderate drinkers. In other words—doctors warned insistently—poverty generated alcoholism, and alcoholism trapped drinkers in poverty. Moreover, heavy drinking affected not only the drinkers themselves, but also their progeny. The most obvious consequence was

---

296 Ibid., 107–8.

the smaller number of children in the families of alcoholics. Doctor Possa calculated the average number of children in the families of moderate and heavy drinkers. His data are conclusive: in the county of Botoşani, there were 2.03 children on average in the families of moderates, compared to 1.50 in families of alcoholics. In Fălciu, the gap was even wider: 2.22 children for moderates, and 1.37 for alcoholics. The examples were numerous. In addition, the children of alcoholic parents, doctors found, inherited their parents' "worst habits." They frequently absconded from school or, when they attended, displayed "bad behavior and no desire to learn." In this area, too, statistics are revealing: in Dorohoi, only 11.76 per cent of children from families of moderate drinkers caused problems at school, compared to 70 per cent of the children of alcoholics. The figures were more balanced for Tutova County, where 10 per cent of turbulent children came from moderates' families, and 51 per cent from families of heavy drinkers. Schoolteachers were also asked to estimate how many of the children they deemed to be alcoholics had been born to alcoholic parents. The figures are shocking: the lowest, 62 per cent, was recorded for Dorohoi County, and the highest, 82 per cent, for Suceava.[297] Schoolteachers appear to have shared the doctors' belief that alcoholism was hereditary.

The data produced by this survey must be analyzed critically. Rural schoolteachers, who were supposed to know their villages well, supplied the primary data. This is positive. But one may ask: what was the difference between a "moderate" and an "alcoholic," and when did a "moderate" turn into an "alcoholic"? Even nowadays, these are difficult questions to answer. The survey aimed to divide the population between these two categories. All the other criteria used in the questionnaire played around these two fundamental categories. I wonder what Leonida Colescu might have said about doctor Possa's statistical survey, and I think I know the answer. I wonder, too, what results Colescu himself might have obtained, had he had the means and the time to organize a statistical survey on this scale on the topic of alcoholism in Romania. Because there are no other large-scale studies, we must content ourselves with doctor Possa's results. What they show with some certitude is that, by the end of the nineteenth century, the medical discourse on the threat of alcoholism had reached the rural intellectuals. From the members of the Higher

---

297 Ibid., 104–5.

Medical Council to the village schoolteachers, in 1899 everybody was convinced that alcoholism posed a serious threat to Romanian society.

The debate on alcoholism followed the course of the hygienist discourse on other themes of public health in the rural world: there came a point when one had to transition from collecting impressions to measuring the phenomenon. Those who studied it proceeded from literature to science: making statements was no longer enough, and one had to be able to support one's claims with statistical evidence. We have seen that, whereas data on morbidity and death were rather shaky, they were more precise on the production and consumption of alcohol. The state's fiscal interests required quantifiable data on consumption, and these, in turn, offered a more accurate picture of the rates of alcoholism in the Kingdom. Therefore, both doctors and tax authorities tried to collect data on the consumption of absolute alcohol per capita. But here, too, data varied, often significantly. In 1894, M. C. Haret was one of the first to make this calculation: he came up with 9.980 liters per capita.[298] For a while, this was the figure accepted in medical circles, too. However, as the number of official statistics increased, some doctors attempted their own calculations of alcohol consumption. Doctor Possa concluded that Haret's data were under-evaluated and that, in fact, the annual consumption of absolute alcohol was 11.7 liters per capita.[299] Doctor Adolf Urbeanu came up with an annual value of 12.5 liters of absolute alcohol per capita.[300] However, doctor Urechia calculated an average for the years 1896–1900, which came close to the figure advanced by Haret, namely, 9.2 liters per capita annually.[301] A consumption rate of 9 liters of absolute alcohol per capita placed Romania in fifth position among European countries in 1895,[302] which was not too high, but not low either. This value might explain some of the less alarming assessments of the situation in 1895. Doctor D. D. Niculescu, for instance, was one of the last observers who could seriously claim that the "rate of alcoholism [...] in Romania was not excessively high."[303] I believe that, after 1900, such a view became indefensible.

---

298 Haret, *Impozitul și beuturile alcoolice în România,* 161.
299 Possa, "Alcoolismul," 56.
300 Urechia, "Cercetări asupra alcoolizmului în România," 191.
301 Ibid., 192.
302 Possa, "Alcoolismul," 56.
303 Niculescu, *Alcoolismul în România,* 78.

More refined statistics compiled in the early twentieth century allowed for a revisionist approach to the entrenched stereotypical belief that alcoholism was mostly affecting the rural population. In an article jointly published by two well-known medical journals,[304] doctor Urechia demonstrated that alcohol consumption was in fact higher among the urban population. He wrote:

> The urbanite drinks more wine, more beer, and more raki. So, who is the real alcoholic? I think it is time to shatter the old "rural = alcoholic" cliché, and admit that the real alcoholic in Romania is the urbanite. With an annual consumption of 7 liters of wine and 5 liters of raki, it is difficult to concur that "our peasants are alcoholics in their overwhelming majority." But with the 31 liters of wine, 6 liters of beer, and 17 of raki, it is most probable that many city-dwellers will eventually become alcoholics.[305]

Responding to Urechia, the venerable doctor Iacob Felix attempted to mitigate some of the more uncompromising statements of his opponent. But even he was forced to admit that "our urban population certainly drinks more alcohol than the rural inhabitants."[306] It is a clear example of how statistics, even in its imperfect early days, and with all the approximations criticized by contemporaries, could lead to a more nuanced view of the rural/urban divide in modern Romania.

## "Alcoholism: From Birth till Death"

Having reviewed briefly the medical views on the spread of alcoholism based on post-1895 statistical data, I shall now analyze the imagery and ideas deployed in this discourse. I shall attempt to identify the hazards of alcoholism at both the individual and the societal levels, and the ways in which this social virus propagated. Let's first define our terms: how did doctors define alcoholism in the late nineteenth century? Doctor Ştefănescu believed that it was a "chronic disease, meaning an ailment that progressed gradually. It was an artificial condition, triggered by abusive drinking by anyone who con-

---

304 Urechia "Cercetări asupra alcoolizmului în România."
305 Ibid., 194.
306 Felix, "Alcoolismul poporaţiunei rurale în comparaţiune cu alcoolismul poporaţiunei urbane," 4.

sumed liquors in immoderate amounts, thereby causing a slow, progressive poisoning of their body.[307] Doctor Niculescu regarded alcoholism as a "composite condition produced by an abuse of liquor; it is made up of a number of varied ailments connected by a shared origin."[308] In his turn, doctor Căplescu talked about alcohol poisoning when he referred to the condition as "a state of intoxication of the body through alcohol."[309] The condition could be acute or chronic, but the doctor also mentioned an intermediary state, which he termed "latent alcoholism." Acute alcoholism, in doctor Căplescu's view, was the state of ordinary drunkenness, which he associated with the lower echelons of society. He reiterated its well-known consequences, as repeatedly mentioned and emphasized in the medical discourse: "[A]cute alcoholism is the state of drunkenness you have often seen among ordinary folk—and it is revolting. The drunken man is a beast without judgment, without emotion. He loses his balance, he insults, swears, is violent without reason—causes fracas—kills. [...] The drunken man is a hideous, degraded creature, often seen falling over and lying in ditches and in mud, before going back home where he beats up his wife and children, who try in vain to abscond in terror."[310] It is noteworthy that doctor Căplescu insisted on the violent manifestations of drunkenness, its antisocial aspects, which fits with the anti-alcohol discourse of his time. This was also the approach of a pamphlet published a few years earlier by the Romanian Anti-Alcoholic League. With an introduction by the indefatigable doctor Cuza, the pamphlet was a compilation of alcohol-related incidents gleaned from the press and presented, with all the trappings of scholarly discourse, as "social documents."[311] When doctors wished to foreground the "evils" of contemporary alcoholism, produced by alcohol distilled from cereals (in Romanian: *bucate*), they compared it unfavorably with the merry drunken revelries such as the ones occasioned in the past by grape harvests. For example, doctor Istrati reminisced nostalgically: "Who fails to remember the times when, in the autumn, thousands of carts, laden with the still fermenting must, drove one after another, from Focşani to Iaşi, and to Botoşani, and so on. Drunken folk often surrounded the carts, forming marching rounds

---

307 Ştefănescu "Vindecarea beţiei ca remediu contra alcoolismului," 343.
308 Niculescu, *Alcoolismul în România*, 10.
309 Poenaru-Căplescu, *Alcool şi Alcoolism*, 21.
310 Ibid., 22.
311 Cuza, *Victimele alcoolului*.

of dancing people, who accompanied the carts, singing and jigging along for miles!"[312] Oh, the charm of the good old times!

In time, regular alcohol consumption became a chronic condition, which destroyed the drinker physically as well as mentally. More often than not, those "victims of alcohol" who did not meet an early death ended up in lunatic asylums or became numbers in statistics of suicides. As an "alienist," doctor Alexandru Şuţu was well placed to understand the symptoms. "The drunkards' physiognomy expresses his moral degradation," he wrote. And further:

His need to drink becomes compulsive, and he will resort to all means, even the most humiliating ones, to satisfy a passion which devours and tortures him endlessly. He becomes maniacal, irritable, violent, hitting those around him mercilessly; he loses all respect for others, as well as all self-respect; impassable and unconcerned, he stands amidst the turbulences he himself has caused, and is indifferent to the downfall of his own family. In some, their conscience might eventually awake, and they will realize their decline; disgusted and angry with themselves, they will find that their only salvation is suicide.[313]

In 1872, doctor Şuţu estimated that, at the Mărcuţa hospice, out of 100 cases of "alienation" (mental illness), 20 were caused by alcoholism. Curiously, in my view, this was identical to the rate of alcohol-related mental illness recorded at the same time in France by Morel, Marcé, and Contese.[314] However, a few years later, the doctor offered an estimate of 40 cases out of 100 at the same hospice.[315] If doctor Şuţu is right, this means that from 1872 to 1877 the rate of alcohol-induced dementia doubled, at least at the Mărcuţa hospice. This can only be interpreted as corresponding to a rise of alcoholism in Romanian society as a whole. Another well-known alienist, doctor George Mileticiu, studied the role of alcoholism in the pathogeny of mental conditions starting from data in the same hospice. His conclusions were similar to doctor Şuţu's: in the early 1870s, between 15 and 17 per

---

312 Istrati, *O pagină din istoria contimpurană a României*, 295.
313 Sutzu, *Alienatul în faţa societăţii şi a şciinţei*, 125.
314 Sutzu, "Băuturile alcoolice şi alcoolismul," 173–74.
315 Sutzu, *Alienatul în faţa societăţii şi a şciinţei*, 125.

cent of cases were alcohol-related, a proportion that rose to 39.3 per cent in 1880. The situation appeared to stabilize over the next decade and a half. For the 1891–1894 interval, doctor Mileticiu studied patients at the Madona-Dudu hospice in Craiova, and calculated that in 38.9 per cent of cases alcohol played a "causal role."[316]

As mentioned, everyone who wrote about the destructive effects of alcoholism used a series of stereotypical images. Sometimes, these stereotypes were embedded in a personal discourse, for example in life narratives. Quite often, for instance, doctor Ştefănescu asks his readers to join him on journeys across alcohol-soaked rural areas. Here is an example:

> I urge you to take a journey through the country's villages. Your coachman will be the first to initiate you into the secrets of drinking in our country. Along long, tedious routes, he will show you things that you may have never asked to know. He knows, for instance, which places sell good wine, which tavern sells plum brandy (in Romanian: *ţuica*) worse than kitchen-sink slop, he knows where the "gents" (in Romanian: *persoanele*) drink and where the peasants drink, and so on. Once outside the city, this man will have you stop at all the taverns; his horses stop there of their own accord, they are so used to it. Winter or summer, the man's thirst for liquor never abates.[317]

The first contact with the rural world, as mediated by the coachman, tells us a lot about the lifestyles of the rural population, at least of significant sections of it. The village in Ilfov County, described by doctor Ştefănescu as a realm of "poverty and ignorance," peopled by alcohol-soaked creatures, is a vivid picture of the ravages of alcohol in the peasant environment:

> One day I was visiting a village in Ilfov Country. It was far from Bucharest, in an isolated place. There were about one hundred souls living there, all poor and sad, as they are in many parts of the countryside. The entire village was impoverished: you should have seen the houses, the roads, words fail to describe them! There was no church to enchant the eyes a little, no school, nothing for the eyes to rest on. This was the monotonous picture of poverty

---

316 Mileticiu, *Studii psihiatrice*, 26.
317 Ştefănescu, "Vindecarea beţiei ca remediu contra alcoolismului," 406.

and ignorance. And yet, in truth, there was something [...] it was the home of a deputy mayor of the village. I wanted to meet this rural notable, I wished to speak to him, but I found it impossible to awake him from his alcoholic torpor, in which he was often immersed. The village I am talking about lacked in everything, and yet, it had acquired a temple of liquor, a tavern, a foundation of the self-same deputy mayor![318]

Doctor Ștefănescu focused on the general picture of the village and some of its denizens. Other doctors chose to enter the desolate home of the alcoholic peasant. In general, rural homes were impoverished and one may wonder what you could possibly add to an already negative situation in the rural habitat? And yet, some doctors attempted a description. Here is doctor Poenaru-Căplescu:

The home of the alcoholic peasant is a heap of rubbish. The interior is dirty, the walls unpainted, the windows broken, the door cracked; the courtyard is desolate, there is no tree, no cattle, no poultry; his children walk around with no clothes, because he spent everything at the tavern, and he still owes payment in labor. Most peasants' households are like this one, for most peasants are alcoholics.[319]

Ultimately, doctor Căplescu's description is not too different from the well-known outlines of the rural habitation by doctor Istrati and others. Everywhere, the universal scourge, alcohol, brought about poverty, disease, and decay.

The tavern was a site of perdition and as such occupied an important place in the medical literature. Descriptions of taverns were obligatory *topoi* in antialcohol writings, a convention observed by most authors. Doctor Ștefănescu, for example, commented on the multiple social roles of the tavern:

Everywhere in the countryside, the tavern is also the village general store, catering for all rural residents as well as for the lowliest of peasants; here he proceeds to drink, although he first entered the place to buy something else.

---

318 Ștefănescu, "Vindecarea beției ca remediu contra alcoolismului," 375.
319 Poenaru-Căplescu, *Alcool și Alcoolism,* 33.

The tavern is the only public place in the area: here, one can buy refreshments, meet people, gather for enjoyment and for exchanging information; the village notables, the officials, the priest, the schoolmaster, and whoever breathes in the rural world, they all come here, filing past the tavern-keeper.[320]

The picture is more tragic in writings with an obvious antisemitic agenda, such as those by A. C. Cuza. He cites a letter by the district practitioner Ioan Şoneriu, who lived in the market town Suliţa in Botoşani County:

That the raki is the cause of all misfortunes is easy to see for anyone who, on a holiday, enters a village tavern, or any of the thirty taverns in this town. All are full of Romanians of both sexes and all ages; moreover, amidst the throng of people, one can see women nursing babies, carousing with all the others. Here, you can see in all its nakedness the state of physical and moral degradation produced in man by alcohol.[321]

Owing to Cuza, doctor Şoneriu's letter became a celebrated text in the anti-alcohol literature.

Unwittingly, doctors identified an anthropologically verified fact: the consumption of food, especially of alcohol, is the necessary, one might even say obligatory, accompaniment of all forms of sociability, alcohol being a key ingredient. From this perspective, the district doctor Iosef Weissberg attempted an explanation for widespread alcoholism in the peasant environment:

Alcoholism haunts the peasant's life step by step, from birth until death. Alcohol is consumed to celebrate his birth and his christening; mothers give spirits [in Romanian: *basamac*] to their children, alas, even to those of a tender age; the peasant has alcohol at work, when he is ill, with his meals, when he gets married; he performs the reproductive act when soaked in alcohol; he seals a trade deal with a drink [in Romanian: *adălmaş*]; finally, he is killed by alcohol and is surrounded by it even after death as others drink at this wake for the good health of his soul.[322]

---

320 Ştefănescu, "Vindecarea beţiei ca remediu contra alcoolismului," 409.
321 Cuza, *Monopolul alcoolului*, 27.
322 Weissberg, "Alcoolismul în Ialomiţa," 348.

It would be a mistake to believe that doctors only highlighted alcoholism in the rural environment. Equally frequent references were made to the abuse of alcohol in an urban setting. Doctor Poenaru-Căplescu, for example, speaking to a distinguished audience at the Romanian Athenaeum, reproduced the argument of his colleague Weissberg, almost point by point, but adapting it to urban milieus and adding his own annotations:

The young drink, and the old drink, we drink in the *summer* to cool down, in *winter* to warm up—all very natural! We drink in the morning to toughen up. We have an aperitif, we drink with a meal and after a meal, we drink in the evening, too. We drink to rejoice when *a child is born*, we drink to mourn when someone dies. We drink at engagements and weddings, and on name days: Ioniță, Ghiță, Costică, Mitică, Mișu, Nicu, Basile, and so on, we celebrate them all. We drink on the day of the Forty Martyrs [in Romanian: *Mucenici*], we drink on all the festival and feast days, at Christmas, Easter, etc., at all the family and public gatherings, at charitable events. After each successful transaction, business deal, and bargain we have a round of drinks [in Romanian: *adălmaș*]. On election days, alcohol flows. Men and women drink, laborers drink for strength, lazy folk drink to pass time, and professionals drink too, writers, artists, poets, lawyers, professors, army men, politicians, all, without exception. *Nowadays, even churchmen drink with a vengeance, bottle after bottle!*[323]

Doctor Căplescu's comments on drinking among the professional classes are surpassed in dark humor by doctor Ştefănescu's observations in a similar vein:

One can often hear people exclaim: the poor peasant is drinking himself to death! This is true, but, on closer inspection, all professions now count many drunkards in their ranks. [...] For example, Romanian tavern-keepers, who, without appearing to do so, poison people with their drinks, start by first poisoning themselves. They deserve to be ranked at the top of the alcoholics' hierarchy. [...] The tavern-keepers—who, in fact, have an unfair advantage in the contest—are followed, in order of consumption, by butchers and

---

323 Poenaru-Căplescu, *Alcool și Alcoolism*, 29.

cooks; coachmen, cart-drivers, and fiddlers; priests, mayors, notaries, and office clerks; vineyard laborers and coopers, who drink more than machinists, blacksmiths, and millers; and finally, many of us, who drink more than the sellers of millet beer [in Romanian: *braga*], lemonade, and rahat lokoum, and so on. There is a tacit emulation among the—more or less liberal—professions, from the cart driver who punctures the vessels he is carrying to the market to sip the spirit (I saw one myself in the centre of Bucharest), to the custodian of the natural science museum who drinks the alcohol from the specimen jars he is supposed to guard.[324]

These doctors, and many of us today, still appear unable to speak about drunkenness and alcoholism without a touch of humour. Few of those who addressed the topic managed to keep a straight face.

## *The "Hazards of Alcoholism"*

Besides poverty—which is serious enough—what were the other dimensions of what doctors called the "hazards of alcoholism"? What were the medical and sanitary dangers of alcoholism? In the first place, we know from doctor Istrati that "drunkards are the ones contributing the most to the spread of epidemics. They seem to be the most vulnerable to all the endemic and epidemic maladies, and mortality is higher amongst them."[325] In other words, alcoholism became a key cause of the high rates of morbidity and mortality in modern Romania. To combat this, the state mobilized all the resources of its public health system. In addition, saying that alcoholics were more predisposed to illness than others was a way of hitting back at the old, but still popular, faith in the healing powers of alcohol. Doctor Ştefănescu, for example, wondered rhetorically:

How many are those, even among the poor, who do not have a bottle of raki carefully secreted away in some cupboard? Everybody has some stowed away, for himself and his family, or for gifting to others, as is the custom, under the pretext that a little brandy, grain raki, grape liquor, or rum cures

---

324 Ştefănescu, "Vindecarea beţiei ca remediu contra alcoolismului," 426.
325 Istrati, *O pagină din istoria contimpurană a României*, 290.

everything from bruises to pains in the heart, colics, indigestions, and other digestive ailments. Liquor is believed to be this universal medicine, this panacea for external, and especially for internal, use, which can be administered to everybody, from children to the elderly.[326]

Doctor Ștefănescu also documented the—typically urban—belief that alcohol was better than water, which recent bacteriological research had found to be a seriously pathogenic medium.[327] And, if we do not trust doctor Ștefănescu, we may prefer to heed doctor Possa's comments about the "prejudice that alcohol is an antiseptic, which kills microbes and protects humans during epidemics," a belief he himself considered evidently to be "a totally bogus claim."[328] Doctors had much trouble with these "prejudices," because in popular culture alcohol was considered to possess almost miraculous powers: it warms up the body, increases stamina, and can be included among foodstuffs rather than poisonous substances. But these "prejudices" were not solely shared among the rural population. Doctor Adolf Urbeanu, for example, knew from experience that many members of the elites, such as the country's lawmakers, shared them. In 1900, Parliament voted on the so-called "plum brandy law" (in Romanian: *legea țuicii*), which doctor Urbeanu himself had initiated and promoted. He summarised the ideas and opinions canvassed in the debates on this occasion. Some alleged that "plum brandy [in Romanian: *țuica*] is a healthy food, a wholesome food, a health drink,"[329] despite the widespread concerns of the medical profession. The only beverage to be considered poisonous was *basamac*, grain raki, which was associated with the Jewish tavern keepers, as noted with sad lucidity by the doctor:

It is not just experts in the matter, but also poets and literary men who, having adopted the belief that basamac is "poisonous," and "a bane," write about the "accursed" drink. The consequences of drinking basamac are so obvious, and so terrifying, that no one could ever imagine that the misfortunes of so many families were caused only by [basamac], without other noxious substances. Therefore, in the popular imagination, we can see that basamac

---

326 Ștefănescu, "Vindecarea beției ca remediu contra alcoolismului," 410.
327 Ibid., 425.
328 Possa, "Alcoolismul," 11.
329 Urbeanu, *Țuica și basamacul,* 19.

has been firmly associated with poison; and who else but the Jew could handle it? In the popular conception, the trinity basamac, poison, and Jew is one and undivided. When you say basamac, you mean the poison sold by the Jewish tavern keeper; when you say Jewish tavern keeper, you say poisoned basamac; when you say poison in the village, you say basamac prepared by the Jew. In fact, basamac is closely linked to the Jew. The Jew brought it here, the Jew prepared it, the Jew faked it.[330]

This text is a good guide to the public discourse in Romania at the start of the twentieth century. But perhaps more dangerous was the idea that alcoholism could be transmitted genetically. In 1895, doctor D. D. Niculescu reviewed all the medical theories concerning the genetic transmission of alcoholism before concluding:

Alcoholism can be passed on from parents to children either directly, or as *dipsomania,*[331] idiocy, mania, epilepsy, hysteria, etc., etc. For a child to be born with any of these predispositions it is not necessary for the parent to have been an inveterate alcoholic. Research has shown that it was enough for the progenitor of such children to be drunk at conception. This is because in alcoholic individuals, virility is weakened, the genital organs are flaccid, testicles can degenerate to almost complete atrophy, and, moreover, alcohol can have a harmful influence on the spermatozoa. If the mother is an alcoholic, it can lead to miscarriages, just like syphilis, resulting from the premature death of the embryo or the fetus. And, just as hard-drinking individuals in time deteriorate and reach a state of manifest weakness, nations of abusive drinkers reach an analogous state of debility known as *degeneracy.*[332]

Obviously, alcoholism was considered a key factor contributing to racial degeneracy. All the conditions that were construed as being transmitted genetically were active factors in degeneracy. They killed off not just the affected individuals, thereby posing a threat to the present of the nation, but also the progeny, the future of the nation. Racial degeneration was the darkest nightmare in the period's medical dystopia.

---

330 Ibid., 39.
331 Italics in the original.
332 Niculescu, *Alcoolismul în România,* 133.

## Against Drunkenness

Individuals, as well as the entire society, mobilized against a danger of such magnitude. Thus, modern Romania's temperance and anti-alcohol movement was born. All the medical writings I have used as sources for this chapter stemmed from research on alcoholism, but they can as easily be subsumed under the category of temperance and anti-alcohol literature. Doctors were among the first to alert society to the dangers of alcoholism. The anti-alcohol propaganda produced attitudes that are still recognizable today. Doctor Ştefănescu documented one such attitude:

> [P]easant women are exasperated by the excesses of their spouses. They search for some remedy, some drug—often just another drink—and so, for 10 *lei*, they end up purchasing in Bucharest a phial of *Antibetina* (a drug prepared by the Hungarian pharmacist Vertes from Lugoj, a charlatan's remedy, based on an active ingredient that is an emetic, therefore it provokes vomiting), which they secretly add to their husbands' food to wean them off drink! Poor souls, in their naivety, they imagine that drunkenness can be treated with drugs, like one treats fever with quinine.[333]

What is interesting in this passage is the adaptation of a modern notion that one can "treat drunkenness" as one of many other illnesses; the fact that the drug was a "charlatan's remedy" is a different matter. One must situate this in its context: many of the period's drugs were in fact "charlatan's remedies," prepared and sold in pharmacies. However, the rural world had its own solutions, which were perfectly integrated in their own environment and of which I know from my own experience. For instance, there was the so-called "bind by the priest" (in Romanian: *legare la preot*), a solemn vow of abstinence consecrated in church whereby the drinker pledged to abstain from drink, at least for a specific period. It is still practiced in my hometown today. I think that this type of oath must have a history, even though I could not find the evidence in the medical literature.

This is how doctor Ştefănescu characterized Romania's anti-alcohol movement in 1896: "Romania is a quasi-virgin territory with respect to at-

---

333 Ştefănescu, "Vindecarea beţiei ca remediu contra alcoolismului," 375–76.

tempts at curbing drinking and combating alcoholism."[334] However, only
five years later, doctor Urechia assessed the situation in the following terms:
"[T]oday, Romania has no reason to envy Western countries: its anti-alcohol army has trained cadres, troops, and even its own mercenaries."[335] Did
anything change in Romania's anti-alcohol movement between 1896 and
1901, or is Urechia's a very subjective assessment? The truth must have been
somewhere in the middle: doctor Urechia's study was directed against A.
C. Cuza and against the *modus operandi* of the Romanian Anti-Alcoholic
League, which prioritized action in the rural world. But doctor Urechia kept
trying to prove that alcoholism was primarily an urban phenomenon in Romania. In 1904, doctor Poenaru-Căplescu, addressing his "distinguished
audience," was confidently stating that "so much has been written, and so often, on the topic of alcohol consumption, that many of you, ladies and gentlemen, already know what I am going to say."[336] This must have been more
than a mere attempt at winning the listeners' goodwill. By the turn of the
century, alcoholism had become, indeed, a much-debated topic in Romania's public arena. The "fight against alcoholism" entered a new phase on
May 4, 1897, when the Romanian Anti-Alcoholic League was founded in
Iași, with A. C. Cuza as its secretary-general. In 1900, the League's periodical, *Antialcoolul*,[337] was launched, with doctor M. Minovici as its editor. This
publication was the main channel for conducting the campaign against alcoholism in Romania until World War I. To some extent, therefore, doctor
Urechia was right.

After 1894, the main methods for combating the social effects of alcoholism were radical measures, such as, for example, abstinence. In contrast,
until then the medical corps focused mainly on disseminating information
on healthy culinary habits. The recommended methods were much more
modest and included a reduced consumption of distilled liquors in general,
and especially of grain-derived spirits, and a ban on the sale of adulterated
or impure alcoholic beverages. The harmfulness of beverages was evaluated on a scale that opposed distilled drinks to drinks obtained by fermentation. As a general principle, the noxious effects increased with the alcohol

---

334 Ibid., 452.
335 Urechia, "Cercetări asupra alcoolizmului în România," 189.
336 Poenaru-Căplescu, *Alcool și Alcoolism*, 3.
337 The complete title was *Antialcoolul. Organul Ligii antialcoolice, secțiunile Iași-București* [Anti-alcohol: The organ of the anti-alcoholic league, Iași and Bucharest Sections].

content. Therefore, distilled spirits are at the top of the toxicity table, followed by wine and the relatively innocuous beer. The public health battle concentrated on distilled spirits, which were, in turn, classified and ranked according to the chief ingredient used: distilled spirits made from fruit (for example the national drink *țuica*, plum brandy) were considered healthier than those made from grain. As was to be expected, the earliest sanitary measures were taken in Bucharest, where doctor Felix ran the public health services. In 1882, he proposed a ban on the sale of unrefined spirits. This launched a major campaign against distilled spirits. The first victory was obtained in 1886, when a ban was placed in Bucharest on the sale of "raki produced from unrefined spirits."[338] It was followed in 1893 by a change in the Health Act, which saw the addition of Art. 156. It stipulated that "only perfectly refined ethyl alcohol was acceptable in the manufacturing of spirits. [...] It had to have a content of minimum 95 per cent per volume at 15 degrees Celsius."[339] This article extended the regulations of 1886 from the Bucharest area to the country's entire territory. Article 156 of the Health Act was expanded in the new "Regulations on Hygiene in the Manufacturing and Retail of Food and Drinks" of 1895.[340] From a legislative point of view, this was a triumph that ensured that the hygienic requirements in the production of spirits were met. However, the distance between norms and practices was not always easy to bridge. Even with the health legislation in place, alcoholism remained a problem that required a tougher approach. At the end of the nineteenth century, the "question of alcoholism" was a growing social anxiety that was difficult to control through normative and rational action alone. The specter of racial degeneration haunted Romanian society, blocking the inhibiting mechanisms of alcoholism, while constantly magnifying its virtual dangers.

338 Niculescu, *Alcoolismul în România*, 141.
339 Șuta et al., *Legislația sanitară*, 121.
340 "Regulament asupra privegherii sanitare a fabricațiunii alimentelor și băuturilor și a comerțului cu alimente și băuturi," Ibid., 511–15.

5

"PELLAGRA, THE TRAGEDY OF OUR PEASANT":
AN ILLNESS IS BORN

When doctors spoke publicly about the "hygiene of the Romanian peasant" and described the rural homes and alimentation, they did so chiefly to explain the high morbidity and mortality rates among the rural population. Most of the medical conditions affecting peasants were not specific to the rural environment: scarlet fever, diphtheritic angina, malaria, and smallpox decimated the population without regard to location, class, or wealth. Popular sayings demonstrate a general awareness of the equalizing role of death. But even popular wisdom had not reckoned with a strange condition that appeared in the last four decades of the nineteenth century. This condition affected the peasant population almost without exception. It was undoubtedly an illness caused by poverty, like many others, but it mainly affected the rural mainly. This was pellagra, called *jupuială* (skin peeling) by peasants in Moldavia and *pârleală* (burning itch) in Muntenia. It was referred to everywhere as the "disease of the poor" or the "disease of poverty."[341]

## *The Illness and Its Representations*

First, here is an introduction to the terrifying disease that attacked Romania's villages towards the end of the nineteenth century. What were the manifestations of this disease? Doctors left many descriptions of the symptoms. Here is a female patient, as described by doctor Nicolae Popescu:

> Mira Petre Radu Drăghici, age 32, from the village of Gratia, was seen in June 1887. No pellagric hereditary antecedents. Alimentation based on *mălai* [polenta]. The condition first appeared in the spring of 1887 with a slight erythema on the back of the hands. She is tall, well built, with a good physique, which can be considered typical; the only sign is a purple erythematous desquamation on the back of both hands. She does not mention any other source of suffering, but is worried because she saw many people who have the condition deteriorate and eventually develop mental illness and die. All I could

---

341 Neagoe, "Studiu asupra pelagrei," 283.

do was to recommend a good diet and tell her to give up the corn porridge [in Romanian: *mămăligă*], which, she said, was difficult as they were poor and did not have much else to eat. In the spring of 1888, around the month of June, she comes again at my office at the village hall, but now, instead of the cheerful woman with a well-proportioned body, we see this tall, lanky figure, with a sad, plaintive countenance, bent over, and the complexion of an ashen hue; the epidermis is stretched and shiny along the cheekbones and on her forehead skin scales which come off easily. The backs of the hands upwards to the third of the forearms are erythematous, with some shiny and some flaky areas. She suffers from headaches, vertigo, pain in the limbs and the spine, lack of appetite, stomach pain, and diarrhea. Her gait is heavy. All these symptoms appear in the spring and last through the summer before disappearing in the autumn. In 1889, the woman we had seen two years earlier was hardly recognizable. All the symptoms of 1888 were there, added to which she was also now thin, anaemic, and walked with difficulty.[342]

The doctor presaged a "fatal outcome" for Mira, which is undoubtedly what happened.

In the medical literature on pellagra, the following is a somewhat celebrated case. It was the first of such cases to be described, and the author is none other than the equally celebrated doctor Iacob Felix. He introduces us to Achim Radu, a wheelwright from the village Românești. In June 1859, suffering from the effects of "clap acquired a long time ago," the man met with doctor Felix at the hospital of Mușcel County. This is the doctor's report:

The patient, 48 years of age, stated that *mămăliga* was his only nutrient, as bread, meat, milk, and cheese appeared less than twenty times per year on his table, and even onions were rare; he said he liked plum raki, but for lack of means, it was only rarely, when he had some money, that he could afford a shot; he also said that in April 1859 he started feeling considerably weak and could not work, that he had headaches and occasional burning pain in the joints, he could not sleep and did not have an appetite. In the month of May, his hands and cheeks became swollen, the swelling caused only a little pain and passed after three weeks, but the cracked skin peeled off and became

---

342 Popescu, *Pellagra,* 89–90.

"black like a Gypsy's." The patient's weakness became such that he could no longer look after his household.[343]

These were the obvious symptoms of pellagra, which doctor Felix diagnosed very precisely. After nineteen days in hospital, the patient regained his appetite and his condition generally improved. He left the hospital some time between July 19 and 22, 1859. Doctor Felix saw the wheelwright Achim Radu again a few months later, as he noted:

In January 1860, my professional duties took me to the village Rumânești, where I found our pellagra sufferer again. The skin on his face and hands was pigmented as before [...], the patient declared that he was fit to work, but that he became tired sooner than two years before; but his regular sleep and appetite had returned. I gave him some sulphuric quinine powders which I had on me and urged him to visit me again in Câmpulung. On this occasion, I also saw the patient's spouse and children, who were all in good health. After that, I only saw the patient again on June 10, 1860, when my duties took me back to the village Rumânești. The patient told me that the symptoms of 1859 had returned in April and May 1860; although the swelling in the face and hands had retreated [...], he had a coin-sized blister on the back of his right hand, which was filled with a little reddish fluid. The patient refused hospitalization, which he blamed for the return of the illness; I gave him twenty powder doses with 3 grams of quinine sulphate each for the next twenty days and recommended nutritious food. Almost ten months later, on March 28, 1861, I saw the pellagra sufferer from Rumânești again at the hospital. I could hardly recognize him. Although only 50 years of age, he looked 65 [...], he could not keep any of the food he ate, he was constantly thirsty and had a light diarrhea, pain in the spine and occasional numbness in his limbs. [...] By March 30, the sickness and diarrhea had stopped, by April 4 some of the ulcers had healed or looked cleaner; the patient, feeling better, and although he was still weak and still had pain in the spine and limbs, did not want to stay hospitalized. He was so melancholic that I let him leave, armed with a free prescription for iron carbonate and quinine sulphate. I also gave instructions to the district under-surgeon to keep the patient under observation and report

343 Felix, "Observațiuni asupra pellagri în județul Mușcel," 23.

to me. I learned from him that, two weeks later, the patient succumbed to dementia, without intermission, and died in the early days of May this year.[344]

How did doctors in the second half of the nineteenth century perceive and describe the condition? In 1887, the young doctor C. Constantinescu considered pellagra a "generalized, cachectic malady," most probably caused by "slow intoxication with altered corn: immature corn, stored in unsuitable conditions, could be affected by mold fungi or fermentation."[345] Over a decade later, in her doctoral thesis in medicine and surgery, Elena Manicatide considered pellagra "a specific illness, brought about by intoxication with a substance present in altered corn, and which acted mainly on the nervous system."[346] Her mentor, doctor Victor Babeş, used a more accessible language in a book published in the interwar period and aimed at a wider readership: "Pellagra is a poisoning caused by corn which has gone bad; it can remain unnoticed for a long time, and manifests itself in a body that is weakly either from birth or from starvation, illness or degeneration."[347] It is noteworthy that doctors described the condition in general terms by inclusion in a specific nosological group (intoxication/poisoning), establishing an aetiology (consumption of altered corn), or foregrounding, like doctor Babeş, certain individual predispositions. Although doctors were not generally an impressionable lot, the physical and mental degradation of the terminal phases of the illness often terrified observers. Doctor Felix was one of the first to observe the effects of this terrible disease:

In some villages of Ţara Românească,[348] one can see living corpses covered in raw wounds, with cracked or hardened skin on their limbs, dragging their feet in the streets. The last manifestation of the souls of these wretched creatures is a lethal madness. In his simplicity, the peasant calls this disease "pârleală" [burning, itch] in some regions and "pecingine rea" [bad sores, impetigo] in others. Science has called it "pellagra."[349]

---

344 Ibid., 23–24.
345 Constantinescu, *Contribuţiune la studiul pellagrei*, 74.
346 Manicatide, *Contribuţiuni la studiul etiologiei pelagrei*, 22.
347 Babeş, *Pelagra*, 12.
348 Ţara Românească and Muntenia are interchangeable names for one of the historic provinces of Romania. Wallachia is an older name for the same region.
349 Felix, "Despre nutrimentul ţăranilor," 366.

Other doctors also commented on the striking "aspect" of pellagra sufferers. In 1887, doctor I. Antoniu considered that the "horrible" aspect of pellagra sufferers could not fail to touch "even the most apathetic of humans."[350] This was indeed, everyone agreed, a terrifying illness that often ended in death.

Having identified the new malady, doctors resorted to the already considerable specialist literature published abroad. Aligning itself with the period's approach to the sciences, the medical profession ordered and created hierarchies of symptoms, established 'stages' and 'degrees' in the evolution of the disease, and studied the aetiology of the new malady. In other words, the new condition was being constructed and contextualized. Today's historians cannot ignore this new scientific approach to the emergence and 'invention' of pellagra. Doctors followed two complementary paths. One of these involved establishing nosological categories for the principal manifestations of the illness, i.e. erythema, poor digestion, and nervous symptoms. Alternatively, these symptoms were linked to stages of the illness, usually three, to which were added the "prodroms," the supposed early symptoms announcing the onset of the illness. I shall use the latter descriptive model because it is more comprehensive and associates symptoms to stages. The first symptom of pellagra is pellagric erythema, which appears as "various degrees of purple reddening of the cutaneous surface [...] especially of areas exposed to the sun, such as the face and neck, the chest and the backs of the hands and feet; the erythema continues with the desquamation of the affected areas."[351] In other words, the skin reddens and, over the course of a few weeks, becomes dry and can easily be peeled off, or "flaked off," the expression peasants used when talking about the condition. Once the erythema disappears, the affected areas of the skin change color, turning a deep red, almost black. Some of doctor Nicolae Popescu's patients described this symptom as "charring" (in Romanian: *pârleală neagră*) and "attributed it some serious characteristics."[352] Characteristically, erythema appeared in the spring, around March, and returned every year in the same period, but in increasingly serious forms. However, doctors identified an earlier stage before erythema. Signs included acute tiredness, headaches, insomnia or leth-

350 Antoniu, *Traité de la pellagre*, 63.
351 Manicatide, *Contribuţiuni la studiul etiologiei pelagrei*, 26.
352 Popescu, *Pellagra*, 40.

argy, "mouth ulcers," and depression.[353] However, as these symptoms can be associated with diverse other conditions, many doctors denied this stage in the onset of pellagra. The early stage was usually identified with the appearance of erythema, which made diagnosis unproblematic. Once a doctor had seen a pellagric erythema, he would never forget it. This stage also included digestive troubles: the loss of appetite, or its opposite—a "real bulimia"—a burning sensation in the mouth descending towards the oesophagus, diarrhea, and, in almost all cases, a "pain in the stomach, like burning or fire, extending towards the oesophagus."[354] These symptoms were complemented by "nervous" manifestations: headaches, dizziness, and pain in the torso or limbs. Pellagra was a disease with a long development, which could evolve over as long an interval as ten years, but which usually reached its terminal phase within three or four years.[355]

The second phase of the illness was characterized by the aforementioned symptoms, but in aggravated form. The digestive troubles became violent, the diarrhea became "dysenteriform," and the nervous symptoms turned into pellagric mania and paralysis. At this stage, patients were bent over and walked with a characteristic shuffle; many attempted suicide. The nature of the illness even dictated the manner of the suicide: drowning. Doctors vied with each other in describing such cases.[356] The third, and last, phase of the condition marked the patient's final degradation. Diarrhea "becomes involuntary, and cannot be stopped by any therapeutic means."[357] Mental alienation was accompanied by paralysis, which could be total. In the end, the patient died, at the center of a terrifying drama of total physical and mental collapse. In the accounts of the elites, pellagra appeared like an illness of the peasant, in the very image of his miserable and brutish life.

### An Illness of the Poor

Having seen how pellagra evolves and how tragically it ends, I shall now proceed to a survey of the main contributions of Romanian doctors to the study of the disease. The earliest reference to the condition appears in the

---

353 Neagoe, "Studiu asupra pelagrei," 389.
354 Popescu, *Pellagra*, 41.
355 Ibid., 53.
356 Ibid., 43–47.
357 Ibid., 47.

doctoral dissertation of doctor Constantin Vârnav. Published in 1836, he documented a new illness in Moldavia which he called "dropsical disease or dropsical blisters" (in Romanian: *boala trânjilor sau rana trânjilor*), the symptoms of which are most certainly pellagric.[358] It is probably no accident that the condition was first documented in Moldavia, which was to become the main focal point for endemic pellagra up to World War I. Interestingly, doctor Constantin Caracaş did not mention it in 1830, but most probably pellagra appeared in Ţara Românească a few decades after Moldavia. The French doctor Joseph Caillat,[359] who visited Ţara Românească in 1847, wrote that he never encountered a single case of pellagra there, but that he knew of a similar condition that had occurred in northern Moldavia.[360] To cite one last example, pellagra—also in Moldavia—was described by doctor Iuliu Theodori in his inaugural thesis at the University of Berlin.[361]

But the disease was first introduced into the scientific medical circuit by doctor Iacob Felix. In 1862, as the doctor of Muşcel County, he published his first observations on pellagra in the official newsletter of the health system, *Monitorul Medical al României*.[362] Once the two principalities[363] were fully united,[364] the young Romanian state had to face a new social scourge, a strange coincidence. Although references to pellagra continued to grow apace, before the 1880s the condition was not perceived as a major hazard. As some doctors put it, it had not yet become "our national malady,"[365] the "terrifying scourge haunting our countryside."[366] And yet, besides the study of doctor Vârnav, doctor Felix reviewed no less than 22 medical titles that mentioned pellagra in 1882.[367] His interest in the condition went further. One of the earliest doctoral theses he supervised at the School of Medicine in Bucharest, thesis no. 5, dealt

---

358 Vernav, *Rudimentum physiographiae Moldaviae*, 62.
359 Joseph Caillat, a French doctor who lived in the Romanian Principalities from 1845 and 1848 and published a memoir of this time in 1854.
360 Felix, *Prophylaxia pelagrei*, 21.
361 Ibid.
362 Felix, "Observaţiuni asupra pellagri în judeţul Muşcel."
363 Ţara Românească (Muntenia) and Moldavia.
364 The Romanian Principalities, Ţara Românească and Moldavia, were united in 1859 under the same ruling Prince, Alexandru Ioan Cuza, and formed a new state under the name the United Principalities of Ţara Românească and Moldavia. The unification process was finalized in 1862 and the new state acquired its modern name, Romania.
365 Sufrin, *Câteva reflexiuni asupra etilogiei pelagrei*, 4.
366 Bejan, "Raport asupra activităţii secţiunei a IV-a de ambulanţă militară-rurală Botoşani-Dorohoi," 481.
367 Felix, *Prophylaxia pelagrei*, 21–24.

with pellagra.[368] Significantly, until 1900, no less than eight doctoral theses written at the medical schools of Bucharest and Iaşi were about pellagra.[369] After 1880, the number of studies increased in accordance with the incidence of the disease or, at least, with the growing interest in it among the medical profession. At the start of the decade, the ubiquitous doctor Felix, as a representative of a country where pellagra was endemic, was the key speaker at section I of the Fourth International Congress on Public Health in Geneva.[370] His conference report on the aetiology and prevention of pellagra was published in Romanian the following year. Doctor Felix maintained a constant interest in pellagra. The first volume of his *Tratat de hygienă publică şi poliţie sanitară* (A treatise on public hygiene and health policy) of 1870 includes a section on pellagra.[371] However, by 1889, pellagra was missing in the second volume on diseases and patients.[372] The absence might be explained by the fact that, in the post-Pasteur era, the study only dealt with transmissible diseases, not with intoxications, as pellagra was considered at the time. A few years earlier, doctor Istrati had devoted a section of his much-cited study to the role of corn in the peasants' dietary habits and included a few pages on pellagra.[373] The same decade saw the publication of the first overview of the disease by a Romanian doctor, the district chief medic I. Antoniu. Antoniu earned notoriety with his admission that, as district doctor in Vaslui in 1870, he had conducted experiments on a few inmates at Dobrovățu prison. The experiments, conducted without the subjects' consent, proved indisputably that the consumption of altered corn could cause pellagra.[374]

Gradually, as the number of cases increased, the medical profession developed an obsessive interest in the condition, as will be seen below in the statistics of pellagra in Romania. A milestone in the medical literature was the publication, in 1888, of the *General Report on Pellagra* [in Romanian: *Raport general asupra pelagrei*], presented to the Home Ministry by the Director-General of the Public Health System, doctor Sergiu. It was the first attempt at a systematic, statistical study of pellagra in the Kingdom.[375] In the same year, doctor

---

368 Ciobanoff, *Despre pellagra*.
369 Crăinician, *Literatura medicală românească*, 366, 371, 390, 394, 402, 409, 462, 46.
370 Felix, *Sur la prophylaxie de la pellagre*, 4–5.
371 Felix, *Tractat de hygiena publică şi poliţia sanitară*, 148–51.
372 Ibid.
373 Istrati, *O paginǎ din istoria contimpuranǎ a Romániei*, 239–45.
374 Antoniu, *Traité de la pellagre*, 206–7, 233–35.
375 Sergiu, *Raport general asupra Pelagrei presintat domnului Ministru de interne*.

I. Neagoe, who became the top expert on pellagra in the pre-World War I period, went on a personal "mission" abroad to study the measures taken against the disease by other European states.[376] Doctor Neagoe seems to have specialized in studies abroad: he went on a second research mission between December 1893 and February 1894.[377] The last decade of the nineteenth century belongs to doctor Iacob Felix, who between 1892 and 1899 was the head of the General Directorate of the Romanian Public Health Service. His reports in this capacity never failed to mention pellagra. Finally, in 1899 the Third Congress of the National Medical Association [in Romanian: *Asociația Medicilor din Țară*] took place. The Kingdom's acknowledged expert on pellagra, doctor Neagoe, presented a report on the disease, which was the highly topical theme selected for that year. Significantly, in the following year, doctor Neagoe won the Adamachi Prize of the Romanian Academy, and his work, the second overview of pellagra in the country, was published in the series "Publications of the Vasilie Adamachi Foundation" [in Romanian: *Publicațiunile Fondului Vasilie Adamachi*].[378] In 1902, as pellagra became a national malady, the Romanian Academy intervened by organizing a contest for original research on the disease. No study was put forward in the first five years after the announcement. The contest was announced again in 1907, and had a late outcome: in 1912, doctors Aurel Babeş and Vladimir Buşilă received the award for their study *Cercetări originale despre pellagră în România* (New research on pellagra in Romania).[379] Doctor Neagoe's study from 1900 had been of the history and aetiology of the disease. The new study of 1912 was based on pure science, the result of research on animals and chemical analysis in the laboratory. This shows how, within a decade, the medical discourse on pellagra moved from narrative to science. It was a shift that occurred in all areas of medical research on the peasant and the rural world, and was largely due to the overall and rapid transformation of modern medicine from an "art" into a science in the late nineteenth century. This was largely made possible by new developments in bacteriology and chemistry, which turned medicine into what it was always meant to be: the science of healing.

---

376 Neagoe, *Raportul d-rului I. Neagoe asupra misiunei sale în străinătate pentru a studia mijloacele de combatere a pelagrei din numitele țări.*

377 Neagoe, *Pelagra în România,* 9–10.

378 Neagoe, "Studiu asupra pelagrei," 279–527.

379 Babeş and Buşilă, *Cercetări originale despre pelagra în România.*

## A Sarabande of Statistics

If one is to fully grasp the place of pellagra in the medical discourse of the late nineteenth century, one must resort to a real sarabande of figures. The end-of-century statistics reveal a large-scale psychosis, which extended from the medical profession and engulfed society, due to the rapid increase in the number of pellagra cases. For the interval 1859–1861, doctor Felix estimated the number of cases in Muşcel district to be around 80 to 90 in a population of 80,000,[380] which amounted to 1 to 1.1 per one thousand inhabitants, not a particularly high percentage. The same doctor Felix did the earliest calculation of pellagra cases starting from hospitalization numbers and records of conscription in 1882. He came up with a figure of 4,500 cases of pellagra across the entire country.[381] Doctor I. Antoniu was less optimistic: a year before the first census of pellagra patients, he stated that, having observed a sample of 10,000 patients as district doctor,[382] he had found "many thousands of pellagra cases,"[383] an impressive result. Doctor Antoniu also claimed that, from his hospital in Bârlad, he had solved once and for all the thorny problem of the causes of pellagra. It may sound far-fetched, but doctor Antoniu's fantasies were indirectly supported by the Ministry of the Interior, which, in the period 1884–1887, adopted further measures for enhancing the public health provision in rural areas in the shape of the so-called rural military ambulance service. In 1884, two such ambulances were deployed, one in Vrancea, the other in Oltenia. In 1885, there were four (in the counties of Gorj, Argeş, Bacău, and Neamţ).[384] Their usefulness was amply demonstrated by the increased number of consultations. By 1886, fifteen such ambulances, one for every two counties, were in service.[385] 1887 was the last year in which military ambulances operated in rural areas. This was also the moment when an astounding number of patients with pellagra symptoms showed up for consultation. For example, in the counties of Botoşani and Dorohoi, doctor V. Bejan reported 2,081 pellagra cases per 8,960 consultations

---

380 Felix, "Observaţiuni asupra pellagri în judeţul Muşcel," 16.
381 Felix, *Sur la prophylaxie de la pellagre*, 31–41.
382 Antoniu, *Traité de la pellagre*, 33.
383 Ibid., x.
384 Spiroiu, "Ambulanţa militară rurală din judeţul Mehedinţi," 193.
385 Possa, *Ambulanţa rurală Roman-Iaşi*, 384.

facilitated by the ambulance service.[386] Pellagra topped the total number of diagnosed conditions. One might conclude that, mercifully, pellagra was endemic only in Moldavia. However, in Muntenia, too, in Ilfov and Ialomița Counties, doctor Eraclie Clement found that, in the same year, 1886, among "the most serious and frequent" diseases, pellagra also came first, with 235 cases diagnosed in a single month.[387] In contrast, the military medic Al. Spiroiu, attached to the ambulance service in Mehedinți County in 1885, found 22 cases of pellagra, which he dismissed as not important enough. He believed that "paludism is here the main, if not the single, cause of morbidity and degeneration among the rural population."[388] On the one hand, therefore, the system of consultations *in situ* facilitated by the ambulance service identified more pellagra cases than the figures advanced in the official estimates. On the other hand, this greater diagnostic accuracy buttressed the psychotic fear of the impending demographic crisis caused by the new malady. In 1887, the number of consultations offered to presumed pellagra sufferers by the rural ambulance service rose to 19,000. Faced with increasing figures in the early twentieth century, even the moderate doctor Felix was compelled to admit that the figure of 5,000[389] he had advanced in 1882 had been an underestimation. He cautioned, however, that "the number of consultations was not a sufficient basis for calculating the real number of pellagra sufferers in the entire country."[390] It was becoming increasingly clear that there was a need for more accurate statistics. This was brought home by doctor Sergiu, who commented on a growing current of opinion:

[C]ounty and district doctors who, by nature of their function, are in close contact with the peasants, report annually the growth of pellagra in our country. The reports of ambulance service chiefs contain thousands of cases of this wretched affliction. In theses, monographs, and other studies, authors often exaggerate the disasters produced by the spread of pellagra. Such exaggerations are then circulated, by the spoken word or in writing, by persons

---

386 Bejan, "Raport asupra activității secțiunei a IV-a de ambulanță militară-rurală Botoșani-Dorohoi," 430.
387 Clement, "Raport științific asupra cazurilor constatate și tratate precum și despre modul funcționării ambulanței rurale Ilfov-Ialomița," 286.
388 Spiroiu, "Ambulanța militară rurală din județul Mehedinți," 196–97.
389 In fact, as discussed above, he had advanced an even smaller figure of 4,500 consultations.
390 Felix, "Pelagra în România," no. 30, 2.

with no expertise in medicine or by the newspapers, and thus the terrifying effects of pellagra are aggrandized.[391]

When he became head of the General Directorate of the Public Health Service in 1887, doctor Sergiu took on the self-assumed task of producing the much-needed statistics. Quite obviously, doctor Sergiu thought that doctor Antoniu's catastrophic visions were mere exaggerations and was convinced, even before the pellagra statistics were published, that the situation was not as dramatic as it looked. In May 1887, when he initiated the collection of statistical data, the journal *Spitalul* (The hospital) published his clinical lecture on pellagra, presented at the children's hospital in Bucharest, where he wrote: "There have been doctoral theses at the school of medicine on pellagra, alcoholism, etc., which, instead of conducting scientific research on the topic and educating the public, were mere scare-mongering writings, which simply showed that the Romanian nation is declining at an alarming rate."[392] He added that, having inspected some 200 villages, he had "made efforts, with the support of the local authorities, to see with my own eyes the patients with pellagra in those areas; I say this to you: the picture I formed of the reality was not as terrifying, I did not see as many cases of pellagra as described in many publications."[393] He continued by outlining all the other conditions with similar symptoms that could be misdiagnosed as pellagra. The survey of pellagra cases, which doctor Sergiu finalized in June 1888, yielded fewer cases than expected: 10,626 patients across the country—except Dobrudja, which seemed pellagra-free. This meant a ratio of 1.96 cases per one thousand inhabitants. For doctor Sergiu, the conclusion was self-evident:

> The number of 10,626 pellagra sufferers in the whole country demonstrates that it is an exaggeration to say that our population is being decimated by pellagra. Many doctors, carried away by the opinions of those who saw the ills greater than they are, depicted the most terrifying tableau offered by the victims of pellagra among our peasants. But now [...] we must stop lamenting and imagining ourselves as the nation most haunted by the diseases of poverty.[394]

---

391 Sergiu, *Raport general asupra Pelagrei presintat domnului Ministru de interne,* 5.
392 Sergiu, *Pelagra,* 178.
393 Ibid.
394 Sergiu, *Raport general asupra Pelagrei presintat domnului Ministru de interne,* 8.

The counties of Moldavia were the most affected, but looking at districts by geographical area and type of cultivation offers interesting data. Thus, in the "mountainous areas," the incidence of the disease was 1.92 per one thousand inhabitants. The situation was worse in the "hilly and vineyard regions," where the ratio was 2.38 patients per one thousand inhabitants. And finally, the "low-lying regions of the plains" had the lowest number of pellagra sufferers: 1.63 per one thousand inhabitants.[395] Of the 10,626 pellagra cases, only 91 were not peasants.[396] It was a triumph for doctor Sergiu, but it was short-lived. Gradually, having been held in check during the directorship of doctor Felix, the social angst around pellagra returned with a vengeance in the early twentieth century. In his attitude towards the various medical anxieties of the period, doctor Sergiu was part of a category of doctors that might have included doctor Felix, but not doctor Istrati or doctor Antoniu. However, their isolated voices, despite coming from the top of the medical hierarchy, were lost in the alarmist clamor of the rest of the medical corps.

In 1892, doctor Felix became the head of the General Directorate of the Health Services. For today's historians, this is good news. The hard-working doctor performed all the professional tasks dictated by his role with unflinching devotion. This included compiling and publishing detailed annual reports on the state of the Kingdom's public health. Pellagra was one of the subjects he did not fail to include. In 1892, doctor Felix admitted that the data on the number of pellagra sufferers were only partial, because there had been no census after 1888. Therefore, in 1892, the number of cases was established by centralizing the cases reported by social assistance services, which yielded 16,488 cases. Doctor Felix was obviously aware that "this number [...] gives us a very approximate picture of the proportions of this endemic disease,"[397] as some patients could attend several consultations, while others were not able to do so. In addition, accurate statistics for pellagra were difficult to compile also because the early signs of the illness—erythema—appeared "in the second half of summer." This meant that census data were better collected in May and June, something doctor Felix himself suggested in 1893. However, the census for this year, complete with nominal lists, only

---

395 Ibid., 11–12.
396 Ibid., 15.
397 Felix, *Raport general despre igiena publică și despre serviciul sanitar ale Regatului României pe anul 1892*, 66.

yielded 7,091 pellagra sufferers, a number even doctor Felix doubted. "[T]he real number is higher than 7,091," he wrote,[398] and cited the evidence. In 1893, 157 pellagra patients were hospitalized in the rural hospital in Slatina (Suceava County). Consultations and medicine were offered to a further 272. And yet, the census only recorded 78 patients for that county. There were similar situations in Vâlcea, Mehedinți, Neamț, and Tutova.[399] The figure of pellagra sufferers recorded in the census for the following year was even lower: 6,694.[400] There were additional anomalies: in Putna County, 449 cases were recorded in the 1893 census, but this number dropped to only 157 in the following year; in Argeş County, 61 cases were listed in the census for 1894, compared to 267 the previous year.[401] The system of nominal census records was retained in 1895, and the results were appropriately 7,531 pellagra sufferers.[402] In 1895, doctor Felix expressed his belief that a nominal census would "give us data which are precise enough."[403] However, the following year, he changed his mind and complemented the nominal census with "lists extracted from hospital registers and tables of patients in the care of county medical officers and district doctors." We do not know what linkages were made between the nominal lists and the tables of county and district doctors' patients, as the latter only recorded the number of patients. What we do know, however, is the important fact that, with the use of the new methodology, the number of pellagra patients increased spectacularly: 17,912 in 1896, and 19,796 in the following year.[404] It is obvious that, during his directorship, doctor Felix constantly searched for the perfect method of calculating the number of pellagra cases, but this proved elusive, for various reasons. Significantly, the nominal census records, which produced verifiable, yet less than accurate data, were constantly criticized and did not last more than three years. The mixed variant, used after 1895, was equally inaccurate, but, because it yielded higher figures, was more credible in a society obsessed with the growth of pellagra as a social ill. Therefore, it was never

---

398  Felix, *Raport general asupra igienei publice şi asupra serviciului sanitar al Regatului României pe anul 1895*, 95.

399  Ibid., 95–96.

400  Felix, *Raport general asupra igienei publice şi asupra serviciului sanitar al Regatului României pe anul 1895*, 66.

401  Ibid., 67.

402  Felix, *Raport general asupra igienei publice şi asupra serviciului sanitar al Regatului României pe anul 1895*, 104.

403  Ibid.

404  Felix, *Raport general asupra igienei publice şi asupra serviciului sanitar al Regatului României pe anii 1896 şi 1897*, 173.

questioned, and even those who used it never expressed reservations. Ultimately, the moderate doctor Felix, along with the entire medical profession,
gave in, and they were forced to acknowledge the growing threat of pellagra.

During the following years, all "doctors in public positions" made nominal lists of pellagra sufferers, which, cumulated, amounted to "a kind of annual census."[405] At the turn of the century, the number of pellagra patients
continued to grow apace, from 21,282 cases in 1898 to 43,687 cases in 1904.[406]
In 1905, the total number of pellagra sufferers increased by over 10,000 to
reach no less than 56,637 cases in the entire Kingdom, pushing the scale
of the disease beyond the psychological threshold of 50,000.[407] From this
point onwards, the number of cases appears to have stabilized, with a minor
regression in 1906 to 56,282 cases.[408] In 1910, however, with 58,403 cases,
the ascending trend resumed.[409] The census of pellagra cases proved to be a
tough nut to crack for the Health Directorate's office of statistics. A decision
was taken to stop the centralization of data after 1906. In addition, a suggestion was made for "a commission to be set up to review and resolve the
situation."[410] Doctors Aurel Babeş and Vladimir Buşilă best summarized
the issues around the collection of statistical data on pellagra in Romania in
their prize-winning work of 1912:

> A census of pellagra cases is, in our view, no easy task; in fact, it is perhaps
> impossible. Here are some of the hurdles. First, sufferers in the early stages
> of the disease do not complain of anything and perhaps they do not even
> know that they are ill. The doctor cannot go from house to house to examine
> all the residents, and even if he did, he might not be able to identify a disease
> that is not easy to recognize initially. As for the individuals who have had the
> disease for a long time, the doctor may not always be sure whether they still
> carry the illness. Consequently, even when a census of pellagra cases is done
> conscientiously, it will only skirt around the truth, without ever attaining it.
> When the data are collected in a superficial manner, by individuals who may
> not recognize their importance or who do not know how to collect them, one

405 Obregia, *Raport general asupra igienei publice şi asupra serviciului sanitar*, 209.
406 Ibid.
407 Ionescu, "Pelagra în România în 1905," 440.
408 Ionescu, "Pelagra în România în 1906," 111.
409 Babeş and Buşilă, *Cercetări originale despre pelagra în România*, 191.
410 Ibid., 172.

can easily imagine the outcome. And this is where the collection of statistical data on pellagra stands in our country.[411]

This leaves little to say on the subject. The impossibility of obtaining a precise figure for pellagra cases allows the imagination to run free, which makes anything possible. One and the same figure can be interpreted in a restrictive or in an alarmist manner. For example, the number of 19,000 consultations offered to some sufferers by the rural military ambulances in 1887 was considered by some doctors as an exaggeration because the "recording was not performed rigorously." Others thought that it was too low because in the months of July and August, when the ambulances were in service, the early signs of the disease disappeared, peasants no longer required medical assistance, and, consequently, "the ambulance registers do not provide an accurate image for the spread of the disease."[412] Both arguments are reasonable and contain a dose of truth. But there was a great deal of public pressure in favor of admitting that the number of cases was increasing and that, generally, the official statistics were under-evaluated. In 1906, doctor Neagoe was persuaded that the real number of pellagra sufferers was "at least" double the official figure: "All of us doctors know it in this country, from the director-general to the humblest doctor X."[413] In his acceptance speech at the Romanian Academy, in 1906, doctor Gheorghe Marinescu admitted to being increasingly worried by the growing number of pellagra cases, which he placed at 100,000 in 1905. We do not know where the figure came from, and neither did doctor Neagoe,[414] but it helped doctor Marinescu demonstrate the progression of pellagra in Romania: "In the eight years from 1897 to 1905, the number grew five times," he said, before concluding, "It is absolutely terrifying. How this will progress in the future, only God knows, but the disaster is awe-inspiring."[415] In a motion in Parliament presented in early 1906, the famous surgeon and deputy Thoma Ionescu advanced a figure of 150,000 pellagra cases.[416] This is almost four times as high as the offi-

---

411 Ibid.

412 Felix, *Raport general despre igiena publică și despre serviciul sanitar ale Regatului României pe anul 1892*, 66.

413 Neagoe, *Pelagra și administrația noastră*, 5

414 Ibid., 6.

415 Gheorghe Marinescu, "Progresele și tendințele medicinei moderne," in *Despre regenerarea și ... degenerarea unei națiuni. Discursuri inaugurale medicale in vremealui Carol I, 1872–1912*, 257.

416 "Discursul dlui Thoma Ionescu, rostit in ședința de la 27 ianuarie 1906" [Speech by Mr Thoma Ionescu, in the session of January 27, 1906], in *Desbaterile Adunărei Deputaților* [Debates of the Chamber of

cial figures. At the end of 1910, doctor Victor Babeş estimated the number of pellagra cases at 80,000. However, being less of an alarmist than his colleague, Gheorghe Marinescu, he admitted that most patients suffered from mild forms, which meant that "the great number of pellagra sufferers does not mean as many degenerates, mentally deficient [people], and manpower lost to agriculture."[417] It is certain that, in the period considered here, pellagra was regarded as a real social danger, and that the anxiety caused by the increasing number of cases was palpable.

We may never know the real figures for pellagra cases in modern Romania, but we do know that the number of individuals diagnosed as having the disease increased constantly in the second half of the nineteenth century and the early twentieth century. This increase was undoubtedly due to a better management of the rural health services and of closer contacts between the beneficiaries of the medical act and its professionals. It is quite possible, too, that rural communities developed a greater awareness of illness in general, and adopted new attitudes towards the body, illness, and healing. All these changes (added to the gaps in statistics) led to the reporting of increasing numbers of cases. However, one should not underestimate the impact of representations of pellagra on the period's collective imaginary.

### "Pellagra: An Illness Caused by Rotten Corn"

If the real number of pellagra cases remained an enigma, so did the origin of the illness until later in the twentieth century. Starting with the identification of the disease in the eighteenth century, theories on its causes varied, but a link with corn consumption was established quite early. Pellagra became known as the illness of corn eaters, and even more so as the illness of impoverished corn eaters. In Romania, the disease was identified in the mid-nineteenth century, so theories on its causes belonged within the general ethos of the period's medical science. The maize-derived theory on causes was almost generally accepted during the nineteenth century, although its proponents were soon divided into two main camps: "One [camp] believed that corn in general, not just altered corn, was responsible for the disease be-

Deputies], 1906, no. 38, 542.
417 Babeş, *Studii asupra pelagrei*, 1.

cause of its lack of nutrients such as nitrous substances and gluten; members of the other camp believed that the disease was caused solely by rotten corn."[418] The latter theory was the most widely adopted in the second half of the nineteenth century and gained the greatest number of adherents among Romanian doctors. Only doctors Iuliu Theodori and I. Neagoe supported the idea that corn was to blame irrespective of whether it was healthy or altered. To our knowledge, doctor Theodori never wrote anything on pellagra after his inaugural thesis in Berlin in 1858, so he can be left out of the present discussion. This leaves doctor Neagoe as the only proponent of a single, maize-related cause. He never gave up on the theory that, without doubt, "the cause of pellagra was an abuse of both healthy and rotten corn in consumption; with rotten corn, of course, eating it will lead to pellagra much more quickly."[419] The single maize-derived cause had the disadvantage of leading to the inevitable conclusion that the only solution was excluding corn from human consumption. However, apart from doctor Neagoe, no one believed that eating high-quality corn could produce pellagra. Doctor Istrati, for example, was convinced that "[p]ellagra is not due to corn as such. It is due to rotten corn, in the same way that moldy bread causes mouth ulcers and gastro-enteritis, which can often be fatal."[420] In 1895, doctor Crăiniceanu was also reluctant to endorse a single maize-related cause for the illness: "[P]ellagra is a hideous disease caused by the consumption of rotten corn."[421] Peasants themselves sided with doctor Neagoe. Doctor Nicolae Popescu testified that, when talking to his patients, they responded that it was not rotten corn that made them ill, "because when they ground it, it was good to eat."[422] We now know that the peasants were right. Doctor Neagoe was aware that such a widespread disease could not simply be caused by altered corn flour for the simple reason that the peasants themselves would have rejected the resulting foul smelling and foul tasting corn mush. Doctor Neagoe knew the peasant well:

I have lived with him, I shared his food when I called unexpectedly; I saw the fare he took in his bag when rafting on the rivers Bistriţa, Mureş, Gurghiu,

418 Felix, "Pelagra în România," no. 30, 3.
419 Neagoe, "Studiu asupra pelagrei," 331.
420 Istrati, *O pagină din istoria contimpurană a României*, 243.
421 Crăiniceanu, *Igiena ţăranului român*, 241.
422 Popescu, *Pellagra*, 25.

Arieş, Sebeş, and Tisa—but I never had to eat mămăligă which I, considered a difficult eater, *would have been loth to swallow*; I saw his victuals as he labored in the field, digging, threshing, mowing, grazing his cattle [...]; I saw his food in the forest in the autumn and winter, as he worked on the roads and railways, I saw it among the poor rather than the rich [...] but I never saw them eat mămăligă or corn mush made from flour gone bad: *I never sensed that foul smell of rotten corn or flour, when it starts turning black or a purple-green-golden hue.*[423]

These are reasonable, common sense comments. So were the observations of doctor S. Sufrin, who, writing in 1899 about his time as district doctor, said that "this food was never missing on my table,"[424] yet he never became ill with pellagra. But why did pellagra strike the rural population almost exclusively? And why especially poorer peasants? Why, in the same family and subjected to the same diet, did some become ill and others did not? Why were the numbers of pellagra cases different in mountainous districts compared to those in low-lying areas? These were questions that medical theories had to address. One did not have to be a doctor to find answers that favored the dominant theory of toxic corn being the main agent: pellagra was predominantly a rural disease because corn was a staple in the nutrition of peasants and because, among poorer peasants, corn was consumed almost exclusively and excessively. It was, therefore, logical for the poorer villagers to become the first victims of the disease. But there had always been poverty in the rural world, as peasant patients themselves often pointed out: "In the old days when there was no food, our forefathers ate tree bark and roots and their skin did not come off."[425] It was, admittedly, a sound argument. There was poverty in towns, too, yet there pellagra was very rare. That was because, as theorists in the opposite camp pointed out, the poor urbanite did not have a diet that was as corn-based as the poor village dweller. Only in exceptional circumstances did pellagra strike cities, even major cities such Bucharest, for example during the German occupation in World War I. During that time, doctor Babeş treated "numer-

---

423 Neagoe, "Studiu asupra pelagrei," 380–81.
424 Sufrin, *Câteva reflexiuni asupra etilogiei pelagrei*, 15.
425 Popescu, *Pellagra*, 32.

ous cases of pellagra."[426] Comparative research has shown that alimentation may explain why, in one and the same population, the disease affected only certain groups. As an example, doctor Nicolae Popescu, who studied the village Clejani, noted his astonishment upon learning of the great number of slaughtered cattle:

> [...] I tried to find out who the consumers were; I learned that normally the consumers were the Gypsies, the peasants eating meat only exceptionally. [...] Being aware that a good diet did not cause pellagra, I tried to find out if there were pellagra sufferers among the Gypsies—the result was negative, but I found 20 cases among the Romanians. (The population of the village is 1,404, of whom 168 are Gypsies). I then tried to see whether there were any notable conditions of hygiene, home, cleanliness, labor, etc. among the Gypsies, and found that the majority were one step behind the Romanians. The only difference was that, comparatively, they had a healthier diet: what they earned, they ate. Many work as fiddlers, and some go to Bucharest or elsewhere in the summer to work, and as such, understandably, they have a better nutrition. Finally, I tried to find out whether Gypsies in other villages where they are numerous, such as Obislav and Căscioare, were also affected by pellagra, given their sanitary conditions, which I compared to the population in Clejani. I found that the Gypsies were lazier than those in Clejani, their lifestyle, alimentation, and hygiene were deplorable, and, as a result, they were affected by pellagra in the same way as the other inhabitants.[427]

The fact that a varied and corn-free diet kept pellagra at bay was a universally accepted truth. The best proof was that the counties of Dobrudja, where, as we have seen, the peasants' diet was based on bread, were free of pellagra. But the doubters still wanted an explanation for the fact that often, in areas where pellagra was endemic, not all members of the same family became ill. In 1903, doctor G. Proca collected statistical data in what he called the "pellagric focal point in Roman County," the village Doljeşti, one of the sites with the highest incidence of pellagra cases in the country. After a survey of 68 families with 335 members, he found "only one pellagra pa-

---

426 Babeş, *Pelagra*, 4.
427 Popescu, *Pellagra*, 28–29.

tient in 73.6 per cent of the families, and two or three cases in the remaining 26.4 per cent."[428] These findings led doctor Proca to conclude that "individual predispositions must have a predominant role in producing pellagra."[429] For doctor Proca, the most obvious of these predispositions were related to age and gender, while doctor Babeş linked them to alcoholism, malaria, and syphilis.[430] One did not have to be a doctor to know that a malnourished body, weakened by disease, labor, and excesses, was a favorable terrain for pellagra. However, the precarious hygiene of the peasants' lifestyles favored all conditions, not just pellagra. In addition, statistical data show a higher rate of pellagra in mountainous areas compared to the plains. What was the explanation? The champions of the toxic corn theory said that people in mountainous areas consumed altered corn because weather conditions in those areas did not allow maize to ripen.[431] Others believed that, in mountainous areas that did not favor the cultivation of maize, the inhabitants purchased cheap, low-quality corn grown in the plains and became ill with pellagra.[432] Despite these beautiful, logical inferences, doctor Sufrin was in a quandary. Experience had taught him something else: as district doctor and then county officer in Iaşi, as well as in the mountainous district Lovişte in Argeş County, he had come to believe that the incidence of pellagra was higher in the plains than in the mountains. And, if the number of pellagra cases was inversely proportional to the degree of "peasant squalor," the theory was verified, because "in the mountains I noticed that the material situation of the peasants was much better than that of the peasants in the plains."[433] But the statistics did not support this conclusion. In his practice in Vlaşca, doctor Nicolae Popescu tested and verified another hypothesis that supported the toxic corn theory: the years in which the weather had been less favorable to the cultivation of maize were followed by a noticeable increase in the cases of pellagra.[434] Lacking firm data on the aetiology of the disease, doctors constructed scenarios based on existing theories. Even when affiliated to the toxic maize theory, doctors had critical minds

---

428 Proca, "Cercetări asupra pelagrei," 672.
429 Ibid., 673.
430 Babeş, *Studii asupra pelagrei*, 2.
431 Felix, *Prophylaxia pelagrei*, 25.
432 Antoniu, *Traité de la pellagre*, 163–64.
433 Sufrin, *Câteva reflexiuni asupra etilogiei pelagrei*, 23–24.
434 Popescu, *Pellagra*, 25.

that often made them skeptical even of a theory they had once espoused. Thus, doctor Manolescu believed that in 1985 the issue had "not yet been resolved."[435] Even doctor Felix, who, as an "avowed advocate of the toxic maize theory, considered rotten corn as the principal cause" of pellagra,[436] admitted in his conclusions that "the only fact determined with any precision was the connection between a diet based predominantly on corn and this disease."[437] Ultimately, it was doctor Valerian George Negrescu who offered perhaps the best summary of the aetiology of pellagra in 1886: doctors seemed to "know much and make many assumptions about pellagra, but we do not possess any positive facts."[438]

## Against Pellagra

Pellagra became, or was described as such, a deadly national calamity in the last two decades of the nineteenth century and the start of the twentieth. What was the nation's riposte to this agent of "racial degeneration"? The most salient feature of the response was the curative rather than preventive nature of the measures taken, but this had always been the case in the Romanian health services. The main effort was directed to identifying and treating cases rather than preventing the occurrence of the illness. In this outline, I shall also foreground the *curative practices* and present the *preventive guidelines* second. The earliest known measure dates from 1852, when a hospital was founded in Moldavia, at Dărăbani, specifically for the treatment of pellagra cases,[439] but it was short-lived. The next anti-pellagra action was documented by doctor Sergiu, who mentions a "lazaretto for pellagra patients," added to the county hospital in Dorohoi in 1876, and apparently still in service in 1882.[440] In 1900, special curative establishments—"hospital sections of 20 beds each"—were annexed to existing hospitals in ten counties "where pellagra was found to be most widely spread."[441] Two years later, attempts were made to cure pellagra with mineral baths. Two provisional

---

435 Manolescu, *Igiena țăranului*, 272.
436 Felix, *Prophylaxia pelagrei*, 7.
437 Ibid., 42.
438 Negrescu, *Contribuțiune la studiul pelagrei*, 3.
439 Neagoe, *Pelagra în România*, 12.
440 Sergiu, *Raport general asupra Pelagrei presintat domnului Ministru de interne*, 16–17.
441 Obregia, *Raport general asupra igienei publice și asupra serviciului sanitar*, 221.

ambulance services were set up at Băile Govora[442] and at Băile Căciulata.[443] Romania also attempted to introduce special hospices, on the Italian model, called "pellagroseries," or "asylums for pellagra patients." In the aftermath of his "mission abroad" for the study of pellagra, doctor Neagoe wrote a report, published in 1889, in which he suggested the creation of asylums modelled on the establishment he had visited at Mogliano di Veneto. These were supposed to be curative institutions with model farms associated to them. The aim was to offer peasants an environment where they could be healed in body and in mind, as the period's doctors would have said. They could learn modern agricultural practices at the farm and acquire other skills in adjacent workshops: the women would learn cooking, and men would be trained to weave twigs into wicker objects and learn "basic notions of metalworking and joinery."[444] These asylums were meant to be school-hospitals. To doctor Neagoe's disappointment, of the four such establishments he proposed, only one was created, much later. This was the Asylum for Pellagra at Păncești-Dragomirești in Roman County, inaugurated in May 1896 and attached to the School of Agriculture. It was the longest surviving specialized curative unit: it was still in service in 1912, when, along the 48 beds in use in the main building, 60 more beds were added in the two "cabins" set up for the summer, when the number of pellagra cases increased.[445] The first medical head of this establishment, doctor Petru Flor, wrote two reports in which he described all the limitations of the new institution. He noted that, in the first place, it could not fulfil its projected mission as a school-hospital on the Italian model, because the director of the School of Agriculture did not permit this. The doctor would have preferred a modern, fully functional institution, independent of the School of Agriculture. His reports take his readers on a tour of the building, describing the corridors and rooms and pointing out their drawbacks, the most obvious being the lack of ventilation, which produced a perpetual "heavy, foul smell in all the halls and wards."[446] The asylum also suffered from the perpetual problem of the period's hospitals, the latrines, as described by Flor:

442 Zorileanu, "Dare de seamă de rezultatul obținut cu tratarea bolnavilor de pellagra," 226–29.

443 Obregia, *Raport general asupra igienei publice și asupra serviciului sanitar*, 222.

444 Neagoe, *Raportul d-rului I. Neagoe asupra misiunei sale în străinătate pentru a studia mijloacele de combatere a pelagrei din numitele țări*, 60–62.

445 Babeș and Bușilă, *Cercetări originale despre pelagra în România*, 129.

446 Flor, "Azilul de pelagroși 'Păucești-Dragomirești' din județul Roman," 352.

The latrines are badly built, they are situated to the north of the main building and, as a result, the wind and the defective manner in which they are constructed cause a lot of problems: first of all there is no Water Closet[447] system, but still the same wretched "à la turque" model, without doors, with insufficient ventilation, all of which make the stay in the hospital difficult, especially in damp weather, and eventually will render it impossible.[448]

There was no kitchen, and the food was prepared in the school's kitchen instead; there was a bathroom, but it lacked the necessary plumbing and amenities, so the patients had to use the school bathroom, where only cold baths could be had. There was no mortuary, no fountain, no wood shed.[449] Doctor Flor's despair is easy to understand. Whether any improvements were ever made in the asylum's lifetime, we do not know. By the time doctor Flor left the institution, in May 1899, nothing had changed.[450] One decade after its inauguration, doctor Neagoe described the asylum at Pănceşti as "a public health and administrative disgrace."[451] The next establishment of this type was the "pellagrosery" of Doljeşti, also in Roman County, in service from 1903 to the autumn of 1904.[452] A pellagrosery that opened in 1904 in the hamlet Brăteşti (the village Paşcani, Suceava County) appears to have had an equally short life.[453] In 1912, doctors Babeş and Buşilă mention only two such specialized establishments: the older "hospital for pellagra sufferers" at Pănceşti, in Roman County, and the "pellagrosery" of Coşula, in Botoşani County, which was "more of a mental hospice, because it treats only pellagra patients with mental disorders" and was described as a "primitive institution."[454]

Doctors knew that a healthy, nutritious diet in hospitals had a therapeutic role on a par with medication in pellagra cases. As a result, 1906 saw the experimental introduction of what doctor Alexandru Obregia called a "temporary dietary service for the sufferers of pellagra," to function alongside the 26 specialized hospitals. In practice, this meant that, between May 1 and

---

447 In English in the original.
448 Flor, "Azilul de pelagroşi 'Păuceşti-Dragomireşti' din judeţul Roman," 352.
449 Ibid., 351–53.
450 Flor, "Spitalul de pelagroşi Pănceşti-Dragomireşti," 92–94.
451 Neagoe, Pelagra şi administraţia noastră, 21.
452 Obregia, Raport general asupra igienei publice şi asupra serviciului sanitar, 222–23.
453 Ibid., 223.
454 Babeş and Buşilă, Cercetări originale despre pelagra în România, 133.

September 1, 1906, each patient with pellagra arriving for consultation on a Sunday received a voucher that entitled him or her to food from the hospital kitchen: "sour chorba[455] [borsht] with pieces of meat and a fresh loaf of bread, which he could eat in the hospital itself or in its courtyard. Patients found out to have been drinking at the pub were not allowed food."[456] These "pellagra lunches" were a success, according to doctor Alexandru Vasiliu, the chief medical officer of Roman County, largely because they brought the population to hospitals. For example, at the hospital in Bâra, until August 13, 295 pellagra patients had been given lunch vouchers.[457] This state-sponsored model was also adopted by private individuals "who showed an interest in the inhabitants of villages." The Health Directorate officially acknowledged these charitable activities and the donors in its newsletter, *Buletinul Direcției*. For example, Adela Vasile Lascăr received thanks for "kindly donating substantial amounts of food on several Sundays and on festival days to patients treated at the hospital at Darabani, in Dorohoi County." So did Constantin Miclescu, for donating food twice a week to pellagra sufferers in the hamlet Stolniceni, in Suceava County.[458] These lunches for pellagra patients could be seen as the Romanian variant of the Italian soup kitchens.

In terms of prevention, there were numerous proposals. Almost every author on pellagra suggested solutions, some more imaginative than others. What they had in common was the toxic maize theory on the causes of the disease, and therefore they all proposed the elimination of altered corn from human consumption. This could be achieved in a few ways. The most obvious way was by cultivating high-quality maize and harvesting it at the right time, when it had ripened properly. Next was storing the harvested corn adequately, which was not possible if the peasant did not have a well-aired, elevated barn. Corn flour could go bad if ground in large amounts, which did not allow for aeration and drying. There were dangers lurking everywhere. One of the earliest preventive measures was proposed in 1885, with the recommendation for ovens to be built next to mills. Here is doctor Nicolae Popescu, summing up the outcomes of this project: "I have never seen any

---

455 From the Turkish *çorba*, which means broth.
456 Obregia, "Circulara no. 7.283 din 19 aprilie 1906," 142.
457 Vasiliu, "Mesele pelagroșilor," 335.
458 "Mesele pelagroșilor" [The pellagra lunches], in *Buletinul Direcțiunei Generale a Serviciului Sanitar* [Bulletin of the General Directorate of the Health Services], year XVIII, 1906, nos. 17–18, 336.

ovens built next to mills."[459] However, at the initiative of doctor Felix, the Health Act of 1893 was amended with an additional article 155, banning the milling and retail of rotten corn and corn flour for "human consumption."[460] The outcome was nil. All these proposals, and many others, were published but never acted upon. Pellagra was an eminently societal disease, and therefore its eradication was also a societal issue. We can only agree with doctor Felix's early insight of 1892, when he wrote:

> Pellagra is going to disappear from our country apace with the progress of civilization, as it disappeared in other countries, the same as leprosy disappeared. When the peasant will have better nutrition, and live in a healthy home, when his cattle will shelter in a clean stable and his grain will be stored in dry sheds, when he will labor the land with skill and produce other good-quality foods alongside maize, when he will take better care of his cow so she produces plentiful milk, when the Romanian peasant will be thriftier and will manage his household well, then pellagra will cease being an endemic disease in the entire territory of the country, and will only strike occasionally and rarely.[461]

Indeed, pellagra disappeared from the nosological map of Romania only with the eradication of the country's major foci of rural poverty, in the late twentieth century. At the end of the interwar period, even though the causes were better understood and an efficient treatment was available for sudden bouts of the disease,[462] pellagra, far from disappearing, evolved "steadily and, apparently, seems to be on the increase."[463] Indeed, the number of patients with pellagra registered in Romania in 1938 reached 84,106.[464] After the war, in 1957, the authors of a major monograph on corn in Romania claimed that in rural Moldavia and Muntenia, the average daily consumption of corn per capita was 400 grams, but could still be as high as 600 or even 800 grams in "many places."[465] This suggests that pellagra was still around. For the com-

---

459 Popescu, *Pellagra*, 72.
460 Şuta et al., *Legislația sanitară*, 120–21.
461 Felix, *Raport general despre igiena publică și despre serviciul sanitar ale Regatului României pe anul 1892*, 62.
462 Claudian and Gruia Ionescu, *Pelagra. Patologie. Sociologie*, 696–703.
463 Ibid., 20.
464 Ibid., 42.
465 Săvulescu et al., *Porumbul. Studiu monographic*, 167.

munist period, data on diseases and patient numbers are erratic and hard to find, but there is information, often marked "for internal use only." In 1962, pellagra still appeared in statistics, although the number of hospitalized patients was very low: 1,317.[466] The disease seemed on the wane.

I cannot close this chapter without making sure that the disease has really disappeared in Romania. A brief online search takes us to the headline: "Pellagra Strikes Again" in Moldavia. And the article does not speak about isolated cases. Doctor Gheorghe Duțescu from the County Hospital in Focșani claims that in May and June 2002, 16 patients were diagnosed with pellagra and hospitalized. He suggested the inclusion of the disease in a national programme, so that free treatment could also be offered to patients without health insurance, who formed the majority.[467] Pellagra, therefore, remains an illness of the poor peasant, an illness of rural, underprivileged areas, and that starts, as doctor Babeș suggestively wrote, "when the peasant is no longer able to give his body enough food to recover what it lost through labor."[468]

---

466 Ion Lăpușan, Petre Neaga, Emil Tureanu, Eufrosina Săndulescu, Filofteia Seciurean, Elena Georgescu, and Florica Burlacu, *Bolnavii ieșiți din spitale. 1962* [Patients discharged from hospitals, 1962], Ministerul Sănătății și Prevederilor Sociale, Institutul de Igienă și Protecția Muncii, Secția statistică sanitară și demografie [Ministry for Health and Social Security, Institute for Hygiene and Work Safety, Section Health Statistics and Demography], Bucharest, no date, 8.

467 Ramona Jachianu, "Pelagra lovește iarăși" [Pellagra strikes again], http://www.ziaruldeiasi.ro/focsani/pelagra-loveste-iarasi~ni2l1s [last accessed June 3, 2013].

468 Babeș, *Pelagra*, 5.

# 6

## The "degeneration of the race and the decline of the nation": Demography and Its Anxieties

Today, the period from the second half of the nineteenth to the early twentieth century looks like a prosperous time in modern Romanian history, almost like a triumphal stage in the national saga. Within seven decades, Romanians achieved their national goals: the first union, of Moldavia and Țara Românească, in 1859; in 1866, a constitutional monarchy; in 1877, independence from the Ottoman Empire, gained on the battlefield; in 1881, the proclamation of the Kingdom; and in 1918, the Great Union.[469] These were events of historic proportions, and they were perceived as such even as they unfolded. However, as the historian becomes more familiar with the period, he or she cannot overlook the fact that, in the second half of the nineteenth century, Romania also experienced the dark side of progress. At the time, participants and witnesses perceived the evolution of Romania with its shadows and lights, dark corners where the dreams and fears of a nation taking a shortcut to modernization lingered. However, twentieth-century historiography foregrounded only the optimistic version of events, pushing the national catastrophes and the apocalyptic visions into a corner or filtering them through a revisionist grid. However, national catastrophes and apocalyptic visions have a way of leaving their imprint on historical agents, who acted under their influence, and in so doing blur the distinction between vision and reality. Imaginary constructs are in fact as real as hard social facts, and the development of modern Romania cannot be understood without them.

## The Beginning of the End

1859 was not simply the beginning of the Romanian nation-building project. In only a few decades, this year acquired an extra meaning. This is what doctor Codreanu, a doctor working in Tutova County in 1880, wrote about it:

---

469 In Romanian historiography, the Great Union (in Romanian: *Marea Unire*) refers to the moment in 1918 when, in the aftermath of World War I, the Kingdom of Romania integrated territories from the former Austro-Hungarian and Tsarist empires.

Oh, the year 1859! [...] This is the year from which many of us start counting the regeneration of Romania, the period of happiness and consolidation of the Romanian state; in a word, it marked the beginning of the era of "reorganization"; but the same year, the year 1859, also marks the beginning of high mortality among the Romanians, of their disappearance from this earth, of their decline and physical degradation![470]

In this vision, it was the beginning of the end. But even one decade earlier, doctors had started sketching a physical portrait of the Romanian peasant in a palette that grew darker and darker. Doctor Gheorghiad Mihail Obedenaru, the local expert on malaria, was one of the first to tackle the subject. His peasants, ill with "miasmatic debility," were not in very good shape:

The women, children and many of the men have complexions of a peculiar and characteristic yellowish hue. They have but little muscular strength (little energy); they are immensely lazy, but it is a laziness for which they are not to blame, because it is a laziness born of illness, the result of poisoning, as the miasmas, which have penetrated their bodies, act like poison. These debilitated bodies have so little strength that they cannot keep themselves erect. Rather than sit, these people recline, languishing, as though they try to spare their strength. You have only to look in the countryside at groups of women together, and you will see that they cannot stand, but are bent over, putting all the weight on their knees, or with their backs propped up against a support; and they do not dart their glance quickly from one sight to another, but stare and then slowly move their heads in a different direction; their arms hang limply, as though they are made of rags. We do not mean here the peasant women from the mountains, those ruddy, sturdy, healthy women, but the women from the low lands, with their gaunt, wan faces.[471]

The doctor, an urbanite born in Bucharest, who studied medicine in Paris,[472] looked on with his severe gaze, saw everything, but understood lit-

---

470 Manicea, *Consideraţiuni asupra mortalităţii generale în România*, 35–36.
471 Obedenaru, *Despre friguri*, 1873, 8–9.
472 Gomoiu, Gomoiu, and Gomoiu, *Repertor de medici, farmacişti, veterinari (personalul sanitar) din ţinuturile româneşti* vol. I, 305.

tle: a simple female gathering, as one can see even today at the corner of a country road, is turned into a clinical case study. Quite clearly, doctor Obedenaru's peasants have not mastered the new codes of the bourgeois body language of their time. The text, written in 1871, had several editions and became very popular. The short treatise on ague, of which it formed a section, first appeared in French in 1871,[473] followed a year later by a Romanian-language edition in a well-known scientific journal, *Revista Şciinţifică*, edited by P. S. Aurelian. It was immediately serialized by the newspaper *Românul* (July–August 1872), and published as a volume in 1873, 5,000 free copies of which were distributed to all the "local authorities in the country."[474] In 1883, a new print-run of 5,000 copies was distributed to the same authorities.[475] Presumably, it was the most widely popularized work by a Romanian doctor in the late nineteenth century.

Towards the end of the 1870s, the young doctor Nicolae Manolescu was, for a short time, district doctor in Buzău County. Only a few days after taking up his new post in the village Pătârlagele, he was invited to a wedding, which served as his introduction to the rural world he was called upon to administer:

It was an important wedding, attended by many people. I had under my eyes significant numbers of representatives of all classes of that society and I saw something I did not expect to see at a wedding: of a group of 58 lads, half of them had the gaunt, discolored, and wrinkled complexions caused by insufficient nutrition. They had the skin of prematurely aged men, and no sense in their faces or limbs of any youthful exuberance. These men stood out in the multitude of dancers, all the more visible in their contrast to a few robust men, a shepherd, or the son of an inn-keeper or a village mayor, under whose feet the earth was rumbling. In this wedding tableau, the women were even more lacking in youthful countenances and vigorous bodies, and the children were all cachectic—as for people of very advanced years, I saw none.[476]

473 Obédénare, *Fièvres des marais.*
474 Obedenaru, *Despre friguri,* 1873, 2.
475 Obedenaru, *Despre friguri,* 1883, 2.
476 Manolescu, "Aparatul de încălzit camerele ţărăneşti în plaiul Buzău," 553.

In this wedding tableau, doctor Manolescu sees the same anaemic, malnourished, ill peasants, with a few exceptions. Even doctor M. Roth described the Romanian peasants in the same terms:

> Looking at our peasants, they generally produce the impression of individuals who carry the germs of a hidden cachexia; their complexions do not have the brown tan of a man who works outdoors under the sun, but an ashen (or muddy) hue, with an icteric touch; their mucous membranes are anaemic, their eyes have no spark, no excitement; their gaze is indifferent and tired; the movements of their bodies slow [...]. The peasant spouse is an old young woman: the hard work, insufficient nutrition and chronic maladies have left the mark of premature ageing on her; stooping, livid in the face and faded, she looks 30 years older; neither men nor women will reach an old age in any of the country's districts.[477]

Whereas doctor Obedenaru attributed the peasant's physical decline to a precise pathology, doctors Manolescu and Roth took the representation one step further, turning it into the typical image of the Romanian peasant. On the eve of the War of Independence, no member of the medical profession would describe the peasants as robust and healthy. From this moment onwards, the rural world became fraught with poverty, physical and mental suffering, illness and death. Any positive features the peasant physique might once have possessed now belonged firmly in the pre-1859 past.

## Degeneration, Depopulation, Antisemitism

In the second half of the nineteenth century, doctors were the first to launch one of the worst dystopian representations of the Romanian population into the public arena, which was going to haunt society until World War I, and even beyond: the fear of racial degeneration among ethnic Romanians.[478] Initially, when I was not yet sufficiently familiar with the period's medical discourse, I was under the impression that racial degeneration was just one

---

477 Roth, *Memoriu asupra cauzelor mortalității populației româno-creștine*, 133–34.

478 There are two outstanding studies on racial degeneration and the eugenics movement in Romania: Bucur, *Eugenics and modernization in interwar Romania*, and Turda, *Eugenism și antropologie rasială în România. 1874–1944.*

theme among others in this discourse, and that doctors spoke about bodily hygiene and the hygiene of clothes, households, and food in the same way they spoke about alcoholism. I was wrong. The theme of racial degeneration produced a medical discourse of its own. In the last decades of the nineteenth century, there was an explosion of hygienist literature in Romania. One reason for this was the doctors' belief that Romanians were degenerating racially and that something had to be done to halt this process and encourage regeneration. To be able to do this, one first had to define and then study the "hygienic ills" of the rural world.

I shall attempt to identify as closely as possible the moment when the concept of racial degeneration was launched in the public arena, and then follow briefly its evolvement in the period leading up to World War I. The first doctor to mention racial degeneration explicitly was Gheorghiad Mihail Obedenaru. In his study of 1871, he explained that palustral fevers combined with "bad" nutrition not only prevented the multiplication of the population, but also led to the "physical and intellectual degeneration of the race.".[479] Two years later, another doctor, who later built a brilliant career in the health services of the Romanian Kingdom, tackled the favorite theme of the medical discourse of the late nineteenth century: the hygiene of village dwellers. This early contribution already contained the main tropes of the discourse on peasants and the rural world. But what is more interesting in this case was the concern expressed by doctor Grigore Romniceanu for the general situation of the peasantry. He observed that, whereas the lifestyles of urbanites were improving noticeably, the peasant was "abandoned to his primitive state," as evidenced in the quality of the dwellings and nutrition among this population. Left to live in the current conditions of hygiene, the peasant was bound "to degenerate altogether, and the only ones left are going to be mere sickly weaklings."[480] The situation was not yet irreversible, but was bound to become so, largely due to the heavy drinking habits of the Moldavian peasantry and the unbalanced diet of the peasant population in general. "Thus, the Romanian people are degenerating, illnesses multiply and become more severe, and the number of deaths is becoming disproportionately higher than the births," wrote doctor Romniceanu.[481] Clearly, by

---

479  Obédénare, *Fièvres des marais*, 23.
480  Romniceanu, "Igiena săteanului," 51.
481  Ibid., 155.

1873, doctor Romniceanu had already established a link between degeneration and depopulation.

Ioan G. Bibicescu was not a doctor and does not appear to have been familiar with doctor Obedenaru's work. Nor did he, apparently, read *Revista Contimporană*. In an article he published at the end of 1874 in the newspaper *Românul*, Bibicescu cited a report of the military doctor Miloteanu about conscription in Mehedinți County. Miloteanu had written that he had seen with his own eyes the degree of "degeneration in that district."[482] In the same article, he noted that, starting from the statistical data for 1873, in Bucharest the ethnic Romanian population showed a higher rate of deaths than births, and that only the Jewish population managed to maintain a higher birth rate. The author naturally wondered about the causes of this situation: "[W]as it racial degeneration that had rendered us unfit to fight for our survival?"[483] He retained this question as a working hypothesis for some of his subsequent work. Only a few years later, doctor A. Mihail Petrini published "On the Improvement of the Race," in which he, too, made fleeting references to the "physical degradation" of humans[484] and the "degeneration of peoples."[485] The concept of degeneration gradually crept into the medical discourse. It did not become a cliché overnight, but it did so eventually, in a specific social and political context, and with the endorsement of one author and his work. This author was C. I. Istrati, who published his study *O pagină din istoria contimpurană a României din punctul de videre medical, economic și național* [A page in the contemporary history of Romania from a medical, economic and national viewpoint] in 1880. This study, entirely devoted to the theme of degeneration, imposed the concept onto the Romanian public debate. In 500 pages, doctor Istrati tried to find an answer to one simple question: "Is the Romanian race in our country degenerating or not?"[486] Needless to say, doctor Istrati held the *a priori* belief that racial degeneration was real. The terms "degeneration" and "degeneracy" appear no less than 55 times in this work, designating the organizing concept of his analysis.

1880 was a milestone in the development of the concept of degeneration. An impressive number of writings was published almost simultaneously on

---

482 Bibicescu, "Mișcarea poporațiunii Capitalei în 1873," 1128.
483 Ibid.
484 Petrini de Galatz, *Despre ameliorațiunea rasei umane*, 21.
485 Ibid., 17.
486 Istrati, *O pagină din istoria contimpurană a României*, 106.

the theme of racial degeneration and the consequent depopulation of Romania: the aforementioned work by doctor Istrati, the text of a conference by Bibicescu on population trends in Romania,[487] doctor Iacob Felix's induction speech at the Romanian Academy,[488] also on depopulation, and, finally, the works of the Jewish doctors Roth[489] and, a little later, Solomon Mendelssohn.[490] By 1880, the theme of degeneration had become very topical.

In Romania, as elsewhere in Europe, the language of racial degeneration has been constructed and re-constructed endlessly by the social sciences and is applied to a wide range of concepts and objects.[491] Degeneration depends on social context and has national variations. In Romania, the issue of racial degeneration cannot be dissociated from other major social issues of the second half of the nineteenth century, such as the "peasant question" and the problems of the country's Jewish population. Likewise, it cannot be understood outside the debates on depopulation. Depopulation has been said to be the specific feature of racial degeneration in France.[492] But the anxieties of depopulation were equally constitutive of debates on degeneration in Romania. In Romania, however, demographic competition was internal rather than European. The threat to the native population was said to come from the "aliens" within, particularly from Jews. This was the specific variant of the theme of racial degeneration in the Romanian context.

We have seen that, after 1870, doctors initially identified the decline in the physical type of the Romanian peasant as a harbinger of racial degeneration. But degeneration is not individual; it is a malady of the societal body and, as such, it has specific causes and symptoms. We know from the preceding chapter that identifying the symptoms and establishing the aetiology of a disease are minimal pre-conditions for seeking treatment. The same approach can be used for social maladies. The medical discourse of the latter half of the nineteenth century allows us to reconstruct the causes and manifestations of the anxiety of degeneration, which haunted the Romanian nation. What were the criteria used by doctors? Firstly, a population is said to

---

487 Bibicescu, *Mișcarea poporațiunii în România de la 1870 până la 1878.*

488 Felix, "Despre mișcarea populației României," in *Despre regenerarea și ... degenerarea unei națiuni,* 41–69.

489 Roth, *Memoriu asupra cauzelor mortalității populației româno-creștine.*

490 Mendelssohn *Câteva considerațiuni asupra mișcării populațiunii României.*

491 Pick, *Faces of Degeneration,* 7–15.

492 Jorland, *Une société à soigner. Hygiène et salubrité publiques en France au XIXe siècle,* 153.

be degenerating when its demographic trends languish. The first sign is the stagnation or, even worse, the decrease of the population. But the earliest population censuses in Romania were organized in 1860 and 1899. In 1905, when he published the final results of the 1899 census, Leonida Colescu stated: "[F]or various reasons, Romania still does not possess a systematic and precise calculation of its inhabitants."[493] Unfortunately, even the census of 1899 was not an "operation of absolute precision,"[494] its own coordinator was compelled to admit. However, he added, it was clearly superior to the 1860 census in terms of method and accuracy of results. Colescu was even more dismissive of the tax censuses of 1884, 1889, and 1894, which he considered to be "very weak."[495] Consequently, the vacuum left by the shaky statistical data allowed for all kinds of manipulations of the official figures and bred all kinds of social anxieties. Colescu also informs us that even the subsequent analysis of the 1860 census by Petrescu was unsound. In his characteristically caustic style, Colescu dismissed Petrescu's calculations:

[T]he locum-tenens of the head of the office for statistics in 1865 [had] accepted the calculated population of Muntenia as 2,400,921 inhabitants, but considered that, standing at 1,463,927, the calculation for Moldavia was too low; having performed himself calculations according to a method which remains a secret, he reaches the conclusion that, to produce an accurate figure for the population of Moldavia, one must add 28 per cent to the above-specified figure. This, he says, is the percentage of omissions in the census "caused by the difficulty in counting the exact number of the populations in areas overwhelmed by Israelites and servants, especially in urban villages." But Petrescu is not consistent in what he says. The census results, published by Negruzzi for Moldavia and by Martzian for Muntenia, and those accepted by Petrescu, show that, for the Moldavian counties, the latter augmented the numbers of Romanians, not of the Israelites, by 33–40 per cent, without a valid explanation for variations from one county to another. In this manner, Petrescu established the population of Romania in 1859 as 4,424,961 inhabitants, which for a long time was taken to be the correct official figure.[496]

---

493 Colescu, *Analiza rezultatelor recensământului general al populației României de la 1899*, 8.
494 Ibid., 17.
495 Ibid., 9.
496 Ibid., 7–8.

Manipulations of statistical data such as the above were done by top governmental officials in 1865. If it could be done at that level, what can be expected from doctors, who did not have the expertise or the skills to skew data? In their hands, such figures were there to be remolded according to the day's agenda, and sometimes they did so even at the expense of logic and common sense. There were only two censuses during the last four decades of the nineteenth century, but this does not mean that no statistical data were available. Most ministries had their own offices for statistics: the Ministry for Home Affairs had one, so did the Ministry for Justice, from 1889 onward, the Ministry for Agriculture, Industry, and Trade, from 1883, and the department of Finance, from 1903.[497] As the century reached its end, statistics permeated public debate, as well as the methodologies of science and administration. The medical discourse was no exception. Here, I am less interested in the truth value of the period's statistics than in the ways in which they could and were manipulated to suit various agendas.

Let's remind ourselves that the main signs of racial degeneration are the stagnation or decrease of the population, or at least of certain social categories. Already by 1873, doctor Gr. Romniceanu had linked the theme of the degeneration of the Romanian population to that of Romania's depopulation. Fearing what he believed to be a real rural demographic hazard, he wrote: "Left to their own devices, as we see them today, they [the peasants] will perish day by day, in numbers incomparably higher than the births, and this decrease of the rural population will be harmful to the Romanian state, not only from a national viewpoint, but also from that of its economic interests."[498] Admittedly, for doctor Romniceanu the decline of the rural population was a matter of belief rather than a scientifically or statistically proven fact. However, in 1870, I am persuaded, this belief was nevertheless credible. The earliest alerts regarding the distressing decline of Romania's population came from a surprising source: an analysis of demographic trends in Bucharest. The first text to discuss this problem[499] on the basis of statistical data was the article by Bibicescu on population trends in the country's capital in 1873, in the newspaper *Românul*. Statistical data re-

---

497 E. C. Decuseară, "Organizarea statisticei în România," [The organization of statistics in Romania], *Revista de drept public*, IV, 1929, nos. 3–4, 538–40.

498 Romniceanu, "Igiena săteanului," 51.

499 Only a comprehensive study of the period's periodicals—which I have not undertaken—will establish with any precision the date when demographic anxiety became a topic in the press.

vealed a painful reality, which, the author wrote, "awakens vivid fears for the future of our nation": an excess of 3,000 deaths above the number of births. A brief glimpse into the past also shows a constant negative natural growth starting in 1867. The conclusion is self-evident, according to the author: "We are going through a terrible crisis, one of those crises from which nations rarely emerge triumphant."[500] An analysis of death and birth rates by religious affiliation reveals what was going to become a much-repeated trope in the demographic discourse of late-nineteenth-century doctors: all confessional communities, except the Israelites, had higher indices of mortality than of natality. In other words, leaving aside population shifts due to immigration and emigration, the number of ethnic Romanians declined, while that of Jews increased. This simple fact, Bibicescu wrote, should "curb the enthusiasm of those who announce every day that we are making constant progress and that Romania is blessed with every imaginable felicity."[501]

Bibicescu's pessimistic vision was a perfect fit for the political vision of a liberal oppositional newspaper in 1874. But reducing the debate to a sideshow of the broader political game would be a mistake. The medical discourse in general, and especially the discourse on racial degeneration, could be used and abused by conservatives and liberals alike. But the "battle" for Bucharest went on. In his report on public health in the capital city in 1875, doctor Felix reminded his readers that "there have been frequent public expressions of the fear that the population of Bucharest is in decline because of disproportionate ratios of births and deaths."[502] But he confessed that he did not share this fear, which he attributed to errors in the statistical recording of births—i.e. statistical under-evaluations of births and over-evaluated numbers of deaths, partly due to the inclusion in the city records of deaths in the Bucharest garrison. In the following year, the series of negative population increases came to an end, and doctor Felix was happy to report that the "population statistics for 1876 show that there is no cause to fear that the Romanian population of Bucharest increases through migrations from other districts rather than through births."[503] But doctor Felix's optimism regarding the growth of the Romanian population was premature. In August 1878,

500 Bibicescu, "Mişcarea poporaţiunii Capitalei în 1873," 1128.
501 Ibid.
502 Felix, Raport general pe anul 1875, 62.
503 Felix Raport general pe anul 1876, 63.

the minister of the interior, the Liberal C. A. Rosetti, expressed his concern about the population trends of Bucharest. Dismissing the small increases of 1876 and 1877, he was also aware of the problems in statistical recording, such as the under-recording of births and over-recording of deaths in the capital city. He deplored the "terrible reality" of a constant excess number of deaths compared to births. Consequently, he instructed the Higher Medical Council to study the causes of the "terrifying mortality in Bucharest, particularly among children of the Romanian population."[504] The minister for the interior was obviously less concerned over mortality among the Jewish population. Doctor Felix, at the time chief medical officer in Bucharest, responded to the official request the same year, with the publication of a report in which he downplayed the minister's alarm. He wrote of his belief that the "source" of the high mortality rate in Bucharest was "deep, and could only be eliminated gradually as civilization spread through education and moral instruction, and as society rid itself of harmful habits."[505] In his view, public hygiene was not necessarily conducive to a decrease in mortality. He cited as evidence the "squalid quarters inhabited by poor Israelites," in which mortality was nevertheless inferior to that of the "suburban, well-aired streets, with well-built houses and large courtyards, inhabited by Romanians."[506] In addition, the doctor added, a comparison with major European cities showed that the death rate in Bucharest was average. Doctor Felix, who knew the population trends in the capital well, concluded that the demographic situation was not as bad as generally believed and that it constantly improved. We do not know whether C. A. Rosetti was happy with the response from the capital's chief medic or whether he ever read the public health reports that the latter dutifully published year after year, starting in 1868.

The demographic situation in the capital, however, was about the leave the front page of public debate and be pushed into the background by the more alarming news from Moldavia. There, the doctors G. Flaişlen and Vasile I. Agappi opened a new battlefront in 1876. The campaign started with analyses of population trends in Iaşi, the capital of that province. In his public health report for 1875, the city's chief doctor, Flaişlen, reached what to us

---

504 Rosetti, "Adresa sub no. 14.757, a D-lui Ministru de interne," 5024–25.
505 Felix, "Mortalitatea în Capitală," 225.
506 Ibid., 226.

sounds like a foregone conclusion: from 1866 to 1875, in Iași, the "Christian element" of the population, i.e. the Romanians, declined through an excess of deaths over births, while the Jewish population increased. His conclusions were far from optimistic:

> These figures tell us that this decrease of the Christian element and growth of the Israelite element are no accident, but a well-observed rule [...] If we look at the results over the last 10 years to make a prediction for the future, we can say that in precisely 50 years there will be no Christian inhabitant in Iași, and the population will consist entirely of Israelites.[507]

In his doctoral thesis, doctor Agappi concurred, even though he did not presage the total extinction of ethnic Romanians in the foreseeable future: "The Romanian element, even if not totally disappearing, will decrease to such an extent that Iași will become a new Palestine through the gradual increase of the Israelite element."[508] But doctor Agappi takes the next step in his analysis, moving from the urban conglomeration of Iași to the county of Iași and then to the entire country. Wherever he looked, doctor Agappi saw the same situation. At county level, his analysis of population trends in the period 1869–1875 yielded a negative result for Christians and a positive one for Jews.[509] At the country-wide level, Agappi trenchantly concluded: "In rural villages, as well as in urban areas, in all seasons, and given the same state of health, the Romanian population decreases, and the Israelite population growths."[510] The danger of depopulation had by now become an unstoppable trope.

However, should one not take doctor Agappi at his word and look at the data he himself had used, you will note something strange: in fact, the numbers show an *increase* in the country's population. They certainly do not suggest either stagnation or the wiping out of the ethnic Romanian population, as feared at the time. To understand demographic trends in Romania, Agappi divided the three decades of the century into two distinct periods: he found a population increase of 847,000 from 1844 to 1859, whereas, over

---

507 Flaișlen, *Consiliul de higienă și salubritate publică din orașul Iași*, 18–19.
508 Agappi, *Cercetări demografice asupra populațiunii României și în special a districtului și orașului Iași*, 15.
509 Ibid., 22–23.
510 Ibid., 37.

the next fifteen years, from 1859 to 1874, the growth was of only around 415,000 persons.[511] While this represents a constant downward trend, one cannot speak of a dramatic decline. On the other hand, it is true that the slight negative growth in the period 1866 to 1873 had an inordinately major impact on the fears of depopulation in Romania.

A year before doctor Agappi's study, the economist Petre S. Aurelian published his well-known monograph *Terra nostra*, in which he addressed population trends among other topics. To the great surprise of today's historian, when Aurelian compares the natural growth for the years 1865 and 1871, he, too, comes up with comments on the "decrease of the population." This was simply because the natural excess of births he found for 1871 was 8,305 units lower than for 1865. It is true that the absolute figures he compared show a decrease: in 1865, the natural excess of births was 38,739 units, and only 30,434 units in 1871.[512] However, both figures are positive, which is evidence of an *increase* in the population. He, too, pointed to the high growth rate of the Jewish population in some Moldavian towns: "In Botoşani, there were 528 births among the Orthodox Christians to 671 among the Israelites; in Iaşi only 1,099 Orthodox to 1,999 Israelites; in Roman, 268 Orthodox and 271 Israelites; in Fălticeni, 126 Orthodox and 275 Israelites, which is two and a half more than the Romanians; in Dorohoi, 198 Orthodox to 322 Israelites. Therefore, in four major cities in the country the births of Romanian children are inferior to that of Israelite children!"[513] It was not just the birth rates that suggested the demographic rise of Moldavia's Jewish population, but also the ratio of mortality and natality in the same towns. This showed that "whereas the Romanian population decreases, the Israelites are growing." Aurelian believed that such figures were no accident and was emphatic that "for us Romanians in particular, the population question is an important matter of national survival."[514]

These examples show that, on the eve of the War for Independence, a growing number, though by no means all, of the intellectual elites aligned themselves with the thesis of the country's depopulation. It was not an optimistic vision of the future, but certainly not as apocalyptic as the afore-

---

511 Ibid., 26–31.
512 Aurelian, *Terra nostra*, 16.
513 Ibid., 20.
514 Ibid., 25.

mentioned views of Bibicescu and doctor Felix. In 1880, in a lecture on Romania's depopulation in the period 1870 to 1878, Bibicescu addressed the
apparently simple question of whether there had been a population increase
in that interval. Uncharacteristically, he started by defining his terms: "By
population increase I mean the result of natural growth rather than an increase through immigration."[515] Following up on his research of 1874, he
started with a case study from Bucharest, where the natural excess of births
was negative. He continued with the country's urban population, where the
demographic trend was identical, and ended with the rural population, the
only section where the trend was marginally positive. He concluded that
the Romanian peasant "maintains the numerical preponderance of the Romanian element through continuing growth. Therefore, we may say that the
peasant represents the "foundation of the national home."[516] Here is another
example that suggests the important role of the peasantry and the central
place of the "rural question" in public debate in modern Romania.

In the same year, doctor Felix was rewarded for his contribution to medical science: he became a member of the Romanian Academy. His acceptance speech addressed the most burning issue facing the medical community at the time: population trends. From the first lines of his speech,
doctor Felix lived up to his reputation for critical, positivist thinking. He
started by saying that he did not wish to contest obvious facts, because statistical data showed clearly that "the population in Romania increases at a
very slow rate, not only through immigration, but especially through births.
Growth through birth rates is observable not only among the general population, but also in part among the Romanian population. Among the Romanians, as well as among aliens who have settled in Romania, there is an
excess of births against deaths."[517] He paid tribute to the rural population,
which, doctor Felix acknowledged, was responsible for the natural population growth:

The peasant, who bears the heaviest weight of public duties, who makes the
greatest contribution to fulfilling the needs of the state in the most comprehensive manner, with his labor, and his blood, is also the one who almost sin-

515  Bibicescu, *Mişcarea poporaţiunii în România de la 1870 până la 1878*, 31.
516  Ibid., 47.
517  Felix, "Despre mişcarea populaţiei României," 42.

gle-handedly maintains the numerical progress of the Romanian nation. In return, society offers him the most deficient administrative and educational assistance.[518]

Such a positive appraisal of Romania's demographic trends must have displeased doctor Agappi. The new member of the Academy was precise in his analysis of the origins and evolution of the trope of demographic anxiety in the previous decade. In his view, previous authors had made unwarranted generalizations on population trends starting from a few specific case studies taken from the urban environment. Secondly, they had constantly compared natural growth rates among the native population and the Jewish population resulting from the same case studies. In other words, the demographic situation in two major cities, Bucharest and Iași, and of a few urban centers in Moldavia, had been fallaciously extended to the analysis of the country's general population.

It was a lucid evaluation of the literature on depopulation that can hardly be matched, even today. Yet, a comparison with demographic trends in civilized Europe led the doctor to the conclusion that the situation in Romania was far from ideal, and the anxieties of depopulation returned, playing havoc with his reasoned, scientific approach:

> The population in Romania grows at a lower rate compared to other countries; therefore, there is a threat of relative depopulation in Romania, which can harm its vital interests. This unhappy situation is still at a stage where it can be remedied, but if it progresses towards absolute depopulation, it could compromise the future of the Romanian state.[519]

It is noteworthy that, even though doctor Felix and the publicist Bibicescu were both reasonable men, endowed with healthy, critical minds and, as such, would have never thought of manipulating statistical data, they were still concerned. Ultimately, they shared their contemporaries' anxieties over the troubled, uncertain future of Romania's population.

---

518 Ibid., 44.
519 Ibid., 68.

As shown earlier, the themes of racial degeneration and depopulation became firmly established in the medical discourse by the publication of doctor Istrati's imposing volume in 1880. But the ethos of doctor Istrati's study is radically different from that of his colleague doctor Felix. From the early pages, the author presents a Romania of light and shades, a country split between progress and decadence:

> We now have a country in her own right, a country which has gone a long way in many respects; we, who until yesterday were an aspiring people, divided and ignored, are now finally a nation. We should be happy, our future should be assured, as the life of the Romanian ethnic element by the Danube should be assured. Yet, looking closely, we can see that we are still paying a tribute, an even greater one. Our existence is still not guaranteed, and tomorrow is still terrifying, because tomorrow we may disappear [...] Moreover, it is not only our political future and our future as a country which is uncertain, but also the future of the Romanian ethnic element, which continues to decline and degenerate as a result of the terrible, massive and incessant migrations of aliens which submerge it![520]

It was not, however, Romania's bright future that doctor Istrati intended to explore in the afore-cited work, but the perils threatening modern Romania, their causes and possible remedies. Firstly, one had to establish whether Romania's population increased, was stationary, or decreased. To do this, the author proceeded to a survey of demographic research in Romania. He was up-to-date with the work of doctors Agappi and Felix, and he did not fail to mention Bibicescu. Of the authors he cited, only Agappi claimed that Romania's population was in decline. Both Felix and Bibicescu spoke of an increase, albeit a modest one. Doctor Istrati was convinced that the latter were mistaken. But how to prove it? He resorted to a simple stratagem: all the authors referenced had analyzed results collected over short intervals, which could skew the overall picture. Consequently, doctor Istrati expanded the timescale and started with the year 1859, for which he found 57.5 deaths per 100 births, ending with 1878, with 101.7 deaths per 100 births. He concluded that the trend was for natural growth to decline. For 1878, it was already neg-

---

520 Istrati, *O pagină din istoria contimpurană a României*, vii–viii.

ative. This led doctor Istrati to state that population decline was a danger to be reckoned with. If the trend persisted, the deaths-births ratio was going to be a terrifying 171 to 100 by 1899. Having surveyed the entire literature on medical demography and having done his own analysis, doctor Istrati reached a clear conclusion, which he explained in a very confusing way:

> [O]ur population is constantly decreasing. An average calculated for any of these years, and even for a series of several years, as Dr. Felix and Mr. Bibicescu have done, cannot be taken as a constant factor of population increase because it is not based on terms which might show a difference between them [i.e. individual years], but only on constantly decreasing terms which can only show the amount by which our population decreases, rather than increases. This is because they are intermediary points linking good years for the prosperity and welfare of the Romanian nation, progressing gradually to grim results, as we approach our own time.[521]

Even though I confess to having lost the logical thread of doctor Istrati's demonstration, it is nevertheless quite clear that, like P.S. Aurelian and doctor Agappi, he turned an increasingly anaemic *growth* into a *decrease* of the Romanian population. All the afore-cited authors, except doctor Felix, held the uncompromising belief that as Romania was emptied of its native ethnic population, it was being repopulated with aliens in general, and especially with Jews. Doctor Istrati summed it as follows:

> This constant decrease in the population of our country is all the more important for us, Romanians, because, while our ancestral land appears to be turning into a graveyard for our own people, it seems to be a smiling garden in which aliens, and particularly Israelites, multiply at a prodigious rate. [...] A few years ago, it was said that Iași would become a Jewish city. It is one now. The same can be said of Bucharest, now swarming with all kinds of foreigners, and especially with Jews [...], the head and the heart of our country being thus alienated, the body, too, will follow. One half of this body is already ill with the Jewish gangrene. The rest is pullulating with Bulgarians, Greeks, Jews![522]

---

521 Istrati, *O pagină din istoria contimpurană a României*, 72.
522 Ibid., 73–74.

Doctor Istrati's antisemitism was visceral, with doctor Agappi and Bibicescu following not far behind. Doctor Felix's texts do not have antisemitic or philosemitic touches, and he remains an example of someone who did not adhere to the antisemitic ideology of the Romanian elites. In his case, there is a simple explanation: he descended from a Jewish family from northern Bohemia. At the start of his academic studies, he declared himself as being of the Mosaic faith, but he converted to Christianity before 1858, when he settled in Ţara Românească. It was a wise decision. Throughout his entire career, he kept an absolute silence on his life before his arrival in Romania.[523] But his ethnic origin was easy to guess because of the surname Iacob. Doctor Iuliu Theodori surmised that doctor Felix was of "Jewish nationality" and was not in favor of him marrying his sister, Olimpia.[524] Doctor Felix, therefore, had every reason to hide his ethnic origin. But it did not stop him in his career. Hard work and support from the influential doctor Carol Davila helped him climb the professional ladder to the very top of Romania's health system.

As we have seen, around 1900 there was an avalanche of titles on demographic trends in Romania. The increasing emphasis on Romania's depopulation and on the gradual displacement of the "autochthonous element" by the "Jewish element," to use the period's jargon, could not fail to trigger a response from Jewish doctors. Indeed, we found two works that can be regarded to some extent as responses to the wave of demographic antisemitism in the period considered here. One of these works, by doctor Roth, attempted to explain things from the other side of the ideological barricade. Doctor Roth did not deny the statistics or the main thesis of the Romanian doctors, but tried to explain in a rational manner why Christians, i.e. Romanians, had such a high mortality compared to the Jewish population. He even went as far as to support the theory of the degeneration of the indigenous race and the eventual depopulation of Romania. Like the Romanian doctors, he was convinced that "it is no exaggeration to state, as many have done, that if things will not improve in the current lives of the peasants, a time will come when this population, the only one representing the pure and unaltered national element, will become extinct [...]."[525] As the theme

523 Brătescu, *Doctorul Iacob Felix. Savantul şi înfăptuitorul*, 11–12.
524 Ibid., 85–87.
525 Roth, *Memoriu asupra cauzelor mortalităţii populaţiei româno-creştine*, 98.

of doctor Roth's study is depopulation and its causes, I shall not dwell on it. Doctor Solomon Mendelssohn's work has a different ambition: it was designed to be a response to doctor Felix's pessimistic conclusions, as outlined in his acceptance speech at the Romanian Academy. Point by point, doctor Mendelssohn dismantled doctor Felix's statistical-demographic construct to reach the following conclusion, which must have ruffled some intellectual feathers at the time. He dismissed doctor Felix's argument in the following terms:

> It is entirely arbitrary and unsupported by statistical data to claim that Romania is threatened by relative depopulation, which could eventually become absolute. I have proved above that, in the last nine years, the population in Romania has grown at least by 3.7 per thousand, despite being harmed by various epidemics in the years 1873 and 1874 and suffering from the effects of the latest war until 1879. I have also further demonstrated that, in the six years between these two dates, themselves not altogether normal years, the excess of births in the population of Romania was proportionally almost equal to the rates in Austria and Italy. Faced with such positive facts, it is incomprehensible to speak of a relative depopulation threatening to become absolute.[526]

Interestingly, doctor Felix's—fundamentally well-balanced—study and outlook were attacked by both Romanian and Jewish doctors. Doctor Istrati, for example, critiqued his all-too-optimistic views on depopulation:

> It appears that the fear of a constant decrease and the possibility of a national calamity have influenced doctor Felix to such an extent, that his conclusion—may the gentlemen allow me to say it—although it appears sad and discouraging, is only a pale reflection of the real and unfortunate state in which we find ourselves.[527]

Doctor Felix's middle-of-the road approach proves once again that, on the issue of the country's degeneration and depopulation, one could only

---

526 Mendelssohn, *Câteva considerațiuni asupra mișcării populațiunii României*, 37.
527 Istrati, *O pagină din istoria contimpurană a României*, 59.

be on one side or the other of the barricade, that is, either in the "national camp" or in the opposite, "Jewish camp." Positioning oneself in the middle meant remaining at the top of the barricade, in the line of fire from all directions. The focus on degeneration shows to what extent the discourse of the medical sciences aligned itself with the period's ambient nationalism. The dominant national paradigm had the extraordinary capacity of hijacking the period's ethos, and the scientific discourse was no exception.

After 1880, the clamor and the anxieties seemed to die down. This does not mean that the theme of racial degeneration and depopulation disappeared from the medical literature. The ninth decade of the century appeared calmer, perhaps also because doctor Istrati's alarming warnings proved to be unfounded: 1878 was the last year with a negative natural growth before World War I. From 1880 onwards, the natural growth of the population was consistently positive and ascending. We should not leap to the conclusion, however, that, with statistics showing increases in the Kingdom's population year after year, social anxieties disappeared. That scenario would be too straightforwardly rational. The Jewish "threat" remained; after the mid-1880s, pellagra emerged as a national malady; the health and social conditions of the peasantry became a locus of concern; and alcoholism was rampant. The fear of degeneration did not disappear, but its expression changed. The last decade of the nineteenth century is dominated by the figure of doctor Felix as head of the Romanian Kingdom's Health Services. I have already noted his balanced views on depopulation and, implicitly, on the Jewish question. Understandably, in the reports he published during his directorship he did not encourage the dissemination of the theme of degeneration and the associated theme of depopulation in the medical literature. And, as a matter of fact, there was no reason for it. The last, and most comprehensive, of his reports closes with the following significant statement:

The most certain sign of material progress in the Romanian state is the evidence of its population statistics, which show a normal rate of growth of the general Romanian population, and especially of the rural population. The statistics disprove the fears, expressed here and there in the press and even in Parliament, of a degeneration of the Romanian race; they show that the gradually improving physical condition of the people ensure not only a fairly numerous progeny, but also the vigorous bodies needed for the defense of the fatherland.[528]

For doctor Felix, in 1899, the problems of racial degeneration and depopulation practically no longer existed. His views were correct, as reflected in the statistical trends of the early twentieth century, when the Kingdom's demographic rise was meteoric: natural growth was positive, expressed in constantly ascending absolute figures. In 1904, it exceeded the magical figure of 100,000 units. Doctor Obregia appeared as satisfied and optimistic as doctor Felix. The statistical data for 1906 were excellent:

> [T]he year 1906 gave us a natural excess of 103,394 inhabitants, with a growth of 15.9 per thousand and a mortality of 24.20 per thousand. From the point of view of public health, this was the best year Romania has had since 1870, surpassing even the excellent year 1900.[529]

The best news was that natural growth "tended to stay in place at 15, which puts us among the European countries with the best population growth rates."[530] And yet, doctor Obregia appealed to reason. A very high birth rate in fact implied that we were not a modern nation, he contended. He also believed that we could look at high natality from the perspective of a

> [...] phenomenon recently described as the pluri-natality of alcoholized populations. This pluri-natality is not something to be rejoiced over. Of the many infants born, many die within their first year, many others are not fit enough for life's struggles, and only a few are normal and healthy enough to contribute towards the progress of the family and the state. And we have a very high mortality for infants in their early years.[531]

From this perspective, the high natality among the Romanian population becomes a sign of economic and cultural backwardness, and, even a worse, a symptom of the spread of alcoholism. Almost overnight, a high

---

528 Felix, *Raport general asupra igienei publice și asupra serviciului sanitar al Regatului României pe anii 1896 și 1897*, I.
529 Obregia, *Raport general asupra igienei publice și asupra serviciului sanitar*, xiii.
530 Ibid.
531 Ibid., xiv.

birth rate, previously thought to be a positive fact, acquires negative connotations. In addition, infant mortality, too, came into focus in the last decade
of the nineteenth century. While the health services had been aware of it
since their inception, infant mortality had remained unquantified for a long
time, and it was only in this period that it became a major public health issue. The above-quoted passage is noteworthy for a new interest in the qualitative make-up of the population, an interest that was possibly influenced
by the rise of eugenic theories in Europe. Nevertheless, doctor Felix's perceptions of Romanian demography at the end of his career remained significantly different from those of doctor Obregia, who belonged to a new generation of medical professionals.

Yet, the more optimistic views of demographic trends in Romania in the
late nineteenth and early twentieth century were not shared by the entire
medical corps, not even at the top. Victor Babeș himself, one of modern Romania's few real men of science, endowed with a remarkably sharp critical
mind, allowed himself to be engulfed by theories of racial degeneration, depopulation, and the consequent antisemitism. In 1900, Babeș believed that,
"undeniably, the Romanian population showed signs of degeneration."[532]
By this he meant general degeneration, which affected not only the peasant masses, but also the country's morally degenerate elites. Moreover, in
his view, the entire social body was caught up in a vicious circle in which
the moral degeneration of the elites led to physical degeneration among the
rest of the population. He was equally negative about the nation's demographic trends. For the years 1898–1899, he speaks of demographic stagnation, "which for a people is identical to stagnation,"[533] because the much-
touted annual demographic growth of 12 to 13 per thousand was not due, in
his view, to the indigenous population, but to the immigration of aliens, by
which he meant the Jews.

Doctor Babeș made no attempt at concealing his demographic antisemitism: like many other doctors at the time, he found that the demographic
battle for Romania's cities was lost as far as the indigenous ethnic element
was concerned. The threat was high, he contended: "If all of them were to
remain in the country, the law of progressive growth says that they would

---

532 Babeș, *Regenerarea poporului român*, 4.
533 Ibid., 12.

soon overwhelm the Romanian race."[534] Like doctor Istrati in 1880, doctor Babeş wrote about an invasion of "Jews, Bulgarians and Hungarians."[535] The Jew was simply the most threatening of the invading aliens. The perpetually unresolved "Jewish question" remained deeply embedded in the spirit of the period, largely due to its perceived demographic implications. The lack of censuses provided a fertile ground for anxieties of invasion, for which a wide range of figures was advanced. The census of 1859 recorded 134,168 Jews,[536] the only value which came close to actual numbers; Fr. Damé estimated the number of Jews in Romania to be 400,000 in 1867; six years later, D. E. Krețulescu pushed the figures downward to 247,034; while doctor Obedenaru adjusted it to 264,800 for 1876.[537] Shortly after the War of Independence, there was a new explosion of estimates: Bibicescu advanced a figure of "over 600,000,"[538] and doctor Istrati, who had not read Bibicescu's study attentively, cited the latter with 400,000 Jews, which he, Istrati, in turn, readjusted to 600,000. By adding all the other foreigners who had settled in Romania, doctor Istrati concluded that, of Romania's 5,000,000 inhabitants, no fewer than 1,000,000 were aliens, which meant "an average of 1 alien per 4 Romanians!" Istrati commented further:

> Let us not dismiss these figures, and I stand ready to be proven wrong. But I do not wish to hear childish objections, according to which the Hungarians, Bulgarians, Armenians who settled here a long time ago, and the Jews—this would be even more ridiculous—and other races are partly de-nationalized. When the number of alien elements will grow in this country, I am afraid that from every Hungarian village will rise a defender of Saint Stephen's Crown, every Jew will grow into a German banker, which is already happening, and every Bulgarian will become a deputy representing the Chamber in Sophia!"[539]

Obviously, doctor Istrati thought that foreigners represented a national threat, because they could not be assimilated. And, even if they assimi-

---

534 Ibid., 14.
535 Ibid., 16.
536 Colescu, *Analiza*, 82.
537 Felix, *Raport general asupra igienei publice şi asupra serviciului sanitar al Regatului României pe anul 1894*, 25.
538 Bibicescu, *Mişcarea poporaţiunii în România de la 1870 până la 1878*, 61.
539 Sophia, for the Bulgarian capital Sofia, in the original. Istrati, *O pagină din istoria contimpurană a României*, 88.

lated—something doctor Istrati did not recommend—the mixing of races was not an advantage. Istrati even referred to a "superior race," by which he meant, naturally, the Romanian race:

> Without being too vain, it is fair to say that a Romania of Bulgarian-born Romanians, for example, would never be a nation which breathes with the true passion in our people' soul![540]

So far, we have established that, around the time of the War of Independence, the fear of foreigners, and especially of Jews, was on the rise. Their numbers were exaggerated, as was the socially diluting impact of their presence. For the period after 1880, we have fewer global estimates of the number of Jews in Romania. In his public health reports from the 1890s, doctor Felix did not advance such estimates. The next census was the one organized by Leonida Colescu in 1899. The results showed that there were only 266,652 Jews[541] in Romania, representing 4.5 per cent of the total population. This was by far less than the earlier estimates of 600,000 or even 400,000 Jews. Indeed, Jews represented 19 per cent of Romania's urban population and 38.7 per cent of Moldavia's urban population.[542] It is equally true that, comparing population growth rates between the censuses of 1859 and 1899 by religion, the rate for the Jewish population (through births and immigration combined) was almost twice as high as the rate for Orthodox Christians: in that interval, the Jewish population grew by 98.7 per cent, while the Christian population had a rate of only 49.8 per cent.[543] Nevertheless, the Jews still represented no more than 4.5 per cent of the country's total population.

The publication, in 1905, of the definitive results of the census of 1899 must have calmed the fears about the demographic relevance of the Jewish population. Yet, in Moldavia, there were still doctors whose thinking had not changed since the pre-1899 periods. Thus, doctor D. Galian from Botoşani published in the journal *Spitalul* (The hospital) a study on the "decline of the population in Botoşani," in which he deployed the language and

540 Istrati, *O pagină din istoria contimpurană a României*, 100.
541 Ibid., 82.
542 Ibid., 85.
543 Ibid., 82.

the arguments used three decades earlier. In the first place, the theme of depopulation remained as overpowering as ever:

> There are towns in the Romanian lands in which, not just by accident, and not just once or twice, but constantly and with almost mathematical regularity, records show an alarmingly large disproportion between the numbers of births and deaths among the indigenous population.[544]

If, in the ten years considered here—from 1898 to 1907—the natural growth of the Romanian population remained negative, while that of the Jewish population remained constantly positive, nothing seemed to have changed, with the sole exception that doctor Galian's study was strictly limited to the town of Botoșani. By 1910, the theory of a general depopulation of Romania was no longer tenable. The only demographic trend still demonstrable was the decline of the indigenous population through natural negative growth in some urban areas, but nothing more than that. The work of Leonida Colescu must have had an impact. In addition—as doctor Galian was aware—the Jews had started migrating from Romania, which led to the decline of the proportion of the Jewish population across the Kingdom. The census of 1912 was about to prove this trend. On the eve of Romania's military engagement in World War I, Colescu chased the clouds from the country's demographic skyline, and used the partial data of the new census to prove beyond doubt that the Jewish population was decreasing: in 1912, the new records showed that there were 239,967 Jews in the entire territory of the Kingdom (excluding New Dobrudja, to be added to the territory by the Treaty of Bucharest of 1913). This figure amounted to 3.3 per cent of the total Romanian population.[545] In the thirteen years since 1899, the growth rate had declined by 26,685 units, which meant a loss of approximately 10 per cent of its population for the Jewish community. In fact, the loss (through emigration) was higher, because between the two censuses, the Jewish population had had a constantly positive natural growth rate. According to Colescu, if this rate was added to the calculation, in 1912 the number of Jews must have totalled 309,822. This meant that, in fact, the loss was of "almost

---

544 Galian, "În cestiunea descreșterii populațiunei orașului Botoșani,"473.
545 Colesco, *La population de religion mosaïque en Roumanie,* 4–5.

70,000 units, or 26 per cent."[546] These figures suggested that the "Jewish question" was about to be resolved.

## Racial Degeneration and the Statistics of Conscription

Let's look at another variant of racial degeneration, which is not of a demographic nature. Like everywhere else in Europe, recruitment records in Romania have been used to prove theories of degeneration among indigenous races. Recruitment statistics offer physical anthropological data (height, thoracic circumference, weight, etc.) and data on pathology (medical exemptions from service) within a specific age group of the country's male population. The sum of these data provides an accurate index of what the medical doctor Zaharia Petrescu called the "military capacity of the country's population"[547] and doctor Felix the "physical worth of the population."[548] Naturally, military aptitude and good physical features are inversely proportional to the degree of racial degeneration in a population. Conscription started in 1864 in Romania. Initially it was supervised by civilian doctors, and only after 1869 did military doctors become involved. The aforementioned doctor Petrescu became the founding father of conscription statistics in Romania. In 1869, when appointed conscription medic in Vâlcea County, he was surprised to find

> [...] a total lack of studies, or of statistical observations on conscription procedures, not only in the district in which I functioned, but in all districts across the country. When, having completed the operation, I wished to report on what I had accomplished in the mission entrusted to me, I looked in the archives of the civilian health service, but found no study to serve me as a basis for comparison.[549]

After 1869, the medical conscription boards were again composed only of civilian doctors. Recruitment examinations were entrusted to military medics again only in 1874. On this occasion, doctor Petrescu managed to collect

---

546 Ibid., 14–15.

547 Petrescu, *O încercare de statistica medico-militară a României*, 3.

548 Felix, *Raport general asupra igienei publice și asupra serviciului sanitar al Regatului României pe anul 1895*, 15.

549 Petrescu, *O încercare de statistica medico-militară a României*, 4.

from all members of the conscription boards data which can now help us re-construct the nationwide statistic tableau of conscription in 1874. Doctor Pe-trescu published his collection of data in 1880 in a study that shows that he was by no means an alarmist. In the county of Vâlcea, in 1869, he found

[...] men of an advanced age, yet very healthy, vigorous and full of life [...] the *muntean*[550] man is robust and happy, the *muntean* woman strong and of a cheerful disposition. The reader might object that I stand in contradiction to my own data, in which he can see far too many lads exempted because of a weak constitution. It is true, but this is only apparently a contradiction; if we consider the 382 young men given so-called legal exemptions, we will find that these men were from the elites, and were among the more robust; this left only the tender, weaker youths available for medical selection. From these *remaindered* young men, I sought to make the best selection possible, and I managed to select 359 recruits, all young, very healthy and robust. From the total of 689 young men who presented themselves, even the 205 with *a weaker constitution* that I exempted were not the wrecks someone might imagine.[551]

This text highlights the traps of this type of assessment and the manipu-lations they could encourage.

Even by 1874, when the waters had been thoroughly muddied in demo-graphic theory, doctor Petrescu found a population that seemed to him to be

[...] in a satisfying health condition, as can be observed from the tables of exemptions for sickness and infirmities; for the numbers of such exemp-tions (190) was small compared to the huge number of young men examined (3,048), and even those exempted only had minor infirmities.[552]

When one moves on to an analysis of conscription statistics for the entire country in 1874, the general tableau becomes more fraught with negative nuances. Not all conscription medics had positive experiences comparable

550 A Muntean is an inhabitant of Muntenia, Romania's historic southern province. See note 59 above. (Italics added.)
551 Petrescu, *O încercare de statistica medico-militară a României*, 8–9.
552 Ibid., 21.

to doctor Petrescu's in his own region: [T]he data in these tables show that diathesic, constitutional, and hereditary diseases were very rare in mountainous localities, but very frequent in the low-lying plains.[553]

This confirms stereotypes of the superior physical type of the peasant in mountainous regions compared to the inhabitants of the plains. It is sufficient to recall descriptions of inhabitants of the rural low-lying regions in the writings of doctor Obedenaru. It is nevertheless noteworthy that, in 1880, the vocabulary of doctor Petrescu does not include the term "degeneration." In contrast, in the same year, doctor Istrati made comprehensive use of conscription statistics to demonstrate the degeneration of Romania's population. Less optimistic than doctor Petrescu, doctor Istrati turned the latter's data upside down. In addition, doctor Istrati could use the nationwide conscription statistics for 1879, which had been "kindly placed at my disposal by Inspector-General Davila."[554] This allowed him to compare data for Vâlcea County over a three-year period (1869, 1874, and 1879) and for the entire country over two years (1874 and 1879). The personal notations on the margins of conscriptions reports by doctors in 1879 were another rich source for the medical professionals. Doctor I. Nicolescu, a conscription medic from Muşcel County, described the reasons for exemption in these terms: [T]hirty-seven young men were excluded because they were less than 1.54 meters; five of them had the appearance of children between 7 and 10 years of age!" The doctoral candidate Spiroiu told doctor Istrati that, in the same county, "in the villages of Nucşoara and Corbii, many recruits at the age of 20 were so short, sickly and degenerate that they had to be *carried* by their mothers!"[555] The imagery in these testimonies left no one in any doubt that the population of Romania was in a "state of malady, suffering, diminution, degeneration, and fatal danger."[556] Nevertheless, doctor Istrati never ceased trying to demonstrate scientifically that his intuitions and assumptions were correct. He found support in the statistics of conscription. By 1879, Vâlcea County was no longer what it had been in 1869: all the indices of the recruits' health had declined: exemptions for infirmity rose from 105.6 per thousand to 168 per thousand; exemptions for debility and

---

553 Ibid., 39.
554 Istrati, *O pagină din istoria contimpurană a României*, 115.
555 Ibid., 138–39.
556 Ibid., 139.

arrested development followed the same ascending trend: 245.5 per thousand (1879) compared to 177.4 per thousand (1869).[557] It was an alarming situation. It was still possible, some hoped, that Vâlcea County was a particularly unhappy case and that, nationally, the statistics of conscription might suggest positive trends. Alas, this was not the case, and the situation in Vâlcea seemed to be replicated across the country. Doctor Istrati did not hide his despair:

> [W]hat in our country is on an enormous scale and cannot be seen elsewhere, is the huge number of feeble constitutions: in 1874, they were 185.2 and in 1879, 177.9. The difference is small, and is rendered even more insignificant as the cases of arrested development increased in only six years from 74.1 to 214, a threefold increase! [...] Thus, the total of weak and poorly developed recruits, which was 259.3 in 1874, doubled over the next six years to reach 392.3. What else do these figures show, but the state of debility, physical degradation and degeneration of our race!"[558]

Doctor Istrati's conclusion was final, his demonstration complete. For him, undoubtedly, the statistics of conscription were perfect even across the country; in his view, between 1869 and 1879, all conscription doctors evaluated cases of debility and arrested development (the foundation of his argument) in a uniform manner; he took it for granted that doctors' exigencies did not change in this interval, and that the only element that changed was the deteriorating physical condition of the recruits.

In the 1880s, other military doctors followed in doctor Istrati's footsteps. One of them was the battalion medic Ioan Dănescu, who, in 1886, defended his doctorate on medical demography and geography. His main sources were conscription statistics, which, for the period after 1879, were complete and covered the country's entire territory. His analysis focused on the five-year interval from 1879 to 1883. What did these statistics reveal to doctor Dănescu? One of his findings was the apparently normal physical condition of recruits, as reflected in features such as height averaging 1.65 meters and a thoracic circumference of 85 centimeters: "Our nation's vigor is still suffi-

---

557 Ibid., 118.
558 Ibid., 123–24.

ciently high, [...] *our race is maintaining itself at normal levels,*" Dănescu concluded.[559] Of the 188,905 recruits he had examined in the five years, only 32,968 were exempt from military service because of disease or infirmity. This represented a percentage of 17.45, which was not alarmingly high, according to the doctor:

> With 17 infirm per 100 strong lads, this is a figure that reflects a more than satisfying health situation, with levels of vigor and virility that show that we can be hopeful for our nation's survival and future.[560]

From the heights of statistical averages, the general picture looked healthy enough; yet, as one's gaze descended to the micro level, the tableau lost its rosy hues as the misery of the sickly, exempted candidates came to the fore. A weak constitution and arrested development were the causes for which over 10,000 young men were rejected. Suddenly, the "excellent qualities of our race started to decline."[561] Compared to 1874, the picture of the physical condition of the population acquired even darker hues: whereas in 1874, the number of rejected recruits stood at 6,317, over the five years considered by Dănescu, and observing the proportions, the number of the rejected should have been 31,585, but in fact it was higher by 1,383 units. Doctor Dănescu concluded that "the country's military capacity, considered from a medical point of view, is in decline."[562] From here, it was only one step to a picture of unmitigated disaster. It was a step doctor Dănescu took when he admitted, for example, that in the village of Iugurul, in Muşcel County, he could only recruit two fit men in five years.[563] In conclusion, six years later, doctor Istrati's rhetorical question on the reasons for the degeneration of the Romanian race received an answer from doctor Dănescu: "[Y]es|! With much regret, we must admit that the Romanian race is degenerating, and it does so at an alarming rate."[564]

Two years later, another military doctor, encouraged by the "success of my comrade [...] Dr. Dănescu's thesis,"[565] picked as a topic for his own doc-

559 Dănescu, *Încercări de demografie şi geografie medicală*, n.p.
560 Ibid., i.
561 Ibid., ii.
562 Ibid., v.
563 Ibid., n.p.
564 Ibid., vii.
565 Gugea, *Contribuţiune la studiul taliei soldatului român*, 11.

toral research a study of recruits' height. The interval was the same as that of his mentor, 1879 to 1883. As was to be expected, the outcome, too, was the same. Doctor Gugea's working hypothesis was that there existed a clear link between the percentage of exemptions from service and the candidates' deficient height, the health levels in their communities, and racial degeneration:

> The men were frequently shorter in counties where poverty was greater. In our country, all these defects in the physical constitution of the population cannot be explained by racial differences. Although, there are indeed regions populated with heterogeneous elements, our personal observations have led us to believe that all these elements have a good level of development, and that physical degeneration caused by unhealthy living conditions only affects the autochthonous population.[566]

Like doctor Dănescu before him, doctor Gugea encountered a methodological problem: the average height among recruits in those five years invalidated the thesis that authors were trying hard to prove:

> [T]he figures in my tables show an average height of 1 meter 65 centimeters for the 224,972 young men who underwent medical examination from 1879 to, and including, 1883. Figures are also upward of this average, with taller men having heights of up to 1.70 meter. We could, therefore, say that our material is in excellent condition and that we can cultivate it by favoring the best environment for its development.[567]

Nevertheless, doctor Gugea remained concerned because, irrespective of what his statistical figures showed, he knew that the Romanian race was degenerating. In these circumstances, he located sites of degeneration in mountainous areas where the number of exemptions on the grounds of height was higher:

> [T]he population of our mountainous localities began degenerating a long time ago, because there, heights of less than 1.54 meter have already reached

---

566 Ibid., 18.
567 Ibid., 28.

maximum ratios of 70 per 1,000, and, in conjunction with some low-lying counties, minimal ratios of 30 per 1,000.[568]

It is difficult to understand why, for doctor Gugea, a minimal proportion of 30 per thousand in exemptions of shorter men should have been a reason for concern and firm evidence of degeneration.

Only one year after doctor Gugea's successful doctoral thesis, in 1889, a younger colleague, Nicolae Soiu, decided to tackle another theme of medical demography in his own doctoral research. Even though the commission for both doctoral theses was chaired by the same doctor Petrescu, their conclusions were rather different. Like his doctoral supervisor, doctor Soiu was an optimist: nothing could persuade him that the race was degenerating. He believed that deficient height, the cause cited in a significant number of exemptions, had been erroneously linked to the unhealthy living conditions of the recruits:

[I]f greater height could justifiably be conceived as representing vigor and good health, it would necessarily follow that shorter heights are a criterion for a weaker constitution and for physiological debility; in that case, the shorter heights and infirmity should obviously go hand in hand.[569]

But, he contended, the statistical data he had collected did not confirm this theory. Doctor Soiu, in fact, followed Paul Broca's[570] theory, according to which height was a characteristic of "race" rather than an indicator of an individual recruit's physical development. It followed that the large number of candidates rejected by conscription boards could not prove anything, because at the age of 21, "the development of the organism was not complete yet."[571] Doctor Soiu was obviously not going to be persuaded otherwise.

In this scientific domain, surprises could crop up from unexpected directions: in 1893, none other than doctor Felix was forced to admit that the average Romanian recruit had a "weak constitution." He used a composite index: the ratio of height and thoracic circumference. It was an "acknowledged scien-

568 Ibid., 39.
569 Soiu, *Valoarea perimetriei toracice în examenul recrutării*, 42.
570 Pierre Paul Broca (1824–1880) was French doctor, anatomist, and anthropologist, best known for his research on the anatomy of the brain.
571 Soiu, *Valoarea perimetriei toracice în examenul recrutării*, 61.

tific fact," he observed, that if the thoracic circumference was half the individual's height plus two to three centimeters, this ratio precisely marked the borderline between a weak constitution and a regular one. He also noted that the average recruit in Romania was located exactly on this borderline: "More than 70 per cent of the recruits we examined have a thoracic circumference of 80 to 90 centimeters and a height of 158 to 173 centimeters."[572]

In addition, in the Romanian recruitment statistics for 1891–1894, doctor Felix identified the same factors doctor Donath had identified in 1894 as prerequisites for the general degeneration of the populations in modern states: while "the number of recruits who pass is decreasing, the number of those exempted for infirmity is increasing."[573] Was it the case that in 1894, doctor Felix reached the same conclusion drawn by doctor Istrati in 1880? This is hard to believe. After this avalanche of bad news, however, the Director-General of the Health Services wished to remind us that it was not all gloom and doom:

[C]onscription statistics do not offer an absolute picture of corporeal development and physical strength in the population, because at the age of 21 the body is not yet fully-formed, and some organs continue to grow even after this age. In our country, and elsewhere, findings show that skeletal development in a significant number of humans sometimes continues after the age of 25, and often growth continues until later.[574]

Doctor Felix appears to have trusted his own intuition more than he trusted "acknowledged scientific facts." In his report on the Kingdom's public health for 1895 (published in 1897), although conscription data did not indicate an improvement of the "physical qualities" of the recruits, doctor Felix's views were much more nuanced. Even though in Romania, the numbers of those considered fit for military service continued to drop year after year—a sure sign of degeneration in the eyes of the "civilian and military hygienists in most European countries"—doctor Felix did not rush to draw conclusions. He did not have enough faith in the ways in which recruitment lists and medical examinations were organized. Statistics showed that the

---

572 Felix, *Raport general asupra igienei publice și asupra serviciului sanitar al Regatului României pe anul 1894*, 42.
573 Ibid.
574 Ibid., 44.

ratio of height to thoracic circumference was the same as two years earlier, and yet, doctor Felix stated, "conscription statistics do not yet confirm fears that the physical strength of the population is in decline and that the population is degenerating."[575] He reached the same conclusion in his report for 1896–1897, published in 1899.[576]

At the end of his career and only a few years before his death, doctor Felix was convinced that the indigenous population was thriving, and that Romania was on the right track as a nation. Not doctor Babeş, who, in a lecture in November 1900 on the regeneration of the Romanian people, expressed his conviction that public health in Romania, especially in rural areas, was in a critical situation. He was, as we have seen, a champion of the thesis of racial degeneration, and could not ignore—without, however, attaching too much importance to it—the fact that "Romanians were in bad shape regarding their vital statistics." The conscription results for 1890–1892 and 1897 show that the percentage of those "rejected" by the conscription boards rose from 5.6 per cent to 8.3 per cent.[577] In the last two decades of the nineteenth century, doctors, some of whom were at the top echelons of the profession in the Romanian Kingdom, gradually rallied behind the theory of racial degeneration. This phenomenon was best captured in the statistics of conscription. We have also seen that not all doctors supported this theory. Doctor Felix was one of them, but he was a special case. Doctor Petrescu, too, only supported the theory partially and unconvincingly. But many others—the majority, we could say—fervently claimed that the Romanian race was degenerating, a claim that became an axiom of the period's medical discourse.

## Infant Mortality at the End of the Century

In the last decade of the nineteenth century and the early years of the twentieth, the medical profession opened a new fight against an old and persistent foe: infant mortality. Infant mortality almost cancelled out the only advantage Romania had over other European states: its high birth rate. It

---

575 Felix, *Raport general asupra igienei publice şi asupra serviciului sanitar al Regatului României pe anul 1895*, 16.

576 Felix, *Raport general asupra igienei publice şi asupra serviciului sanitar al Regatului României pe anii 1896 şi 1897*, 26.

577 Babeş, *Regenerarea poporului român*, 14–15.

was identified as the main hurdle that blocked the demographic explosion so ardently desired by the health authorities. Mortality in general, and particularly infant mortality, once it reached certain levels and started affecting demographic growth, was regarded as an indicator of racial degeneration. Interestingly, doctors' interest in infant mortality remained quiet in the 1870s, a period that included three years—1873, 1874, and 1878—of negative natural growth. Paradoxically, this interest emerged much later, when national anxieties caused by demography seemed to have calmed down. One explanation might be that, when negative demographic trends became visible in the late 1870s, the medical discourse was fixated on the "Jewish question" and used general demographic indices such as natality, nuptiality, and mortality. These were the only indices produced at this stage by the science of statistics. Research on causes of death belonged to a new statistical era, which only started in Romania at the time of the War of Independence, gaining momentum in the last decade of the nineteenth century and especially after 1900. But why would an interest in infant mortality become manifest at the end of the century, at precisely the moment when doctor Felix attempted to allay fears by denying that the race was degenerating, and when, in absolute values, natural growth in the Kingdom was ascending? A possible explanation might be that infant mortality was perceived as the last obstacle to demographic growth in Romania. But, most certainly, it was also the result of the enduring social anxieties about degeneration, which now found another focus. As natural growth rates turned positive and ceased to be a reason for obsessive concern, infant mortality emerged as the new threat against which the medical corps mobilized all its energies.

Let's return to the statistical records, which, after 1871, listed mortality by age group.[578] After this date, all the figures on infant mortality were there for anyone to see, and yet, no one sounded the alarm bells. But mortality data were simply the visible signs of the disease. To cure it, one needed to identify the causes and find a treatment. However, statistics was late in providing the causes of infant mortality. Initially, the cause of death in all age groups was recorded only in Bucharest. It was only after 1886 that the cause of death started being recorded statistically across the Kingdom, and even

---

578 Alesandrini, *Statistica României, de la Unirea Principatelor până în prezent* I, 189–212.

then, the records used very broad categories such as "illness, incidents (accidents), suicide,"[579] which is hardly helpful for our purposes.

Progress was made after the start of the new century, as noted with fine irony by doctor Vasile Sion in a text that, in my view, is the most articulate analysis of state involvement in the provision of health services in Romania. Doctor Sion wonders, with false naivety, what a foreign doctor would do if faced with the high infant mortality of rural Romania:

> A civilized foreigner asking himself this question would look at how things are done in his own country and, aware that Romania possesses a health service run by the state, would search for an answer in the statistical publications of this service. But this would be a very naïve thing to do. Our health service would not be able to provide an answer, for the simple reason that it does not have one. Officialdom only knows of two types of death in rural Romania: violent death (suicide, murder, accident) and death from natural causes. In our country, the need to break down the *death from natural causes* category is still only partly felt. The cause of death is recorded only for epidemics and only starting with 1901, when records started being *published separately* for towns and villages.[580]

This means that, until World War I, the data on causes of mortality in rural Romania are patchy.

Doctors and statisticians vied with each other in criticizing the deficiencies of the statistical methodologies in the Kingdom. They all agreed that much was still to be done in this area. Before we move on to the causes of infant mortality as understood by doctors in the late nineteenth and early twentieth century, we must first spend some time on the more stable ground of general mortality rates and infant mortality rates in modern Romania.

We have only very approximate figures for general mortality in Romania, as expressed in the classic index of number of deaths per one thousand inhabitants. This is because we do not have a precise count for the total population until 1899, and therefore our calculations are based on estimates. In the circumstances, the most accurate index is natural growth, obtained by

---

579 Ibid., 238.
580 Sion, "Asistența medicală în România rurală," 209.

subtracting the number of deaths from the number of births. It was perhaps for this cause that natural increase was the star index deployed in the medical texts of the last three decades of the nineteenth century.

In 1895, when N. A. Alesandrini calculated mortality by age group starting with 1871, the calculation was made not per one thousand inhabitants, but per one thousand deaths.[581] This means that we can break down one thousand deaths by age group. Returning to general mortality, we must note that the indices used for its calculation varied across the period considered here. Again, Alesandrini calculated general mortality between 1859 and 1890 using an index that became obsolete after 1890: the number of living inhabitants for every deceased individual. Using this index, in 1859 we have one death per 59.19 living inhabitants, and in 1890, one death per 34.98 living individuals.

After 1890, the practice of calculating mortality per one thousand inhabitants became generalized. Looking at general mortality between 1859 and 1890, the 1860s stand out. In this decade, there was a constant rise in general mortality, but it remained under the threshold of 30 per thousand, except in 1866, when mortality peaked, at 39.49 per thousand. Over the next decade, from 1870 to 1880, mortality remained high, almost constantly over 30 per thousand, before it stabilized downwardly in the 1880–1890 interval.[582] And, finally, in the last decade of the nineteenth century, general mortality did not differ significantly from that of the previous decade, except for the end of the interval: in 1898 it stood at 26.38 per thousand, and in 1899 at 27.91 per thousand.

General mortality stood at 24.72 in 1900, making it an exceptional year. The trend remained unchanged in the following years.[583] It was firmly established that, in the first decade of the twentieth century, general mortality stabilized around 25 per thousand.[584] The sharp decline in general mortality in the early twentieth century was good news and added to the positive appraisals of that period. And yet, it was precisely at that moment that infant mortality emerged as a new source of concern among the medical profession. This concern is best illustrated by the choice of infant mortality as the theme of the 1902 congress of the National Medical Association [in Ro-

---

581 Alesandrini, *Statistica României*, I, 184.
582 Ibid., 146.
583 Obregia, *Raport general asupra igienei publice și asupra serviciului sanitar*, 12.
584 Colesco, "Le mouvement de la population de la Roumanie en 1911," 647.

manian: *Asociația Generală a Medicilor din Țară*]. The congress papers, later published in the association's official bulletin, are remarkably rich in statistical sources. It seemed as though infant mortality was merely a matter of statistics. But let's remember that in the first decade of the twentieth century, all the major themes in the medical literature, from the hygiene of the home to a healthy nutrition, were buttressed by impressive displays of numerical data. At this stage, capturing social reality in all its variety meant measuring and quantifying it, more so than in the last three decades of the previous century. Statistics became the keystone of all administrative disciplines, and implicitly of medical science.

But what were the rates of infant mortality at the end of the nineteenth century? Doctors say that they were far too high, compared to similar indices in Western Europe. It was a well-known fact that in areas of high natality, mortality rates were not far behind. In the period from 1871 to 1895, between 40 and 49 per cent of the annual numbers of deaths were of children under five.[585] If children up to ten years of age are added to the calculation, then the mortality index rises above 50 per cent. In other words, in the last decades of the nineteenth century, one in two children died before their tenth year. The death of children was a daily reality for all families, from the humblest peasants to the royal family, even though it was not necessarily experienced with the same intensity everywhere. The hecatomb of Romania's children ended up capturing the attention of the medical profession at the turn of the century. However, it was not necessarily treated as a problem *per se*, but as a serious sub-chapter within general mortality, which in its turn was a symptom of racial degeneration among the indigenous population. The discussant of the theme at the 1902 congress, N. C. Thomescu, senior doctor at the hospital for children in Bucharest, placed infant mortality side by side with the other major "causes which decimate our race and send it into degeneration": alcoholism, impaludism, pellagra, and tuberculosis.[586] It was also doctor Thomescu who made a reference to the symbolic representation of children in the period's national ideology: for the state, children became "that part of the population on which depends the future of our beloved homeland; today they give their laborers' arms, tomorrow their

585 Sion, "Asistența medicală în România rurală," 201.
586 Thomescu, "Asupra cauzelor mortalității în prima copilărie în țară și mijloacele de a le combate," no 18, 4.

strong chests to defend her, and always their bright minds to make her famous and guide her on the road to progress and civilization, which are ideals which we all share."[587] In this variant of the image—the most widely circulated at the time—children represented the future social body, the homeland *in nuce*. Their role was to perpetuate the nation: the individual child ensured the perpetuation of the family, and in the same way, children as a social group ensured the perpetuation of the social body of the homeland. In this logic, the high mortality of the children of today means the destruction of the homeland of tomorrow: degeneration in action.

In the same period, doctor Sion conceptualized the relations of child and state from a different perspective. He regarded infant mortality as

[...] a depletion of national energy, a hole through which the shared national wealth is leaked. Once born, a child must be safeguarded as an asset to which is added every day a small part of social capital. Destined to remain untapped for many years, this social capital will in the future yield interest and thus benefit society. Therefore, every child who dies before he can contribute to the community represents a loss of the common wealth. This is especially true of infant mortality from causes that are by no means inevitable: this type of mortality gives the best measure of the waste of life and energy, of the carelessness of an improvident society.[588]

This is obviously an economic interpretation, which offers a new angle on a social problem that remains essentially the same. Whether a child is regarded as an agent of the nation's social and biological reproduction, or as the yet untapped part of the country's social capital, his or her death contributes to the weakening and decay of the nation. No matter which angle it is looked at, death is a loss, a diminution and, implicitly, a threat to the social body of today and of tomorrow.

I shall now turn to the causes of racial degeneration as they were perceived and contextualized at the end of the nineteenth and the early twentieth century. Because racial degeneration manifested itself primarily in demographic rates of stagnation or decline, studying its causes means studying

587  Ibid.
588  Sion, "Asistența medicală în România rurală," 200.

the causes of morbidity and general mortality in the population. As we have seen in earlier chapters, the period's hygienist discourse addressed all these sources of degeneration comprehensively. I shall not, therefore, return to them. Instead I shall focus on the causes of infant mortality as causes of racial degeneration. By the early twentieth century, it had become obvious that the huge rates of infant mortality in Romania were due less to infectious disorders than to "avoidable" diseases, as doctor Sion called them. Smallpox appears to have been completely eradicated by the turn of the century: in each of the years 1900, 1901, and 1903, there was only one death caused by smallpox in the entire Kingdom.[589] Not all epidemic diseases can be prevented by vaccination, but epidemic-induced mortality was fairly low in rural Romania: in the 1901–1903 interval, only 5.1 out of 100 deaths were caused by an epidemic disorder. Despite the weaknesses of statistical methods, doctor Sion calculated an epidemic-induced mortality of 9 units in 100 at most for the 0–5 years age group.[590] This means that the remaining 91 children died from other causes. These were the "avoidable" deaths, and the numbers were significantly high. It was against these deaths that the health system had to mobilize all its forces—and it did.

If analyzed with the tools of medical statistics, the causes of infant mortality would have offered, if not certitudes, at least some fact-based information. But infant mortality was conceptualized by the entire medical profession in these vague terms: infants generally died from "poor care." The general practitioner and the hygienist both knew that infant mortality in Romania had four major causes:

Infection during birth, which often kills both the child and the mother in the early days—because of poor or lack of medical assistance to the parturient woman; 2. Disorders of the digestive system—caused by deficient nutrition—which kill especially in the first two years, but also during the next three; 3. Diseases of the respiratory system, the so-called common colds; 4. Death in the early days or weeks caused by under-development of the fetus in the womb.[591]

589 Obregia, *Raport general asupra igienei publice și asupra serviciului sanitar*, 103.
590 Sion, "Asistența medicală în România rurală," 209.
591 Ibid., 239.

Out of 100 deaths, 91 were caused by these essentially social, and hard to eradicate causes. Let's analyze them together with the doctors, who discussed these causes in their academic publications and congress papers. Neculai Lapteş, a doctor from Covurlui County, was fully aware that children of peasant families had hard lives as soon as they were born:

> [T]he infant sees the light of day in adverse circumstances, born on a pile of straw or on a rug, or at best, on a bed covered with dirty linen, because using a clean sheet would make it dirty; the navel cord is cut with filthy scissors or a rusty old knife, then tied with some soiled rug, with unwashed pieces of fabric or even with household implements.[592]

Often, following such "ministrations," the newborn died of tetanus. What doctor Lapteş did not know—and would not have condoned had he known—was that giving birth on a bed of straw had biblical connotations. Peasant practices were not simply expressions of ignorance and poverty, but often had their own logic, which did not conform to the rational, modern values of doctor Lapteş's world. But why would doctor Lapteş empathize with the peasants, why would he try to understand their customs and practices, when, obviously, these helped maintain a high mortality rate? Doctor Lapteş had a good knowledge of peasant child-care practices and offers detailed descriptions of bathing and swaddling, only to condemn them:

> [T]hey bathe the infant in scalding water, from which he emerges as red as a crab, because they say he sleeps better after the hot bath, so the old village woman pulls him out by the head, with his little body dangling, so his "neck will be longer," she says. She swaddles him in dirty linen and ties him with a girdle, or even with pieces of string, binding him so tightly that it leaves marks on his tender little body.[593]

Also at risk for an early death were the infants listed in medical statistics as having a "weak constitution." The underlying cause of a weak constitution was a genetic propensity to illness, perceived as the main cause of

---

592 Lapteş "Mortalitatea copiilor la săteni," 436.
593 Ibid., 436–37.

racial degeneration. Doctor I. Apostoleanu defined this category of causes with precision: whatever the doctor could not identify was subsumed to the broader category of congenital debility. This became the umbrella term for all the unknowns in the period's medical sciences:

Congenital debility [...] comes from debility in the parents' constitution. This in turn comes from alcoholism, paludism, pellagra, syphilis, tuberculosis, poor living conditions, and a deficient nutrition. All these maladies and ailings in parents manifest themselves as a general weakness and low vital resistance to damaging influences in children. This debility makes them prone to death from even the least harmful causes. [...] You may look at infants who die at the age of a week or even a month and, try as you may, you cannot identify a single sign of a particular malady. Then you see their crumpled, emaciated bodies, you look at the parents, and they are sallow and wizened, and living in the worst possible conditions. What better and more accurate diagnosis can a doctor reach but *congenital debility*?[594]

Once hereditary morbidity was deployed as an explanatory tool and the categories and terms used in the analysis became vague, racial degeneration was bound to rear its ugly head.

If they survived the perils of labor and the early weeks of life, the infants of peasant families were assailed by new dangers, the most lethal of which seemed to have been disorders of the digestive system. These were due almost exclusively to the inadequate ways in which mothers fed their newborns. Here, too, the dangers were manifold and could be caused by breastfeeding practices as well as from the early introduction of mixed feeding. In 1900, Iacob Melcon Iacobovici, a grantee of the "Carol I" Royal Foundation, received the Hillel Award for his study on the causes of infant mortality in Romania. In this study, he offers us a handy summary of all these threats:

[I]n our country, there are no rules on breastfeeding: when the infant cries, his mother will suckle him. At other times, a busy mother will have the infant feed when she finds the time, every two hours, or three, or four, whenever she can. This happens not just among uncultured mothers, but also among edu-

---

594 Apostoleanu, "Mortalitatea copiilor în România," 3.

cated women who have not had the opportunity to learn about hygiene or see it practiced. [...] This explains the huge mortality rates among infants of primiparous mothers. Romanian mothers believe that maternal milk is not sufficiently nutritious and feed their infants anything they have in the home. For example, during fasting, they give them broths made of beans, peas, potatoes, or prune compote, sauerkraut, corn porridge, pretzels, everything. During the rest of the year, an infant will share any food that his parents eat, without distinction. The mother or father holds the baby, if he is young they will chew the food before feeding it to him, if he is past eight months he will partake of any food he finds. And those poor mothers, how happy they are when told that their offspring eats "like a grown-up." Who can persuade them that what they do is a crime and that a huge number of children fall victim to these primitive habits?[595]

Once doctors introduced the theme of infants' nutrition in the hygienist discourse, references started being made to irresponsible parents who subjected their children to fasting from an early age. Doctor Lapteş relates the subterfuge he used to convince a peasant woman to feed goat's milk to her baby during the fast ahead of Saint Mary's feast:

[O]nce an infant has been weaned, he becomes *human*, and there are no prohibitions as to the kinds of food which he is allowed to eat. At the same time, all the rules strictly prescribed by the church apply to the child too. Children observe all fasting periods from the age of two, and even when ill. Doctors find it hard to convince the mothers that a child who is sick should be given milk. As I was working to combat an epidemic of dysentery, during the fast of Saint Mary, a mother was lamenting very noisily the fact that, for the last 4–5 days, she had had to let the milk from her only goat to go bad, while she fed roast peppers to her boy, who was two. I had a hard time citing numberless sayings of popular wisdom and quotations from the Holy Scripture to convince her that she should give the milk to that poor exhausted child.[596]

Nobody knows what happened to that child once the doctor was gone.

---

595 Iacobovici, "Cauzele mortalității primei copilării în România și mijloacele de a le combate,"44.
596 Lapteş, "Mortalitatea copiilor la săteni," 437.

When they tackled the subject of infant nutrition in the peasant environment, doctors endlessly reiterated a few habits that contributed to the high
mortality in these age groups. One was the use of the so-called *moțoc*, the rural equivalent of the modern dummy:

> All these guardians, if they cannot soothe the infant by rocking and sway-
> ing, will put a teether [*moțoc*] in his mouth. In general, this teether is made of
> a rag with a knot in the corner, which contains a small piece of bread dipped
> in sugary water. But this teether is also used to help children develop strong
> gums and start teething sooner. Many of these dummies are sites of culture
> for the bacilli of Löfler,[597] Frankel, Koch, and others.[598]

Lastly, another common theme running through the medical discourse
could be termed, using a misnomer, children's alcoholism. For doctors, this
was the supreme horror story. In all social classes, from the elites to the peasant classes, adults made a habit out of adding alcoholic drinks to the nutrition of infants, as Iacobovici testifies:

> As for beverages, there is no restriction, among the wealthy, or among the
> poor classes. In affluent families, children drink various imported alcoholic
> or alcoholised beverages, syrups, teas, coffee—black or white— among oth-
> ers. Among the middle classes, children as young as one month are given large
> amounts of coffee, teas, and so on. The peasant woman, who cannot afford
> syrups and coffee, gives to her child what she has available, spirits and wine.[599]

The doctors did not approve, and medical disapproval of such practices
has not changed with time. At the time, infants were given alcoholic drinks
as fortifiers or sedatives. But, as doctor Possa believed, the consumption of
alcohol became habitual among children of two and above in Moldavia's rural areas:

> From the age of 2 or 3, all children are given raki, especially on festival days,
> and parents look on in amusement as their drunken, unsteady children hit

---

597 Löfler [sic] in the original of Iacobovici's text. Friedrich Löffler (1852–1915) was a German bacteriologist.
598 Iacobovici, "Cauzele mortalității primei copilării în România și mijloacele de a le combate," 50.
599 Ibid., 49–50.

their heads against the walls. When a boy of 4 or 5 years of age downs a shot of raki, the proud parents rejoice that their lad drinks just like an adult man.[600]

If they survived infection at birth and digestive troubles as infants, children could still die of respiratory diseases: the foul air in rural homes and winter christenings performed in unheated churches increased the likelihood of such an outcome. And lastly, even though infectious diseases were not the killer diseases they had once been, they still proliferated in villages; at least they did so in doctor Possa's Moldavia:

[F]inally, there are infectious diseases and all sorts of disorders which find easy targets in flocks of beings who seem ready to die; epidemics rage on such fertile terrains, microbes mature splendidly, and the result is a cruel harvest. Entire villages are left without a single child: it happened in the mountains of Suceava County in 1893–1894 after a diphtheria epidemic, and it still happens today with scarlet fever and other diseases.[601]

Bad habits form a relentless concatenation: the peasant woman who cannot feed her child or protect him or her from the cold will only rarely, and sometimes only *in extremis*, appeal for medical help when the child falls ill:

[W]hen a child becomes ill, she [the mother] will use all the remedies that she knows of, will seek advice from all the old women in the village, and only as a last resort will she run to see the doctor. These habits are disappearing in the villages close to the residence of the doctor, where medication is also available, as shown in the growing number of Sunday consultations, which the doctors offer in their own homes.[602]

We are faced here with an extremely tenacious stereotype of the medical discourse, which few dared to challenge. As my readings on the rural health system accumulated, I have formed the overall impression that what we have here is a representation that says more about the way in which doctors saw the peasant world (primitivism, lack of education, poverty) than

---

600 Possa, "Mortalitatea copiilor," 7.
601 Ibid.
602 Lapteş, "Mortalitatea copiilor la săteni," 438.

about an actual and consistent *rejection* of modern health assistance by peasants. Finally, I had a revelation in the form of an intuition of what doctor Sion himself had found in 1904:

> If we are honest, we will have to admit that [...] the peasant *does not* receive assistance either in illness, or at birth. Those who believe that the peasant is so dull-witted as to reject the doctor's superior knowledge, or that the peasant woman "does not trust" those who could enlighten her, are wrong. The truth is that those who could enlighten her are not there in her hour of need—it is as simple as that.[603]

I must admit that I was delighted to find a doctor who challenged the dominant image of the peasant as a primitive, almost an animal, who refused the medical assistance so generously offered to him or her by the modern state, who fled the hospitals and opposed vaccination so fiercely. The truth was, in fact, that health assistance was almost non-existent in rural areas. And I must agree with doctor Sion when he says that the state had the

> [...] mistaken belief [...] that the rural population has such an inferior, such an animal-like understanding of the need for health, that the state feels it is entitled to treat the peasants' health as it treats the health of livestock. This view is akin to all the numberless misconceptions that we—the superior classes—have formed of the rural population because of our ignorance and of the distance we are keeping from this population.[604]

I would not be able to put it better. Once I found out about doctor Sion's views, I realized what an exceptional character he was.

I cannot conclude this section without a reference to one of the most important aspects of the theme of racial degeneration and its accompanying anxieties: the issue of heredity. For what else is racial degeneration but a gradual accumulation of degenerative traits in a population? The "hygienic ills" of the rural population, which I have discussed at length, were just as much preconditions of social maladies that, transmitted hereditarily, led to

---

603 Sion, "Asistența medicală în România rurală," 246.
604 Ibid., 247–48.

the progressive decline of future generations. From this perspective, it is important to find out which maladies or features were believed to be transmissible hereditarily in the late nineteenth century. In 1876, doctor Petrini compiled a comprehensive list:

> Mental illness is one of the disorders that can be transmitted via heredity. [...] Tuberculosis, scrofula, cancer, gout, syphilis, arthritis, and eczema can often be passed on to posterity. Of skin conditions, psoriasis is one of the most transmissible. [...] The transmission of talent in art, in music, is well known; but a predisposition to *theft*, *rape*, *murder*, and *suicide*, is also hereditary.[605]

These observations show that, either directly or in diluted form as predispositions, heredity was regarded as omnipotent. In the period's theories, diseases, moral traits, and talent were all heritable. Here, we are witnessing the emergence of eugenics in Romania. For, if the race was clearly seen to be degenerating, doctors knew that it could also be re-generated through a judicious choice of marital partner. A good marriage meant that degenerative traits in one or both spouses could be kept under control and diminish in the next generation.

The young doctor V. Manicea presented an outline of such a "rational" marriage:

> [F]or a rational marriage, one would have to select spouses devoid of physical or moral defects; but, as they say, perfection is not of this world; therefore, the imperfections in both spouses must be combined in such a way that, instead of increasing in the next generation, it may be at least neutralized through a mutually beneficial match. From a physiological point of view, marriage must be a good match of opposites through a neutralization of defects in both spouses.[606]

Only one step separated this view on marriage from proposing a programme of negative eugenics, a step doctor Manicea took in 1880, when

---

605 Petrini de Galatz, *Despre ameliorațiunea rasei umane*, 11–12.
606 Manicea, *Considerațiuni asupra mortalității generale în România*, 59–60.

he suggested a ban on marriages between "persons suffering from scrofula, cancer, or tuberculosis," because such marriages "lead to the degeneration of the human genus."[607] The degeneration was already noticeable to the period's doctors. But it was not only morbid heredity, which contributed to the conception of non-viable progeny with a low resistance to "morbigenous" conditions, to use the period's terminology. Morbid heredity also happened because the rural population lived in dire conditions. Doctor Dănescu highlighted hard work and poor nutrition:

> Parents exhausted through continuous labor of almost titanic proportions, and deprived of the appropriate nutrition, will unfailingly produce offspring who, from the moment of conception, carry the germ of future morbigenous causes. The nutrition of this offspring in childhood consists of the milk of a mother who is herself drained of strength by physiological hardships and at puberty of a less than frugal diet; and then, even before they reach adolescence, children are sent to communal work to sustain the existence of the family.[608]

Ultimately, all medical professionals agreed with doctor N. C. Thomescu's assessment:

> [A] child is as fit as its heredity: vigorous, healthy children can only be born to healthy parents. The foremost causes in determining infant mortality are maladies inherited from the parents.[609]

It is, after all, a sensible axiom. A few years earlier, doctor Manolescu had claimed, and, I believe, the entire medical profession agreed with him, that "in very large numbers, peasants are perpetually ill,"[610] which was a clear sign of degeneration. I would argue that heredity, which had a central role in theoretical conceptualizations of degeneration, had secondary importance in the Romanian medical discourse. It did permeate that discourse in a dif-

---

607 Ibid., 60.

608 Dănescu, *Încercări de demografie şi geografie medicală*, II.

609 Thomescu, "Asupra cauzelor mortalității în prima copilărie în țară şi mijloacele de a le combate," no. 29, 2.

610 Manolescu, "Neputința organisațiunei actuale sanitare în apărarea populațiunei rurale contra boalelor," 100.

fuse way, but it never overshadowed the demographic component, which, in Romania, as well as in France at the time, was co-substantial to the theme of degeneration.

Having reviewed the main manifestations of racial degeneration, as well as the complex set of its supposed causes, we should now try to identify the sources of the social anxiety it generated. Racial degeneration was not a creation of the Romanian scientific community, but rather a medical theme doctors brought with them from abroad or had read about in the scientific literature. It was eventually adapted to the local context, but essentially, it was an import. However, its rapid rise and the degree of its ideological fit with the *zeitgeist* suggest that it responded to an imperious local need. Once the adaptation was complete, racial degeneration turned into an indigenous construct.

In the mid-nineteenth century, the Romanian professional elites were educated predominantly in France, and, after 1870, in Germany. Romanian doctors discovered the theory of degeneration in French intellectual circles. Anyone familiar with the medical literature of nineteenth-century Romania knows that the sources it cited largely came from the French scientific culture. There were, obviously, exceptions, some of them quite remarkable: Victor Babeş and Iacob Felix stand out. If, out of curiosity, one browses the collection of doctors' biographies published by N. T. Ionescu in the early twentieth century, one can easily notice that of the 131 doctors active in 1905, twelve had obtained doctorates in medicine in Paris and two in Montpellier.[611] At that time, Paris was one of the most sought-after academic centers for those intending to pursue medical studies. In addition, it is well known that significant sections of Romania's intellectual elites were French-speaking and Francophile. I. G. Bibicescu was no exception: in 1874, when he probed the hypothesis of the degeneration of the Romanian race, he used the French edition of doctor Eduard Reich's *Sur la dégénérescence de l'homme, ses causes et sa prophylaxie*.[612] A lecture on population trends, which he gave at *Concordia Română* in 1880, was inspired, he explained, by the fact that, only a few days earlier, he "had come across the population question in some French scientific writings."[613] In the same year, doctor Fe-

---

611 Ionescu, *Medicii noştri*.
612 Bibicescu, "Mişcarea poporaţiunii Capitalei în 1873," 1128.
613 Bibicescu, *Mişcarea poporaţiunii în România de la 1870 până la 1878*, 8.

lix, who was very familiar with the "French scientific press,"[614] cited the same population "question." If we take doctor Istrati as our last example, and his study of 1880,[615] which, in our view, launched the debate on degeneration in Romania, we will notice that his entire argument and his comparative data come from the French scientific literature. However, it is noteworthy that the author's fervid nationalism compels him to dismiss everything that is not indigenous, even if it is French. We are, therefore, persuaded that the Romanian medical discourse on demography was influenced by the theme of depopulation in France. Depopulation in Romania was consistently compared to depopulation in France, although some pointed out that the Romanian Old Kingdom did not have a population of the same "quality" as France. In his characteristic style, doctor Istrati expressed his view that

> [...] in our own special way, we are unique! We do not produce children, we do not accumulate capital, we do not possess wealth! But we do kill ourselves, so that [...] others may grow [...] on our grave.[616]

This brings us back to the "Jewish question" and the year 1880. This might be a good moment to start wondering why 1880 became the year when the theme of racial degeneration made such a spectacular entrance on the stage of the Romanian medical literature. As we have seen, although the theme had been lurking backstage since the early 1870s, it did not make much progress until the end of that decade. And suddenly, we have 1880. The explanation is not difficult to intuit. I think I am right in associating the theme of racial degeneration in Romania with the "Jewish question," which was being so assiduously debated in the public arena in the years 1878 and 1879. The Congress of Berlin had demanded a change in article 7 of the Romanian Constitution of 1866 with respect to the emancipation of the Jewish population. The debate around this article became the most important political debate of the day.[617] The "Jewish question" was suddenly everywhere, in the political press and parliamentary debates. The scientific periodical press could not remain on the margins. The medical profession re-

---

614  Felix, "Despre mișcarea populației," 55.
615  *O pagină din istoria contimpurană a României din punctul de videre medical, economic și national*, Typografia Alesandru A. Grecescu, Bucharest.
616  Istrati, *O pagină din istoria contimpurană a României*, 79.
617  Iancu, *Evreii*, 160–90.

sponded to this political and intellectual ambience by conceptualizing the theme of racial degeneration and making it the focus of the medical discourse. I am persuaded that, without the parliamentary debates around article 7, the theme of racial degeneration would not have acquired the importance it did. On the other hand, it is worth remembering that, even though the "Jewish question" served as a catalyst to discussions on demography and degeneration, the sources of these anxieties had been present in the medical discourse long before 1878 and would remain there after 1880. However, once the indigenous elites solved the question so as to meet their own agenda, which was by not offering emancipation, the demographic component of the theme of degeneration entered a stationary phase. Nevertheless, degeneration acquired growing importance at the center of another medical theme: the hygienic hazards affecting the rural world.

In conclusion, the theme of racial degeneration in the late nineteenth- and early twentieth-century Romania has two main components. The first is demographic, and could take many forms, depending on the social and political context of the day. For example, at the time when the "Jewish question" dominated public debate, demographic statistics were used to demonstrate the high natality of the Jews and high mortality of the Romanians. After 1880, when the "peasant question" outpaced the "Jewish question," mortality in general, and rural mortality in particular—especially when caused by maladies such as pellagra—became the focus of demographic statistics. In the early twentieth century, as we have seen, the modern theme of infant mortality suddenly entered the debate. Demographic anxieties came and went in quick succession, acquiring new forms as the socio-political context changed. Yet, they did not form neat series of discrete categories, but overlapping, entangled events brought to the fore of the public discourse by specific contextual shifts. The high natality of the Jewish community, the high mortality of Romanian city-dwellers, the high mortality of peasants living in hardship and deprivation, and infant mortality co-existed in the medical discourse from 1870 to 1914. What changed was the light cast on them as changing historical circumstances demanded.

The second component of the broad theme of degeneration is strictly linked to the "rural question," the term used to designate the living conditions of the peasant population. Whereas other sections of the intellectual elites associated the "rural question" with the issue of landed property, the medical profession focused on what they referred to as the hygiene of the peasants' "living conditions." This was a euphemistic phrase designating the dire living conditions of the rural population. The medical profession constantly attempted to draw the attention of the political classes to the national hazards of this situation. One of these was the danger of racial degeneration.

Georges Vigarello observed, with reference to France, that the emergence of anxieties of degeneration after 1850 ran in parallel with the massive and decisive intervention of the state in the management of public health. The "hygienist, regenerative state" was a compelling self-representation of the state in French society.[618] From this perspective, Romania is perhaps a special case, because state involvement in public health started early, as the theme of degeneration was just emerging. That early involvement was strictly prescriptive. However, once the theme was established, especially in the first decade of the twentieth century, the state made a few—admittedly modest—attempts at intervening in the sphere of urban public health. Public health in the rural world remained pure theory for quite a long time. Doctor Sion is our guide here, and we may ask—and answer—some important questions with him:

> After 30 years of—rather expensive—public health initiatives in the rural world, how many of the 3,000 rural villages have got steady supplies of drinking water? How many have been equipped with an active system of sanitation for waterways, ditches and sewerage, roads, courtyards, homes and refuse disposal, etc., etc.? How many have got even the most rudimentary machinery or installation for disinfection? None.[619]

However, even in France—Romania's cherished model—state action in the crucial domain of drinking water and sewerage installations in the rural world did not make significant progress until the first half of the twentieth century.[620]

Looking back—even if only for a quick glance—at the last two centuries of Romanian history, one finds that there was no period between 1859

---

618 Vigarello, *Histoire des pratiques de la santé. Le sain et le malsain depuis le Moyen Age*, 217.

619 Sion, "Asistența medicală în România rurală," 246.

620 Goubert, *Une histoire de l'hygiène. Eau et salubrité dans la France contemporaine*, 214–17.

and 2013 when demographic anxieties did not become manifest in one form or another. After World War I, Greater Romania was haunted by the specter of the non-assimilation of some minorities and of the decrease of Romanian population, for example in Banat. And let's not forget the qualitative dimensions of the Romanian eugenic theories and practices. The communist period became famous for its pro-natalist policies. After 1989, Romania experienced a dramatic demographic collapse through negative population growth and economic emigration. The results of the 2011 census showed a decrease of approximately 1.5 million persons compared to the earlier census of 2002. In an interview, Vasile Ghețău, the director of the Centre for Demographic Studies of the Romanian Academy, expressed his concern over demographic trends in the last twenty-four years in Romania. But— not unlike the late nineteenth century—the main reason for concern is the future, not the present, as Ghețău pointed out:

I have made calculations based on census data, starting from the assumption that the fertility rate of 1.3 children per one woman will remain constant. Here are the resulting population figures: 15 million in 2050; under 14 million in 2060; and 8 million in 2100. And they do not include emigration.[621]

Vasile Ghețău's latest book is entitled: *Drama noastră demografică. Populația României la recensământul din octombrie 2011* (Our demographic tragedy: Romania's population in the 2011 census). It is a title that speaks for itself.

---

621 Ovidiu Șimonca, "Copilul nu mai este o prioritate în cuplurile românești. Interviu cu Vasile Ghețău" [Having a child is no longer a priority for couples in Romania: An interview with Vasile Ghețău], https://www.observatorcultural.ro/articol/copilul-nu-mai-este-o-prioritate-in-cuplurile-romanesti-interviu-cu-vasile-ghetau-2/, 2 [last accessed: July 19, 2013].

# PART THREE

# MEDICAL CULTURE VS. PEASANT CULTURE

1

## THE POWER OF MEDICAL CULTURE:
## NEW LAWS FOR PEOPLE LOCKED IN THE PAST

*For the Sake of the People's Health: Laws, Regulations, Norms ...*

In early April 1893, Romania's Senate initiated debates on changes to the Health Act, a debate that had been engaging the minds of the medical profession and politicians for some time. The rapporteur, doctor N. Garoflid, presented an articulate rationale for the proposed changes and the role of the health service in a modern state:

> It is on a proper organization of the health service that all the other interests of the population rest, because health and life are the foremost human needs: hygienic and sanitation measures are required so that villages and towns, households and institutions where the tender new shoots of the population are nursed should not become foci of infection; local health services, the study and eradication of localized maladies and of epidemics, the prevention of epidemics, vaccination, health care for the poor in their own homes or in well-organized hospitals, medical assistance and help with difficult parturition (birth). Are these not the first and foremost duties of a government aware of its mission and intent on pursuing it? They are, without doubt.[1]

---

1  *Dezbaterile Senatului* [Debates in the Senate], April 7, 1893, Sesiunea ordinară prelungită [Extended ordinary session] 1892–1893, şedinţa de la 5 aprilie 1893 [Session of April 5, 1893], 656.

This excerpt summarizes the main roles of a modern health system, and they are reiterated in numerous documents, from the text of the Health Act itself to the inaugural circular sent to the medical corps by doctor Iacob Felix when he was appointed General Directorate of the Health Service in July 1892:

> From today, Doctor, we are going to work together, strive together for the improvement of public health, for the elimination of all threats against it, and for the reduction of mortality among the population; we shall offer comfort to the suffering poor who seek the assistance of the medical science and art, we shall present the benefits of medicine to all those who are still unacquainted with them; we shall manage together the physical education of the young and we shall be held responsible before the nation if, instead of a vigorous generation, capable of ensuring the country's moral and material progress, we shall allow a generation of weaklings to grow up, incapable of performing its patriotic duties.[2]

Both texts reflect a mix of traditional conceptions of medicine as charity with the new ideological imperatives of modern health care. But both point to the same ultimate aims of a modern health service: the safeguarding of "life" (doctor Garoflid) and ensuring a "reduction of mortality among the population" (doctor Felix). The underlying ideological challenge is populationist: the state's involvement in the management of a modern health system reflects an obsessive concern for the increase of the population. From this perspective, everything is quantified: the magic index of mortality, which is directly proportional to the index of morbidity, should, ideally, be placed in a position of inverse proportionality to the index of natality.[3]

The creation of a modern health system is inconceivable without a legislative and normative framework, which forms the topic of the present chapter. Even a rapid survey of the health legislation will reveal the massive scale of the modern state's efforts in setting up and managing the health services in the last three decades of the nineteenth century and in the early twentieth century. But what do these prescriptive texts tell us? They pres-

---

2    Felix, "Ordinul circular sub no. 10850 din 4 iulie," 193–94.

3    Naturally, the inverse proportionality should apply only to the pair lower mortality – higher natality, not the other way round.

ent an ideal situation, a this-is-how-things-should-be scenario. Alongside this *Belle Époque* representation of Romanian society as envisioned by health legislators, there is another, apparently very different, picture. This chapter aims to analyze the two images comparatively. I am not, in fact, interested in legislation as a social projection. I want to know what was done to put it into practice and what changed in society as a result. We thus enter the sensitive area of norms versus practice, which remains a minefield for legislators even today.

Let's first define our terms. When we speak of legislation, we mean primarily the Health Acts. Romanian Parliament voted on the first Health Act in 1872,[4] but it was only passed, published, and came into force in July 1874. This was the famous Health Act of 1874, later subjected to a series of changes in 1877, 1881, 1885, 1893, and 1898. Its last variant, in 1898, had very little in common with the text of 1874, but the principles of health care and hygiene it enunciated remained unchanged. New health legislation was debated in both chambers in 1910, and came into force at the end of that year. Apart from the Health Acts proper, there was additional legislation on health provision, which is also included in the broad category of public health legislation. My analysis has also drawn on related regulations, which comprise guidelines for the application of the law.[5] The details they offer are important for an understanding of social realities in the way that generic law texts are not. Ultimately, however, nothing can guarantee *a priori* that they were enforced more strictly than the laws they related to. Therefore, we may have to concede that the regulations may not take us closer to the hard facts than the ideal, "how-things-should-be" legislation. According to article 93 of the 1866 Constitution, regulations were the King's prerogative,[6] which means that they operated like royal edicts. Considering the issuing authority and the recipient, I have divided the regulations into two main catego-

---

4   *Dezbaterile Senatului*, April 7, 1893, 656.

5   Only rarely did the descriptor "health act" or "health legislation" appear in the titles. See, for example, *Regulament de aplicațiune al legii pentru înființarea de spitale rurale* [Regulations on the implementation of the law on rural hospitals], or *Regulament al legii asupra alienaților* [Regulations on the implementation of the mental health act]. The title of the regulations often referred to the specific aspect of the legislation they were supposed to be annexed to.

6   "He issues the necessary regulations for the execution of the laws, but does not have the authority to change or suspend legislation." Adapted from *Constituțiune și legea electorală* [The constitution and the electoral law] (Bucharest: Imprimeria Statului, 1867), 24.

ries, as used by doctor Felix[7]: general public health regulations, issued by the central health authorities and valid across the country, and local health regulations, issued by the local authorities and valid only in the territory of regional administrative units. The local regulations prove to be very informative. As an example, I shall enumerate regulations adopted in the town of Târgoviște up to 1891: *Regulament pentru construcțiuni și alinieri* (Regulations on building and street alignment) (1889); *Regulament pentru salubritatea construcțiunilor și locuințelor* (Regulations on the salubrity of buildings and dwellings) (1890); *Regulament pentru menținerea curățeniei în piețele și stradele orașului* (Regulations on cleaning services in city squares and streets) (1889); *Regulament pentru stârpirea porcilor de pe stradele orașului* (Regulations on the removal of swine from city streets) (1890); *Regulament pentru fabricarea și vânzarea de gaz, spirt, chibrituri și alte materii explozibile* (Regulations on the manufacturing and sale of gas, spirit, matches and other flammable substances) (1890); *Regulament pentru fabricarea de pâine și jimblă* (Regulations on the manufacturing of bread and bakery products) (1890); and *Regulament pentru privegherea prostituțiunii* (Regulations on the control of prostitution) (1890).[8] With his characteristic sense of humor, doctor Felix noted that the town of Târgoviște never lacked in regulations, "only in their application and execution."[9]

The Health Acts, the additional legislation on health provision, and the general and local public health regulations all added up to the legislative scaffolding of Romania's modern health service, which I shall call here, cumulatively, "health legislation." I shall not dwell on the emergence and development of health legislation in the United Principalities and the Kingdom of Romania. However, we need to establish a few preliminary facts. As already mentioned, the earliest modern Health Act was voted in 1874 and remained in force until 1910. It was based on modern principles: the health services were state-run, and they were placed under the authority of a directorate within the Ministry for Home Affairs. Preventative medicine was not neglected: the law had a specific chapter on public health, with entries on industrial hygiene, the hygiene of "public establishments" and of dwellings

---

7   Felix, *Raport general asupra igienei publice și asupra serviciului sanitar al Regatului României pe anii 1896 și 1897*, 59.
8   Felix, "Raportul domnului doctor ~, membru consiliului sanitar superior," 87.
9   Ibid.

and food, measures against epidemics, etc. The provision of health care was placed under the authority of general, local, and special "health authorities" (the Ministry for Home Affairs, the prefects and permanent district committees, under-prefects, and communal mayors). These worked together with general, local, and special "public health bodies" (such as the Higher Medical Council, the county chief doctor and public health council, the district chief doctor and veterinary officer, as well as the doctors and veterinary medics servicing the villages). In sum, the health services relied on cooperation between the central and local health authorities. By law, a rural health service was also created, with the district practitioner (in Romanian: *medic de plasă*)[10] at its center. A new institution, the rural hospital, was added in 1881. The health system created by the Health Act of 1874 was a hierarchical structure, with the village, district, and county at its base. The hub of the system was the Higher Medical Council, which had a consultative role.

The Health Act of 1874 stipulated the future addition of no less than 17 regulations. Some were only completed and added more than ten years later, for instance the *Regulations on the Alignment of Village Streets and the Construction of Peasant Dwellings*, published in 1888. Some were published even later: the *Regulations on the Sanitary Control of the Manufacturing of and Trade in Food and Beverages* (articles 154, 155, 156, and 157 of the Health Act), signposted in article 123 of the 1874 law, was only published in 1895.[11] There are also examples of regulations which had not been anticipated in the text of the law: for example, the Higher Medical Council issued a *Regulament pentru vaccinație și revaccinație* (Regulations on vaccinations and booster vaccinations) only one year after the publication of the Health Act. Such examples show that the elaboration of statutory regulations was a lengthy and complex process. The next Health Act, in 1910, anticipated the publication of 35 additional regulations.

A cursory survey of the health legislation may leave the impression that, at the end of the nineteenth century, Romania had a modern, fully functioning health and sanitary system. However, that impression is misleading: Romania was still far from achieving what we have called modernization in the

---

10  This role, created at the initiative of doctor Carol Davila, was older: the first district practitioners were appointed in 1862.
11  In the title, the article numbers refer to the Health Act of 1893.

areas of health and hygiene.[12] In the early twentieth century, doctors were in agreement that the legislation in force was "excellent,"[13] and would be "perfect, with minor additions,"[14] if only it could be enforced both in spirit and in letter.

### ... And the Impossibility of Enforcing Them

Let's now assess the extent to which Romania's modern health legislation was put into practice. Was it observable on the ground? Were there visible outcomes in the management of public health, or, as a nineteenth-century doctor would put it, in the peasant's home? For answers, we shall have to look at a specific category of documents in which doctors evaluated the operation of the health system, namely, the public health reports, in which doctors evaluated the practical application of the health legislation. Let's start with the doctors' general view, which proves to be highly negative. Doctor Felix, for example, believed that there were improvements in health and sanitation, but that they were minor and "a direct consequence of natural advancements in civilization among the population rather than of the management of our health system."[15] This is another way of suggesting that the state could dispense with a health system, which, in practice, did not bring any benefits to the citizen. Was doctor Felix's appraisal exceptional? It seems that his views are corroborated by his peers in the highest medical body, who, having surveyed the reality "on the ground," came to similar conclusions. Doctor Fotino, for example, wrote that the health service in 1886 was pure "fiction."[16] The examples could continue, and the resulting picture is catastrophic. We shall construct our own catastrophic picture here, starting from a few specific chapters in the Health Act and the relevant additional regulations.

One such chapter was school hygiene, where, doctors agreed, much was left to be done. The hygiene in both rural and urban schools was a disaster. Doctor Felix provides a sharp analysis:

---

12  See Bărbulescu and Popovici, *Modernizarea lumii rurale*, 7–104.
13  Felix, *Raport general asupra igienei publice și asupra serviciului sanitar al Regatului României pe anii 1896 și 1897*, 61.
14  Rigani, "Mersul serviciului sanitar al județului Mușcel în 1905," 80.
15  Felix, "Raportul domnului doctor ~, membru consiliului sanitar superior," 18.
16  Fotino, "Raportul d-lui dr. Fotino... în anul 1886," 1137.

School hygiene exists only in the text of article XX of the Health Act, which was never put into practice. Many schools function in insalubrious buildings, which become media for the transmission of infectious diseases and the spread of epidemics. This is aggravated by the fact that tutors and teachers are not given guidelines on how to deal with contagious diseases once they arise in a village. Errors are made, and basic notions of sanitation are overlooked. Not for reasons of economy or ignorance, but because of sheer negligence. Let me give an example: I found that in many rural and urban schools, desks are arranged in the wrong way, so that the source of light comes from the right-hand side of the pupil, or from the back, rather than from the left.[17]

There were exceptions. In larger towns, such as Brăila, doctor Fotino found that "the private school for girls known as the 'Romaşcanu' school," had premises that could not be faulted "from a hygienic point of view."[18] But appraisals remained generally negative. Doctor Nicolae Măldărescu visited schools in the counties Gorj, Dolj, Mehedinţi, and Vâlcea, and wrote:

From my own observations in all the villages I visited, I can say that school premises are in a state of revolting neglect and squalor. The walls are never whitewashed, and spiders are free to build their cobwebs above the heads of pupils and teachers; the dirty floors are covered in layers of grime a few centimeters thick; the windows are broken, and very often with missing glass panes; very few of these buildings have stoves, and when they have them, they do not work; the furniture is defective.[19]

Such comments on hygiene in schools were ubiquitous.

Let's now look at the area of industrial hygiene, which was allocated an important space in the health legislation, in addition to a general statute created specifically for this subject in 1875. Statutory norms divided industrial establishments into three main classes, according to the degree of pollution they caused, to use recent terminology. The aim was to move high-polluting industries outside of the cities. The main conclusion was that the hygiene of

---

17  Felix, "Raportul domnului doctor ~, membru consiliului sanitar superior," 20.
18  Fotino, "Raportul d-lui dr. Fotino… în anul 1891," 341.
19  Măldărescu, "Raportul d-lui doctor N. Măldărescu," 168.

insalubrious industries was being neglected.[20] Following an inspection in one of the country's largest towns, Ploieşti, doctor Felix concluded:

> In defiance of the prescriptions in the Regulations on insalubrious indus-
> tries, around 20 tanneries have been installed in the city center, with autho-
> rization from the Town Hall; some of these have extensive installations, and
> employ up to 30 workers. It is too late today to ask for these industrial estab-
> lishments to move their premises outside the town, but at least they should
> be requested to observe a few rules of salubrity, which, without harming
> their economic interests, would protect the adjoining suburbs from volatile
> emanations and harmful slop from the tannery works.[21]

At Brăila, doctor Fotino found candle-making and soap-making workshops, as well as butchers' shops, installed on *Strada Regală* (King street),
right in the center of town.[22] Doctors encountered the same problems everywhere. In Vâlcea County, in 1891, one doctor found that

> The Regulations on insalubrious industries are not applied in any of the vil-
> lages. Sludge from the making of hemp forms puddles in the middle of vil-
> lages. There are brandy stills in the inhabitants' courtyards, and plum dregs
> are left there for pigs to feed on. Brick-making kilns and lime kilns are also
> located randomly.[23]

But how were the legal provisions applied in the important domain of the
prevention of infectious diseases? The key norms here made it mandatory to
declare cases as they occurred and to isolate patients. But here, too, it was easier
said than done: these rules were almost impossible to enforce in rural regions.
In 1898, a simple epidemic of scarlet fever caused nightmares for doctor Mihail Cruceanu, who had been allocated the task of eradicating it, as he narrates:

> For almost six months, all we could do was record undeclared older cases.
> Most were discovered when the patients were already cachectic and suffer-

20  Felix, "Raportul domnului doctor ~, membru consiliului sanitar superior," 21.
21  Fotino, "Raportul d-lui dr. Fotino... în anul 1891," 117.
22  Ibid., 338.
23  Măldărescu, "Raportul d-lui doctor N. Măldărescu," 220.

ing from various and serious complications of this infectious disease. Many were found when they were already in agony and some only after death. Even when cases were discovered on time, there was little that could be done, except adding them to the statistics, for the peasants did not heed medical advice and the spread of the epidemic could not be stopped through the usual methods.[24]

The epidemic could not be controlled because uncooperative peasants did not observe the usual medical prescriptions for such situations. In despair, doctor Cruceanu appealed to the military.[25] He tells us what happened next:

Although a small military unit was placed at our disposal recently, the isolation of infected houses still leaves a lot to be desired. Now, as before, when the houses were guarded by villagers, the residents still found the means to communicate with the infected houses, either directly, or by jumping over fences or running out at the back, where they could not be observed, and sometimes they ran over long distances to reach the infected houses. Thus, we found the woman of one Gh. Tichigiu, in whose house two children had succumbed to scarlet fever complicated with diphtheria, and two others were still lying ill, we found her, as I said, distributing pretzels and other foods as alms to children in the village; she was also found giving alms in the house of a villager whose three children also had scarlet fever; and yet, both houses had a soldier at the door.[26]

The world doctor Cruceanu described was very much life-oriented: all Gh. Tichigiu's wife was doing was to try and tame death, in the words of Philippe Ariès.[27] And yet, how anti-modern this taming was, and ultimately how tragic! Doctor Cruceanu's nightmare only ended when, at the initiative of the director-general of the health service, tents were installed for the

---

24   Cruceanu, "Dare de seamă asupra epidemiei de scarlatină care a bântuit în comunele Măgureni și Călinești," 240.

25   Seeking the aid of the military was often recommended in the medical literature for help in isolating contaminated houses.

26   Cruceanu, "Dare de seamă asupra epidemiei de scarlatină care a bântuit în comunele Măgureni și Călinești," 241.

27   Ariès, *Omul în fața morții*.

isolation of the patients. But the experience had left him traumatized, and he recounted the indignation and revolt he had felt when the peasants "concealed their sick children." He was particularly distressed by

[...] the case of the tavern keeper Tanasă Vişoiu from Măgureni, who even denied that he had a daughter called Lina, four years of age; she had been ill for 15 days when we discovered her, after three days' searching; she had anasarca and enormous cervical adenitis. This child has made a full recovery in the meantime. This is a very enlightening case: the tavern keeper denied the existence of the child with the utmost cynicism, in the presence of some 15 villagers, and even of the village's mayor, who had accompanied us to the tavern, and all this because he did not want his house to be isolated.[28]

The passage undoubtedly reveals incomprehension on the part of doctor Cruceanu. As for us, looking back at the peasant world from such a historical distance, we may perhaps be a little more understanding, but probably not that much more accepting of the rules by which this world lived. I will not dwell further on other applications of the health and sanitary norms. Instead, I will briefly look at the doctors' general picture of conditions of hygiene in many Romanian towns and villages. Unsurprisingly, doctors were not happy with many of their findings. Visiting Giurgiu, for example, doctor Felix noted in 1891:

On side streets, one can still see many hovels and peasant dwellings built of mud bricks and wattle and daub; on the outskirts of towns, there are piles of cattle dung in the center of yards, some of which is left there to dry before it is used as fuel. The streets in the center are mostly straight, and sufficiently wide, but the town does not have one single sewer pipe for draining meteoric waters and refuse, which leads to the stagnation of filthy liquids in many yards and in gutters along the streets. Many streets have cobblestones and good pavements, some are paved with gravel, but the stones used are calcareous and friable, so that both cobblestone roads and gravel roads are covered with dust in the summer, and with mud in the spring, autumn, and winter.

28 Cruceanu, "Dare de seamă asupra epidemiei de scarlatină care a bântuit în comunele Măgureni și Călinești," 240.

Many ox-driven and bull-driven carts carrying freight between the town's warehouses and the harbor leave large amounts of dirt in the streets; even in these circumstances, the street-cleaning services, consisting of 10 sweepers and 10 carts, could be up to the task, if they only had to do this one job and if the carts were not also used for transporting paving materials. But the worst is the lack of cleaning in houses and yards, and the town council would be well advised to organize a cart service operating at regular intervals for carrying the refuse out of town.[29]

In smaller towns, sanitary and hygienic conditions were even worse. Drăgășani, recently raised to town status, was downgraded by doctor Nicolae Măldărescu, who observed that it had no cemetery and the dead were buried "around the town churches," it lacked water for "the needs of the inhabitants and for general salubrity," it had no doctor and no vaccination programme. There was no abattoir, and "the slaughter of large cattle and small livestock alike" was "done in the private yards of the inhabitants."[30] It was a desolate picture. Every site, and especially the marketplace, was a focus of infection. The central market in Târgu-Jiu was no exception, according to doctor Măldărescu:

Trading is done by laying out merchandise directly on the ground. The few butchers' sheds are in a state of the most revolting pollution, and they do not have enough room for the display and preservation of the meats. Vegetables, greens and all the other goods for consumption are laid out directly on the soil. All the dregs and scraps, rotten vegetables, refuse and other filth resulting from trade and the presence of crowds are dumped in a small ditch or plot at the back of the marketplace.[31]

As for the hygiene of rural areas, doctor Măldărescu gives us a general picture, which is reiterated almost obsessively by the medical profession:

In villages, the streets and courtyards are covered in the most revolting filth. Rotting corn cobs, dung, every type of refuse, are spread across all areas of

---

29  Felix, "Raportul domnului doctor ~, membru consiliului sanitar superior," 54.
30  Măldărescu, "Raportul d-lui doctor N. Măldărescu," 289–90,
31  Ibid., 215–16.

the village. In some of the inhabitants' yards, the piles of waste grow into hills as tall as the eaves of the house, and in rainy weather, cattle swim up to their necks in those swamps. The inns and taverns are the most squalid holes, and the privies in these establishments, overflowing with filth, defy description. There is no authority to check and ensure the standards of hygiene of these places and that of the nasty wares sold for the consumption of the rural public.[32]

It would appear that the village was a wholesome place to live in only in the writings of the romantics; doctors had an altogether different opinion.

To conclude, the public health reports show that the application of sanitary laws was selective and imperfect. Most often, it was simply ignored. Doctor Gheorghe Rigani contended that the law remained "black letters on white paper."[33] But was this true? We must answer in the negative. Even though the implementation of its provisions remained patchy, the health and sanitary system was in place and working. After 1900, it was improved to meet the citizens' needs more adequately. In other words, it became more efficient. One year before his appointment to the top of the Kingdom's General Directorate of the Health Service, doctor Felix identified the main problem of the state-run system, namely, its emphasis on cure, rather than prevention, which, as we have seen, remained marginal for a long time.[34] But the numbers of hospitals increased in towns. After 1881, the rural population benefitted from the services of their own hospital network of rural hospitals, which developed apace. The number of doctors increased, too. We believe that it is safe to contend that, in 1900, the levels of health care and public hygiene in the Kingdom were much improved compared to 1874, which was, as we have seen, a seminal year. Still, the impression of stagnation was enduring. What were the reasons? It is not easy to explain, but we may venture a few working hypotheses. One cause might be the specific nature of the sources and what I have called their hidden trap: they obviously highlight deficiencies and malfunctioning rather than progress.

As they went on their inspection tours, doctors Felix, Măldărescu, and Fotino reported on what they believed the Minister for Home Affairs had "to act on to take measures for improvement." Their guiding principle was:

32 Ibid., 167.
33 Rigani, "Mersul serviciului sanitar al județului Mușcel în 1905," 102.
34 Felix, "Raportul domnului doctor ~, membru consiliului sanitar superior," 18–19.

while it is wonderful that some things work, those that do not work have to be notified to the authorities so that measures can be taken. However, perceptions of immobility at ground zero in health provision also came from the doctors' personal experiences as they went on their annual inspections. Doctor Măldărescu's exasperation seems justified:

> I take the liberty, Minister, to draw your attention, from the start, to the fact that we, the members of the Higher Medical Council, submit these reports to the Hon. Ministry every year. These reports are published in *Monitorul Oficial* and relevant sections of them are sent to all county and communal local authorities; and yet, when the time of the next inspection comes, we find that none, but absolutely none, of the failings we identified has been acted upon: no emergency measures were taken to improve public health and the hygiene of public establishments, and local authorities failed to support health personnel to fulfil such tasks, and many others. So, we meet again after the last inspection, facing the same facts, which grow ever more threatening in time. We are met with the same objections and, what is sadder, with the same indifference and even ill will.[35]

Doctor Măldărescu was right: from one year to the next, things did not seem to improve. But historians have the advantage of a longer perspective. If we take one decade, for instance, or even better, a generation (20 to 25 years), change suddenly becomes perceptible. This was not, however, the pace of change Romanian doctors wanted to see at the end of the nineteenth century.

One question arises: was modern Romania's health legislation expected to be applied comprehensively and seamlessly from its early days? Let's look at what the documents say. In 1891, the *Regulations for the Prevention of Infectious Diseases* [*Regulamentul pentru prevenirea bolilor infecțioase*] included guidelines for the disinfection of contaminated dwellings. However, the text read, "the prescriptions included in this set of rules will be strictly applied, where their application is possible. When all may not be observed, because of the poverty of the resident or of the village, it is expected that at least some of them will be put into practice, as circumstances will allow." Whenever the

---

35  Măldărescu, "Raportul d-lui doctor N. Măldărescu," 156.

lawmaker had doubts that the guidelines could be applied in their entirety, he resorted to the magical formula: "as circumstances will allow." For example, if a town did not have "specialized disinfection officers," local authorities could appoint "sanitation commissars and surgeon's assistants" (in Romanian: *comisari sanitari; subchirurgi*) to deal with the task[36] "as circumstances will allow." Another example: county councils would pay "a number of midwives, as circumstances will allow," to offer free assistance at birth in rural areas.[37] Resulting from doubts in the legislators' minds, these texts could become rather convoluted. The best example is the only set of regulations aimed exclusively at rural areas: *Regulamentul pentru alinierea satelor și construcția locuințelor țărănești* (Regulations for the alignment of village streets and peasant dwellings). In 1888, the lawmaker was firmly convinced that he could use administrative fiat to ensure that all peasant dwellings in the plains used only "brick for the making of walls and lime wash paint on fences," that only "iron, clay tiles, thin clapboard and reed" were to be used for roofing, and that chimneys were not built higher than 30 centimeters on the top of the roof.[38] Even now, in the village where I live, I can see many smoking roofs where chimneys do not rise higher than the attic, which is a traditional feature of peasant dwellings. The regulations of 1888 do not seem to have been applied.

There were occasions when the legislator enunciated the norms using the "subjunctive" form with an imperative value, as, for example, in the 1890 *Regulations on Measures to be taken for the Prevention and Eradication of Granular Conjunctivitis* [*Regulamentul asupra măsurilor de luat pentru prevenirea și combaterea conjunctivitei granuloase*]. The measures recommended for use by the military are particularly instructive:

Art. 10. Suitable barracks should be built to accommodate the number of troops destined for various garrisons. Art. 11. Superimposed bunks should be dismantled in barracks [...] Art. 13: Ammunition should no longer be stored in soldiers' dormitories.[39]

36  *Regulament pentru prevenţiunea bolilor infecţioase (molipsitoare) dezvoltător art. 9, 12, 13, 128, 129 şi 130 din legea sanitară* [Regulations for the prevention of infectious (contagious) diseases, additional arts. 9, 12 13, 128, 129, and 130 of the Health Act], art. 40, in *Legislaţia sanitară*, eds. Şuta et al., 358.

37  *Legea sanitară din 1874* [The Health Act of 1874], art. 61, in Ibid., 56.

38  *Regulament pentru alinierea satelor şi pentru construirea locuinţelor ţărăneşti. Igiena şi salubritatea lor*, art. 4 and art. 5, in Ibid., 295.

39  *Regulament asupra măsurilor de luat pentru prevenirea şi combaterea conjunctivitei granuloase*, art. 10, art. 11, art. 13, in Ibid., 318.

If further proof were needed that these regulations were meant to be applied in some indefinite future, "as circumstances allowed," I am reminded of the time when, as a young recruit, I was "serving my country" in the Timişoara garrison in 1989. There, in flagrant contradiction to the 1890 regulations, the dormitories had superimposed bunks and the walls were lined with arm racks. Such examples demonstrate, in fact, that the majority of norms in the health legislation should have been applied with immediate effect.

It is worth adding that the health legislation was not applied uniformly in the country. As we move further away from the hub of the Kingdom and the large urban centers, we see that the understanding of the law becomes less precise. Even in one and the same city, the peripheries ignored legislation applied in the center. The center represented modernity, while the periphery was still locked in the past. As a correlative, modernity is associated with the elites, and archaism with the poorer classes. An increasing number of doctors' reports, particularly those on the prevention and eradication of epidemics, document this correlation. In 1899, doctor Vasile Sion, at the time a research assistant at the Institute for Pathology and Bacteriology in Bucharest, was tasked with identifying the causes of a typhoid fever epidemic that had erupted in Galați that year. He quickly abandoned the hypothesis that indicated drinking water as the possible agent for the spread of the disease. The mapping of the epidemic showed that, as he reported, "all the patients whom I have visited live in areas of Galați which I can only call underprivileged."[40] As a result, he suggested, the causes had to be sought in the "hygienic condition of the streets, courtyards, and homes where the patients live, and of the latrines they use."[41] Visits to the homes of those affected convinced doctor Sion that his theory was correct: "In the courtyards I visited—which were usually quite small—I found two or three dwellings of 1–2 rooms each, and each was occupied by several families with children; the yards were strewn with garbage, including animal and human feces."[42] This was an image of absolute squalor, reinforced by his persuasive description of a latrine he saw in a home on Strada Spitalului (Hospital Street), at no. 62:

---

40 Sion, "Referatul d-lui dr ~, asistent la institutul de patologie și de bacteriologie din București, despre cercetările făcute de d-sa asupra originii febrei tifoide la Galați," 283.
41 Ibid.
42 Ibid., 284.

The latrine is around 25 meters away from the well; between the two, and adjacent to the latrine, is a stable, which has no floorboards; instead of floorboards, there is a thick layer of vegetable scraps reeking of urine; only one step and a half separates one side of the stable from the well. In the house itself, a delirious typhoid sufferer lay, covered in flies, a swarm of flies such as I had never seen; and, stepping from the door to the bed, I had to tiptoe carefully through the grime.[43]

These were terrifying images then, and they are even more so today. They led doctor Sion to muse on the contrasts within modern Romania, as reflected in his report to the Director-General of the Higher Medical Council:

Sir, my hotel is situated on a clean, bustling street which, if it does not surpass, at least is not inferior to Calea Victoriei[44] in Bucharest. Those in the suburbs should be guaranteed at least the benefits of cleanliness and the right to live—the denizens of the city center can keep the animation and the lights for their own selfish enjoyment.[45]

Three years later, in 1902, the Bucharest's chief doctor's findings did not differ substantially from doctor Sion's conclusions about the causes of typhoid fever and diphtheria in Bucharest. Typhoid fever, he found, "affects mainly the impoverished population, and especially the laborers, who do not have a permanent abode."[46] Diphtheria could not be eradicated, and became endemic. The medical professionals concluded that the propagation of such diseases

[was] primarily due to the ignorance of the poor, to the superstitions they believe in, to their living conditions and the state of their dwellings, despite all our attempts to provide instructions and distribute special brochures for each disease, and despite all the measures of disinfection and preventive vaccination.[47]

---

43  Ibid.
44  Calea Victoriei was a fashionable boulevard in the capital city, Bucharest.
45  Sion, "Referatul d-lui dr ~," 285.
46  Georgescu, "Raportul d-lui medic-șef al Capitalei no. 2836 din 27 septembrie 1902," 298.
47  Ibid., 299.

The health services mobilized their entire arsenal, and yet, the results remained modest.

In the late nineteenth century, poverty, poor hygiene, disease, and noncompliance with the norms of hygiene all overlapped and converged in two sites: the urban suburbia and the villages. These were the locations which modernity seemed unable to reach. Modernizing processes in Romania appear to have been modelled on the "oil spill" pattern: from one central point or several central points, represented by the urban areas, modernity was supposed to radiate and gradually cover the entire national territory. Still nowadays, the process is incomplete.

To conclude, the health legislation in late nineteenth-century Romania was perfectly aligned with modern European standards. As such, it was perhaps ahead of its time, and bound to remain a project rather than a real possibility. Some aspects of health provision were easier to manage than others, although there was a chronic deficit of medical personnel as well as of ancillary staff throughout the period considered here. In the domain of public health, things were more complex, and the initiatives often pursued goals that belonged to the realm of ideal, even utopian, projection. The period's public health legislation offered the template of a future society; it was an imaginary construction of a future reality as legislators envisioned it. From this perspective, it was pure fiction. However, it was to be hoped that one day *fiction would become reality.*

2

## Two Mid-Nineteenth-Century Case Studies: Marin Vărzaru and Stoian Buruiană

### Empirics, Charlatans, and Ignorance

In the night of January 5 to 6, 1860, a fairly common incident occurred in the hamlet Găureni of Babele village, in Vlaşca district: a rabid wolf entered the village and attacked humans and cattle. Here is a narrative of the episode by the sub-administrator of the district of Neajlov, C. I. Arion:

> As [the wolf] grabbed a piglet from the barn of one villager by the name of Oprea Radu, his wife ran to save the piglet, and [the wolf] rushed upon her and bit her hand and her backside; as she screamed, the villagers rounded up the wolf and killed it; immediately they called a man from the village Roata-Cătun, by the name of Marin Vărzaru Catană, a man known for his skill in treating that disease, so he attended to the woman, and to five other inhabitants and several cattle, which now had rabies, and they were all cured.[48]

So far, there is nothing unusual in this nineteenth-century story: a rabid wolf is on a rampage in a village, and a peasant can heal rabies. The incident became newsworthy, however, once the Health Authority became involved and an inquiry was ordered. The story went straight to the "human interest" column of *Monitorul Oficial*,[49] among robberies and accidents.

Around the same time, the health authorities ordered an inquiry into the case of another peasant healer, Stoian Popa Ion Buruiană from the village Reda, in Romanați district, who had built a reputation for healing mental conditions. He was identified as such by accident, "on the occasion of the census in the village of Reda," as evidenced by the inquiry documents:

> We were given assurances by everybody in the village, among whom priests and other respectable people, that, for a long time, he had offered palpable

---

48 Arhivele Naționale Istorice Centrale, Bucharest; Fondul Ministerului de Interne, Direcția Generală a Serviciului Sanitar (The National Historical Archives, Fonds Ministry for Home Affairs, General Directorate of the Health Services), dosar (file) 8/1860, f. 2r. Hereafter ANIC.

49 *Monitorul. Ziar Oficial al Țării Românești*, March 19, 1860, no. 67, 272.

evidence of his sublime knowledge, which he had inherited from his parents; the villagers recounted how wretched folk, restrained in chains, [...] had been brought to him from as far as Turkey, and they were healed when they left him. The medication he applies consists of some mystical herbs, the salutary effect of which is almost immediate; those with more severe conditions took as little as 20 to 30 days to be cured.[50]

These cases interest me solely because they illustrate the relationship between the dominant medical culture promoted by the modern state and the peasant medical culture. The power relations between the two are not difficult to read between the lines. As I read these files, I tried to go beyond the narrative details and search for the deeper sources of the societal changes we now associate with processes of "modernization." These processes include what has been termed the "medicalization" of society. The term is ubiquitous nowadays, but often remains vaguely defined in the social sciences: it is one of those "catch-all" concepts that owe their success to their intrinsic ambiguity. So far, in the Romanian social sciences, there has been only one attempt at a definition, by Lidia Trăușan-Matu, who wrote that "*medicalization* [...] as a term covers the set of mechanisms whereby the state enforces measures for the maintenance of health among the population."[51] This meaning includes both curative and preventive (public health) medicine. State intervention seems to be the key factor in the medicalization of society as defined above. However, medicalization can also occur outside of state intervention. It might be easier and more useful to define what medicalization *is not* rather than what it *is*. A typical example of a society where medicalization has not penetrated yet is European pre-industrial peasant society. In this type of society, both the doctor as a modern health professional, and medical care in the modern sense, are unknown. Naturally, at least in Europe, no peasant society was ever so isolated as to remain completely unmedicalized. Almost everywhere in Europe, empirical medical practices were contaminated by professional medicine. A perfectly medicalized society, in which all individuals have recourse to modern medical practices, remains a utopia. For as long as medicine has not discovered the

---

50   ANIC, f. 13r.
51   Trăușan-Matu, *De la leac la rețetă. Medicalizarea societății românești în veacul al XIX-lea (1831–1869)*, 356.

secret of "youth without old age and life without death," such a society remains utopian.

Medicalization can only be approached and understood as something
that happens at the intersection of dominant and subaltern cultures. From
the moment modernizing processes started to penetrate the rural world,
peasant culture has remained a subaltern culture. Here, the concepts of modernization and medicalization are used to indicate the results of processes
of acculturation resulting in cultural homogeneity, the cherished aim of the
modern state. In this sense, medicalization is a set of strategies of internal
acculturation deployed by modern states to disseminate the official medical
culture and its associated social practices across society. This process has an
institutional component, often discussed in histories of medicine, consisting
of hospitals, institutions of higher education, professional associations, etc.
There is also a behavioral component, best illustrated by the peasants' resistance to modern medical professionals and practices. Norbert Elias has described the gradual stages through which, in the "civilizing process," behavioral norms prescribed by modern societies are internalized at the level of the
individual, and social discipline becomes self-discipline.[52] In the Romanian
Principalities, in the times of Marin Vărzaru and Stoian Buruiană, the process of imposing norms in society was still in its early stages.

In the mid-nineteenth century in the Romanian Principalities, illness
and healing were in the hands of two categories of agents: the peasant healers—the empirics, as the medical authorities called them—and the medical
doctors, key individuals in the new state-run health system. The following
sections look at the relationships between these two categories of healers.

Peasant healers had always existed in pre-industrial peasant communities, and Romanian villages were no exception. Peasant communities
had their own ways of managing the rapport between illness, healing, and
death. Before the advent of modern doctors and medicine, which in the Romanian Principalities did not happen before 1862, peasant communities resorted to individuals who specialized in the healing of certain conditions,
using nosological categories proper to peasant medical culture.[53] Women

---

52  Elias, *Procesul civilizării. Cercetări sociogenetice și psihogenetice*. First published in 1939 in German as *Über den Prozeß der Zivilisation*.
53  By peasant medical culture I mean here the totality of peasant knowledge and practices related to illness and healing.

in labor were assisted by so-called empirical midwives, who were much ma-
ligned in the period's professional medical culture. There were "orthopae-
dic specialists," and an army of other healers who specialized in individual medical conditions. The above-mentioned Marin Catană, for example,
specialized in rabies, and Stoian Buruiană used his skills to heal mental
conditions. They were just two in an army of spell-casters, enchanters, and
other specialists in remedies against occult aggression: priests, monks, and
witch doctors. In the pre-modern peasant conception, illness was not simply a (humoral or physiological) disorder of the body, but the outcome of
divine punishment or the result of a magic spell.[54] In the peasant world,
healers were omnipotent. In fact, they were the only ones available. Faith
in the healing powers of these personages proved to be enduring: even today, surprisingly, one can find oral testimonies about their activities in the
rural world.[55]

There were categories of empirics operating in the urban environment
as well. In the late nineteenth century, doctor Constantin Dumitrescu
Severeanu met a few empirics working in Bucharest, and he mentioned
those with "a large clientele" in his memoirs. *Moș Rățoi* (Uncle duck), an
orthopaedist, carried "bits of thread, some brick dust, a few eggs and several ends of broadcloth in his bag. With these, he performed every operation on fractured bones."[56] There was also *dascălul Drăgoi* [school-teacher
Drăgoi] from the Văcărești suburb of the city, and the famous *Mățăreasa*
[the gut-washer woman]. The latter's name came from her former line of
work at the abattoir, which she gave up to "take up physics," becoming a
specialist in treating diphtheric angina in the "old-fashioned" way by sending dog's dried feces down the patient's throat. But her skills also included
"tending to sprained joints and broken limbs."[57] In the mid-nineteenth century, everything and anything was possible in medicine. In the town of Severin, a Greek pie-maker turned into a doctor overnight, after a journey to
his homeland. This is how a clearly amused doctor Severeanu describes this
metamorphosis:

---

54  Bărbulescu, "At the Edge of Modernity: Physicians, Priests and Healers (1940–1990)," 550–51.
55  See, for example, Bărbulescu, "At the Edge of Modernity," 549–61, as well as the collections of primary
    oral documents in *Țărani, boli și vindecători în perioada comunistă. Mărturii orale.*
56  Severeanu, *Din amintirile mele (1853–1928)*, 107.
57  Ibid.

Upon his return, some six months later, Kir Tănase had undergone a great change: he wore European-style clothes and spoke in a grand manner. Kirie Tănase no longer made piès, to my great sorrow. [...] "Well, well, Kir Tănase, why have you changed?" And he answered: "My good sir, you know, I am a doctor now, sir," and to prove it, he took me to his room and showed me a box, a kind of satchel with compartments, inlaid with mother-of-pearl; from it, he took out a few small bottles with liquids of different colours and some small glasses, all things you could not find in Severin; to prove that he was a doctor, he started mixing liquids and pouring them into the glasses, so the colour changed: he mixed two liquids as clear as water and obtained a black liquid, or a yellow or blue one. Faced with these miracles, I became convinced that our Kir Tănase the pie-maker had, indeed, become a physician. Throwing his satchel over his shoulder—like a soldier his kit bag—Kir Tănase would go down the streets, crying out his services: "Iatros-Kalos, Kalos-Iatros!" and thus he practiced medicine.[58]

This person was no longer simply an empiric, but a downright "charlatan": with no academic title or qualifications, he employed methods had never been sanctioned by the science of medicine. In a hierarchy of healers compiled from the perspective of the health authorities, the empirics were at the top, followed by charlatans in second place. The practitioners of magic medicine—spell-casters, priests, monks, witches—were not even listed. They were not considered to belong in the category of healers.

## The New Order of Carol Davila

The second category of healers belonged to the dominant culture: the doctors, those who, in the mid-nineteenth century, created the health system of the Romanian Principalities. Their status and activities were validated by specialist academic studies, degrees, and professional titles.[59] Officially, from the time of the Organic Regulations,[60] in the Romanian Principalities,

---

58  Ibid., 35. Kir is Greek for "mister"; iatros means physician or doctor; and kalos means beautiful or good.

59  On the professional status of Romanian doctors in the early nineteenth century, see Trăuşan-Matu, "The Doctor and the Patient: An Analysis of the Medical Profession in the Romanian Society of the 19th Century (1831–1869)," 465–74.

60  The Organic Regulations (in Romanian: *Regulamentele Organice*] were the earliest quasi-constitutional set of laws in Ţara Românească and Moldavia. They were imposed by the Russian authority govern-

and subsequently in the Kingdom of Romania, only qualified doctors were authorized to practice medicine. Theoretically, therefore, they had a monopoly on the arts of healing. I say "theoretically," because by the last decades of the nineteenth century, the war against the other categories of healers had not been won. In fact, it had only just started. Developments in the next century proved the resilience of peasant medical culture and its practitioners. It is enough to look at the considerable ethnographic literature on magic medicine and recent studies, to see that the spell-caster, the priest, the witch, and the empiric participated, alone or alongside the doctor, in processes of healing in the rural world as late as the second half of the twentieth century. I do not think that I am far off the mark when I claim that even today, despite a century and a half of medicalization, peasant medical practices are still thriving in parallel with modern medicine in Romanian society.

In the late nineteenth century, even in cities, empirics found a niche, often working in parallel with doctors: doctor Severeanu, for example, on a home visit to the Fălcoianu family, a "good" family in the capital city, came face to face with Mățăreasa,[61] who had been called upon to treat the old lady Fălcoianu for a fracture of the radial bone.[62] In the town of Caracal, he was called by Mr Stamatopulo, a "major cereal exporter," to treat an open fracture of the tibia after two doctors and two peasant empirics had failed to cure it:

Two local doctors, one Greek, the other Italian, had called two master peasant healers. To consolidate the bones, they mixed oil into powder from the head bones of a dog (they claimed), and poured the mixture round the joint, which they then bound tightly with a ligature. But gangrene set in, and the panicked peasants ran away. When I arrived in Caracal, the gangrene had spread up the shank almost to the knee.[63]

In the end, Mr Stamatopulo was saved, but he lost half of his leg.

On the other side of the cultural barrier—a very fluid barrier at the time—the aforementioned Stoian Buruiană, who specialized in mental con-

---

ing the Principalities after the Russo-Turkish war of 1828–1829. They came into force in 1831 in Țara Românească and in Moldavia in the following year.

61   For Mățăreasa, see above, page 247.

62   Severeanu, *Din amintirile mele (1853–1928)*, 107–8.

63   Severeanu, *Din amintirile mele (1853–1929)*, 12–13.

ditions, had a diverse clientele: he treated not only fellow peasants, but also, for example, "the sister of Mr Costache Prejbeanu from the town of Cara-cal," and even the wife of a high-ranking Ottoman Pasha, the "Kadın of Paşa agi-ali from Rahova."[64] Around the same time, mother Cassandra (in Roma-nian: *mama Casandra*), the most famous herbalist in Iaşi, "was visited every Sunday by the most distinguished society Ladies in Iaşi," who purchased herbs for the bath, hart's tongue fern,[65] and "other weeds which invigorate virility. *Mama* Cassandra had everything."[66] In this context, I cannot fail to mention the witch I knew in my own home village, Corlăţel, in Mehedinţi County. In the 1980s, she was said to have clients as far away as Serbia and she was known to go on business "tours" all the way to Severin and Craiova.

In the early 1860s, Carol Davila re-organized the health system of the United Principalities. One of his first initiatives was precisely to estab-lish which individuals could be officially authorized to practice as state-recognized medics. Before 1860, the Health Authority (in Romanian: *Administraţia Serviciului Sanitar*) held no list of qualified doctors practicing in the Principalities. According to Davila, for the period 1842 to 1854 there was no information about doctors who had settled on the country's territo-ry.[67] July 8, 1860, marked a milestone: *Monitorul Oficial* published the first "Table of all medical personnel: doctors of medicine, master surgeons and patrons of surgery, veterinarians, dentists and midwives, recognized by the Government as having the right to practice their art in this Principality."[68] This table comprised the official healers, i.e. the accepted healers. This must count as the birth certificate of the medical profession in the Romanian Principalities. It should perhaps not come as a surprise that the greatest number of documents on inquiries launched by the Health Authority into the activities of empirics date from the period 1860–1862. At that time, the number of individuals practicing medicine in Ţara Românească included 96

---

64  ANIC, f. 31v.

65  In Romanian, *năvalnic*, an evergreen fern (in Latin: *Scolopendrium vulgare*) with medicinal uses.

66  Leon, *Amintiri*, 32.

67  *Supliment la Monitorul Oficial* [Supplement to *Monitorul Oficial*], July 8, 1860, no. 160, 751. However, lists of doctors practicing in the Principalities had been compiled as early as the 1830s. We know who prac-tised medicine in Ţara Românească in 1833, 1834, 1836, 1837, and 1838: Gomoiu, *Din istoria medicinei şi a învăţământului medical în România (înainte de 1870)*, 253–55, 263, 285–87, 301–2.

68  "Tablou cu tot personalul medical: doctori în medicină, magiştri şi patroni în hirurgie, veterinari, dentişti şi moaşe care se cunosc că au dobândit dreptul de la Guvern de a exersa arta lor în acest Princi-pat," in Ibid., 752–53.

doctors of medicine, 11 master surgeons, 18 patrons of surgery, 7 veterinarians, 5 dentists, 13 midwives with diplomas obtained abroad, and 61 midwives who "studied at the Institute for births in Bucharest."[69] In October 1861, the same newspaper published a new, longer list: the number of doctors of medicine had increased to 98. But the greatest increase was for the number of Romanian-trained midwives: 78.[70] A few months later, after the full unification of the Principalities, *Monitorul* published the final, complete list of all doctors authorized to practice medicine in "the state of Romania."[71]

Since prior to 1875, there were no home-trained medical doctors, the Romanian health authorities had to establish the criteria for Romanian or foreign doctors who wished to practice freely in the Principalities. The first condition was a degree from a foreign university. It would appear that, at least in pre-1836 Moldavia, presenting such a document to the Medical Board was enough. But, from 1836 onwards, because of some irregularities in the procedure, the Board requested the right to examine the candidates.[72] We do not know whether it acquired this right. Thus, in 1862, when doctor Carol Davila chaired the Medical Council, a decision was taken that "doctors wishing to practice medicine in this Principality" had to pass an examination by a commission formed of five academic staff members from the National School of Medicine and Pharmacy.[73] Only twelve years later, the Health Act of 1874 dispensed with the examination and made an addition to article 69:

> The right to practice medicine, pharmacy, veterinary medicine, and midwifery is granted by virtue of academic titles conferred by the Romanian School of Medicine and sanctioned by the Minister for Public Education, as well as of diplomas obtained at foreign universities and verified by the national School of Medicine.[74]

But the law was modified again in 1885, and the examination was reintroduced, this time only for candidates who had obtained their titles

---

69 Ibid.
70 *Monitorul. Ziar Oficial al Țării Românești*, October 4, 1861, no. 218, 871–72.
71 *Monitorul. Jurnal Oficial*, February 3, 1863, no. 25, 103.
72 See Gomoiu, *Din istoria medicinei*, 283–84.
73 *Monitorul. Ziar Oficial al Țării Românești*, May 18, 1860, no. 115, 480.
74 Șuta et al., *Legislația sanitară*, 57.

abroad.[75] In 1893, when the Health Act was modified again, the examination was maintained, but there were further specifications for the composition of the examination boards.[76]

Let's return to 1860, when regulations were introduced in turn for all the sub-disciplines of the medical sciences. Sub-surgeons were granted the right to practice by examination.[77] Doctors who had studied abroad, but had not gained a doctoral degree, were offered the possibility of becoming health officers.[78] Regulations were also introduced for assistant pharmacists,[79] for midwives and dentists,[80] as well as for the different ranks of veterinarians.[81] By the end of 1860, regulations were in place for all medical personnel in the United Principalities. If they complied with these regulations, these health professionals, both the highly qualified and the lower ranks, were licensed to practice.[82] This marked the moment when the dominant medical culture imposed its own norms to separate the *true* healers from the *false*.

The roles of these key medical figures were important: doctors had expertise in the science of healing, but also in the remedies to be administered. They examined the patient, established a diagnosis, and decided on a treatment that often involved prescribing drugs. But the latter were sold by pharmacists, and sometimes by grocers. Under Carol Davila's energetic administration, the Health Authority also issued regulations on the retail of drugs, which created de facto a monopoly of pharmacists by banning the sale of drugs by "other private individuals."[83] In this way, the health professionals obtained the monopoly on the preparation and issuing of remedies. Individuals like Marin Vărzaru, Stoian Buruiană, and all their peers in the healing business remained locked outside the enchanted circle of the health profession. They came from a different world, one with its own illnesses, its own

---

75   Ibid., 75, 81 (art. 22 and art. 70).
76   Ibid., 111 (art. 105).
77   *Monitorul. Ziar Oficial al Ţării Româneşti*, March 18, 1860, no. 66, 268.
78   *Monitorul. Ziar Oficial al Ţării Româneşti*, May 26, 1860, no. 122, 508.
79   *Monitorul. Ziar Oficial al Ţării Româneşti*, June 10, 1860, no. 135, 559–60.
80   *Supliment la Monitorul Oficial*, July 8, 1860, no. 160, 751.
81   *Monitorul. Ziar Oficial al Ţării Româneşti*, June 14, 1860, no. 139, 575.
82   The regulations were codified in 1866 and published as *Regulament pentru examinarea titlurilor şi capacităţii medicilor, farmaciştilor, veterinarilor şi moaşelor din străinătate, care cer dreptul de a exercita în România* [Regulations for the verification of titles and qualifications of doctors, pharmacists, veterinarians and midwives trained abroad who seek the right to practise in Romania], in *Monitorul medical*, year V, 1866, no. 21, 171–74.
83   *Monitorul. Ziar Oficial al Ţării Româneşti*, February 13, 1860, no. 35, 140.

remedies, and its own criteria for validating the healers. The health authorities remained perpetually suspicious of the empirics, and at best tolerated them, waiting for their gradual, but imminent, natural demise.

## The Empirics and Their Remedies

I shall now look at the remedies and practices of the two peasant healers I have chosen as my case studies. Their stories shed light on the ways in which the health authorities treated them. First, it is noteworthy that the inquiries into their activities were initiated not from inside the medical profession, but from the official administration. The early reports were in fact benevolent: the deputy administrator of Neajlov County, who apparently discovered Vărzaru, demanded a reward for him in the first instance.[84] Even the Home Minister, Ion Ghica, deemed it fit to send a copy of the report to the Inspector General of the Health Service, none other than doctor Carol Davila. Ghica asked for the healer's remedy against rabies to be popularized:

> Taking into account that, after all the attempts that have been made, medicine has still not found a method for healing rabies, I thought it my duty to bring this important case to your attention, so that you may seek a way of popularizing it.[85]

In 1860, the Home Minister of the United Principalities believed that the peasant Marin Vărzaru had found a cure for rabies. The criterion he—and most of his non-professional contemporaries—used for assessing the healing act was simply its *efficacy*. If healing was the outcome, this automatically meant that the methods used were appropriate. No other factors were considered: neither the healer's professional status, nor his social background and level of education mattered. Ion Ghica did not yet make a distinction between dominant culture and peasant culture, the distinction that has informed my research.

The Buruiană case was first assessed by two officials, who, having failed to obtain the secret treatment for insanity from the healer, reported to their

---

84  ANIC, f. 2r.-v.
85  ANIC, f. 1r.

superiors on the "real advantage which such a salutary discovery, until now hidden in a remote village, would bring medicine. You may wish to inform the government so that, through parental enquiries, it might find a way to wrest this mysterious remedy."[86] Thus started the inquiry.

The inquiry proceeded with a visit to the village by district doctors and a meeting with the peasant healers. It was a meeting that unsealed the secret therapies used by the healers, but also exposed the essential incompatibility between these healers and their professionally trained peers. The doctors were not as enthusiastic as the officials had been when they found out about the "medicine" used by Marin Vărzaru to cure rabies. Apparently, he used plants and insects:

> The first is called hedge-hyssop (*Rubis Gratiola*), the second is great mullein (*Verbascum*), and small blister beetles (*Cantharides*), which he ground and mixed with raki, and made a scarification under the tongue.[87]

This treatment corresponds to what is known about traditional peasant remedies against rabies. Blister beetles (cantharides, also known as Spanish flies) seemed to have been widely used: ground, boiled, and mixed with water or wine, they were the base for a medicinal preparation given to people and cattle bitten by rabid dogs.[88] The use of cantharides in remedies against rabies is still practiced today. I found it during fieldwork conducted in 2010 in a locality in Cluj County: to prevent rabies after a suspicious bite, locals took five or six "blister beetles,"[89] ground them into a powder, which they mixed with sugar and recommended a spoonful or two of this mixture per day.[90] Another common peasant therapy, also used by Stoian Buruiană, consisted of "incisions in the blood vessels under the tongue" to prevent the occurrence of "blisters,"[91] also known as "rabies blisters."[92]

86  ANIC, f. 13r.
87  ANIC, f. 21r. The Romanian original, with minor errors in the Latin names, reads as following: "Cea dintâi se numește otrava pământului (*Rubis Gratiola*), lumânărică (*Verbatium*), gândăcei (*Chantarides*) pisat și cu rachiu, și făcea scarificație subt limbă." Nicu Mihai transcribed this document.
88  Leon, *Istoria naturală medicală a poporului Român*, 262–64; Grigoriu-Rigo, *Medicina poporului*, 22–23.
89  "Pepti de frasân," the local designation for beetles.
90  Bărbulescu, *Țărani, boli și vindecători*, vol. II, 150.
91  Severeanu, *Din amintirile mele (1853–1929)*, 179.
92  "Căței" or "căței de turbare" in the Romanian original. Felix, *Raport general asupra igienei publice și asupra serviciului sanitar al Regatului României pe anii 1896 și 1897*, 319.

From the detailed inquiry of the district doctor from Romanați we also learn that Stoian Buruiană had learned the "trade" from his father, who "had been known to cure those suffering from that malady."[93] The son had narrowed his specialism to include only the "furious mad, those who caused harm and those who tore their clothes off." Those who "sleep-walked or night-walked he sent to Grandpa Mihail from Negrești, who knew all the herbs to use for sleep-walkers."[94] The complex therapy he used involved the administration of a decoction, fumigations, and a draconic diet. This is the description by the district doctor:

> For three days he gives them [the patients] a decoction of herbs cooked in wine, 50 grams of it three times a day; after that, the sick will start foaming at the mouth and suffer from loose bowels; on the third day, their minds will be clear, and they will fall into a deep sleep which can last up to a week, after which they get up from their sick beds. He [the healer] will keep the sick without food or water for three days, because water especially is very harmful. After three days, food is to be taken very cautiously. Three times a day, when the medicine is taken, he will fumigate the sick with other herbs and will wrap them up with bed linen.[95]

The district doctor, like the authors of the reports before him, was unable to find much about the plants themselves. The healer told him that the decoction was made from the roots of "three species" of plants, and he used one plant for the fumigation, but he did not "know their names, only [that] they grow in forests, and he knows them from the dry leaves left after winter, which he digs up exclusively in the month of March." The doctor could not see the plants, because, the healer explained, he "does not have them here now." Obviously, the peasant did not trust the doctor enough to disclose the popular names of the plants, which might have helped identify them. In addition, on April 20, the day of the inquiry, he did not have with him the plants he collected only a month earlier, which is hard to believe. But the lack of trust went both ways. For Stoian Buruiană, finding the district doctor on his doorstep must have been a bad sign. Yet, trusting in his art, he de-

---

93 ANIC, f. 39r.
94 ANIC, f. 31r.
95 ANIC, f. 31r.

clared that he was ready to go to Bucharest "any minute" and present the Health Authority with "indisputable proof of his knowledge."[96]

The inquiry continued. The local authorities started assembling the documentation requested by the Health Authority. The deputy prefects, who had visited the village where Stoian Buruiană's patients lived, started sending in their reports. In addition, the district medical officer conducted his own surveys. The resulting documentation included information on a total of thirteen patients. Of these, one could not be identified, another denied having used the healer's services, and one (the wife of the Pasha of Rahova) could not be questioned. This left ten verified cases. Of the ten, eight had ended in a cure and only two could be considered medical failures, which is an impressive rate of positive outcomes. However, to obtain a clearer picture of the case, we must look at the unfolding of the therapeutic process and the parties involved. The first observation is that most of the healer's patients were peasants like himself. Only one patient came from an urban background: the sister of Mr Costache Prejbeanu from Caracal, who, however, denied having ever met him or used his services.[97] But among Buruiană's patients we also discover a priest and "the wife of Mr Nicolae Provejanu" from the village Giorocelu in the district of Dolj. In the latter case, because of the family's social standing, the healer was called to the patient's bedside: "They sent for him."[98] In most cases, depending on the patient's condition and the distance to the healer's home, it was not the patients themselves who went to see him, but their relatives: of the ten patients who were questioned as part of the inquiry, only two seem to have met him face to face. The husband, the father, or persons referred to simply as "people," took the remedies to the patient, along with the instructions, and supervised the treatment. All the patients testified that they had received the same therapy, administered in the same way. It was the treatment described by the healer to the district doctor: a decoction of herbs boiled in wine, which had a powerful emetic and diuretic effect, and fumigations with dried herbs. Another detail worth mentioning is the fact that most clients were female: of the thirteen documented patients, only three were men.

---

96  ANIC, 31v.
97  ANIC, f. 36v.
98  ANIC, f. 33v.

In terms of the set of symptoms of the conditions treated, the inquiry reports show that they were diverse and, even given the period's levels of knowledge, not all could be classified as mental disorders. For example, Father Ion, the priest of Măceşu village in Dolj district, described his own condition in these terms: his "malady affected only the head, with pain and dizzy spells and trouble seeing."[99] The district doctor, having questioned a few patients among Buruiană's fellow villagers, identified one condition as "a lesion of the spine marrow caused by trauma," another as *"coup de soleil"* (sunstroke), another as "urticaria," and yet another as *"febris lactea"* (milk fever).[100] These were hardly mental conditions.

In his report, the chief medical officer of the county listed only Buruiană's empirical remedies. All other aspects of the therapy were ignored, probably because they were considered irrelevant for the healing process. Obviously, the deputy prefects engaged less with the dominant medical culture than their medical peers. Consequently, their reports made references to aspects that doctors left out. One was a type of therapy Buruiană had borrowed from traditional magic medicine: as he started the empirical treatment, the patient was required to bury the clothes he or she had been wearing when they became ill.[101] One can penetrate even deeper into the peasant culture in which Buruiană lived and practiced by looking at the testimonies of the elders of Reda village. These reveal further traditional therapies in which the parish priest mediated sacred practices. In this variant, treatment included the administration of

> [...] herbs three times a day, in the morning, mid-day and evening, and in the evening the priest will read the prayers of St. Basil; each time, 50 grams of herbs cooked in wine are given, and fumigations with other herbs are also applied three times. This is done for two days, and on the second day, in the evening, the priest reads the Lord's Prayer and the prayer of St. Basil when the herbs are given. And the vessel in which the herbs were boiled is then thrown into a river and on the third day he [the patient] rests and is given a little unsalted bread and water for a whole week.[102]

---

99   ANIC, f. 33r.
100  ANIC, f. 36r.-v.
101  ANIC, f. 33r.-v.
102  ANIC, f. 40r.-v.

This shows that the therapeutic process used by the empiric cannot be reconstructed from one source only. The historian must use all the documentary sources left by the professionals and officials who formed the cultural and social elites of "modern Romania." At the top of the hierarchy were the doctors, who, as representatives of the dominant culture, ignored the sacred and magic dimensions of the therapy. The mid-tier included officials in the local and central administration, who, by and large, belonged to the mainstream urban culture, but who, at lower levels, still interacted with peasant culture. On the lower rungs of the hierarchy, at the level of the village, a strong, autonomous peasant culture combined empirical and sacred-magical practices.

Now that we have identified the key individuals and established the facts, we are going to look at the—highly predictable—reaction of the health administrators. The key official who ran the inquiry locally was the district doctor. He met and questioned both sides involved—the healers and the patients—and sent his report to the Inspector-General of the Health Service. The judicial process started at this point. The district doctor from Romanați was ruthless in his prosecution of the Stoian Buruiană case:

> As I have shown above, I concluded that the afore-cited individual does not possess the required knowledge for the treatment of mental alienation, but only inherited this after the death of his father who was said to be able to cure the said malady.[103]

The Medical Council's deliberations on Stoian Buruiană's case in December 1860 were based on a wholesale acceptance of the district doctor's conclusions. Its own final report ended with the following conclusions:

> The named Stoian Popa Ion Buruiană possesses no proficiency in the healing of those suffering from mental alienation. Moreover, he is mistaken in confusing physical maladies and mental alienation, which is a psychological malady, which proves his complete ignorance and charlatanism. The Council is hereby instructing the Health Authority to communicate to the honor. Ministry of the Interior its request for banning the aforementioned from the

---

103 ANIC f. 39r.

exercise of this abusive enterprise. In case of non-compliance, he must be handed the harshest penalty in accordance with the law, both to stop him and to offer an example to others.[104]

This was a harsh decision: despite obvious therapeutic successes, the healer was banned from practicing the "trade" because he did not use the concepts and taxonomy upheld by the period's modern medical science. As a result, he was penalized for his "ignorance" as well as for an even worse crime, "charlatanism." Interestingly, the list of accusations did not include that fact that he did not have a doctoral title or a license to practice in the Principalities, accusations levelled against another peasant healer, Manolake, from Ruşii de Vede, two decades earlier. The latter had been banned from practicing the "physician's craft" because he did not possess the "knowledge of medicine and a doctor's diploma, the only certificate permitting this trade." It is also true that Manolake's patient had died during treatment. The victim was the wife of a local notable, the *serdar*[105] Gheorghe Turnavitul, from a southern region of Teleorman County, who immediately reported the case to the Committee for Quarantines.[106]

Ultimately, Stoian Buruiană was blamed for his lack of knowledge of modern medical practices, a knowledge he could only have acquired by studying for a medical degree. Such a title would have been an emblem of the "science of healing," which, in the official logic, could only be acquired at a European university. But Buruiană was not one of the elect! We do not know whether Stoian Buruiană ever gave up on his "trade." Most probably, he did not.

The other case study is that of Marin Vărzaru, who famously treated rabies. His outcome seems happier. I have already mentioned that the deputy administrator of Neajlov County, who had discovered the healer, had demanded a financial reward for him. The Home Minister, too, had been impressed, and it was possibly because of his enthusiasm that, by mid-February 1860, an award of "five hundred *lei* was deemed appropriate for the named Marin Vărzaru Catană,"[107] a considerable sum of money for a peas-

---

104 ANIC, f. 37r.
105 *Serdar* is a Romanian boyar title.
106 In Romanian: *Comitetul Carantinelor.* Gomoiu, *Din istoria medicinei,* 305–6.
107 ANIC, f. 9r.

ant at the time.[108] However, the officials' enthusiasm was not matched by that of the health authorities. On February 9, 1860, the Health Council met to discuss the Vărzaru affair. But without first-hand information collected at the scene, the Council was unable to do anything more than express its lack of faith in the prowess of the healer from Roata-Cătunu. Firstly, the Council concluded, "If we are to allow that the master villager found a cure, we need palpable evidence that the aforementioned wolf really had rabies when he attacked the village Cătunu-Găureni."[109] The incubation period for rabies could be as long as three months, and the Council had met a little over a month after the events. In addition, the report read, for the Council to be able to make a pronouncement on the case, "it would require the presence of the aforementioned master of hydrophobia and a description of his curative method and his medical materials."[110] And finally, the Medical Council doubted that the wolf had been rabid and that its bite could have been dangerous, which in fact was certainly the case. But the wolf had been killed during the events, and the local administration, which offered 6 lei for the killing of a "wild beast," had not been sent at least the animal's "ears and paws," because the "wolf had rabies."[111] All this was the result of a vicious circle, and the reward had been offered before the collection of the evidence. The only solution was to order a local inquiry led by the district doctor and obtain a "formal" testimony from the village of Babele, confirming whether the wolf had rabies and whether Marin Vărzaru had indeed cured those bitten by the animal. The testimony was easy to obtain. The district medical officer, like his peers in the Medical Council, was inclined to believe that the wolf had not been rabid: "[T]he undersigned believes that the wolf was not rabid, because rabid wolves have not been known to take cattle from village barns; but the medicine prescribed is known and has been tested by doctors."[112] Lack of evidence meant that the case could not be prosecuted. Moreover, the doctors

---

108 To illustrate this, let's look at the year 1862, when the position of borough doctor was created. At that time, a borough doctor's monthly pay (salary plus daily allocation) was 500 lei. See *Monitorul. Jurnal Oficial al Principatelor Unite*, March 31, 1862, no. 73, 304. To keep the comparison closer to exchange values known in the peasant world, here is what Marin Vărzaru would have been able to buy with 500 lei in the "cattle market of the Capital city" on January 2, 1862: five cows, each with its calf—ten cattle in total. For prices, see *Monitorul. Jurnal Oficial*, January 22, 1862, no. 17, 72.

109 ANIC, f. 4r.

110 ANIC, f. 4v.

111 ANIC, f. 2v.

112 ANIC, f. 21v.

were right. Marin Vărzaru kept the money and, as I have been unable to identify any sources in the archives of the Medical Council that show that he had been formally banned from practicing his "trade," I think that he continued to offer treatment for rabies. But Marin Vărzaru's case seems to have been an exception. By 1861, things had changed compared to the more relaxed situation at the start of the century: in 1803, a peasant by the name of Ion Turbatu[113] from the village of Rotunda, in Romanați, who also claimed that he could treat rabies, had been allowed to continue his trade and had even managed to obtain a certificate of tax exemption from the ruling prince.[114]

If we place the two above-mentioned cases side by side, we cannot fail to be surprised by the strangeness of the comparison. The inquiry had gained evidence that Stoian Buruiană, who treated mental conditions, had cured eight out of his ten known patients, and yet the Council banned him from plying his "trade." However, Marin Vărzaru, who treated cases of rabies, was not only able to continue his practice, but also received a considerable financial award. This might suggest that in 1860, the Health Authority under Carol Davila was still far from having complete control over medical practices and that there was still room for negotiation and maneuver. It is noteworthy that the publication, in 1860, of the first list of doctors licensed to practice in the Principalities was not accompanied by a corresponding ban with respect to other categories of healers who wished to practice their "craft." It was not until 1862 that the Health Authority intervened by declaring that "according to the legislation in force, no one is free to treat the sick and prescribe medicine, and no pharmacist is free to dispense [that] medicine whose name is not on the published list."[115] To this end, copies of the list of authorized doctors were displayed in pharmacies.

Documents from 1860 to 1862 reveal that there was a continued negotiation between the Health Authority and various categories of healers, who could not be placed on the select list of trained doctors, but who claimed that, before the arrival of Carol Davila, they had been free to practice their "trade." Here is the example of two brothers who petitioned to the Health Authority for the right to practice as

---

113 Like the surname Buruiană, meaning "weed," the surname Turbatu suggests the individual's occupation: in Romanian, it means "rabid, infected with rabies."
114 Samarian, *Medicina și farmacia în trecutul românesc*, 313.
115 *Monitorul. Jurnal Oficial*, February 3, 1862, no. 25, 102.

[...] doctors who had specialized in the practical treatment of rabies, a right which has been guaranteed to us by all former Governments, from Prince Caragea until today, as shown in the Princely Decrees and many other governmental papers in our possession, [as well] as from testimonies from the authorities in places where we treated the sick.[116]

To have their old rights confirmed, they asked to undergo a practical examination consisting in healing one patient. I do not know whether there was any follow-up on their application. Another example is that of Stoica Bălănescu from the suburb Broştenilor in Bucharest, who in June 1860 made an application to the health authorities for the right to treat epilepsy according to his own method, which he had used from 1851 "until today."[117] Cautious as ever, the Medical Council asked him to prove his skills by healing three patients at the Mărcuţa Institute, under medical supervision.[118] From this point onwards, things got complicated for Stoica Bălănescu, who asked for time and tried to find new allies. The patients were taken from Mărcuţa to Colţea Hospital, but the healer failed to turn up and asked for the patients to be moved again, to Spitalul Brâncovenesc Hospital, because, he explained, "I was previously engaged to attend to patients there."[119] But Brâncovenesc Hospital declined to take in patients suffering from epilepsy. Bălănescu decided to make a joint application to practice with a certain N. Apoloni, another healer who specialized in epilepsy. In May 1861, the Council considered the application from Bălănescu & Associates, who this time requested medical supervision, not in a hospital, but in the patients' home. This was rejected because of the nature of the condition. But the petitions continued, and, in October 1861, the Medical Council rejected the application once again and notified the "petitioning gentlemen that, if they do not comply and continue with their treatments of epilepsy, they are going to be found guilty of endangering public health."[120]

We might think that this was the end of the saga of Stoica Bălănescu's petitioning. But in 1865, he renewed his never-ending campaign to obtain the right to practice, this time in association with another empiric, Panait

---

116 ANIC, f. 18r.
117 ANIC, f. 42r.
118 ANIC, f. 44r.
119 ANIC, f. 59r.
120 ANIC, f. 88v.

Stoenescu, who treated rabies. In January 1866, the Medical Council finally decided to end the affair with a trenchant decree:

> [T]he application by Mr Bălănescu and Mr Stoenescu is rejected as without merit and […] the gentlemen themselves as persons with no right to practice the art of medicine, will be stopped from committing such abuse in the future, and will be prosecuted for their past criminal activities and ordered to pay damages to all those whose credulity was exploited by the aforementioned Mr Bălănescu and Mr Stoenescu.[121]

The tactic employed by the urbanite Stoian Bălănescu differed from that of the rural healers Marin Vărzaru and Stoian Buruiană. They were all empirics who had specialized in well-defined conditions, but, whereas the rural healers were discovered by the authorities, Bălănescu seems to have approached them at his own initiative. He was a combative individual and used every means he could think of to have his right to practice recognized. It is quite clear that Bălănescu tried to adapt to the new legal framework of medical practice in the Principalities by starting a war of petitions with the Health Authority, which he ultimately lost. But the war lasted no less than six years, during which the Medical Council did not formally ban his practices. We may wonder whether it might have been more profitable for him to continue practicing clandestinely, like most empirics in 1860s Bucharest. He obviously believed that, in absence of a medical degree, one way of having his art validated was by offering evidence of a successful therapy. Medicine considered itself to be an art as well as a science.

Let's remember that, before the 1870s and the emergence of experimental medicine, medical practice was the arena for a multiplicity of competing medical doctrines, which often contradicted each other, as Lidia Trăuşan-Matu has shown in her well-documented study.[122] It must have been a baffling situation for the practitioner, who had to cut through the noise and reconcile the alternative medical catechisms, often by using his intuition. A medical practitioner must have at times felt that he was nothing more than a gifted soothsayer.[123] In this context, was it not possible that individu-

---

121 *Monitorul Medical*, year V, 1866, no. 6, 44.

122 Trăuşan-Matu, *De la leac la reţetă*, 119–216.

123 Léonard, *La France médicale. Médecins et malades au XIXe siècle*, 122–25.

als outside the medical profession might have devised and used new therapies successfully? The medical authorities did not initially deny the possibility, but became increasingly suspicious of such cases. I have not been able to
find one single case of a healer who managed to persuade Carol Davila and
the members of the Medical Council that he or she had found and practiced
an effective healing method.

As I have suggested, after 1860 the Health Authority started an offensive against non-professional healers of every category. This was the start of
concerted attempts by the narrow circles of medical professionals to obtain
the monopoly of health care in Romania. Almost overnight, all the other urban and rural healers—empirics, charlatans, orthopaedists, and oculists—
turned from honorable individuals into pariahs. Until then, some of these
healers had been integrated and had been operating in the official health
system. Such was the case of a certain Christea Ianotul from the village of
Aleşii Ciocăneşti, in the Ilfov district, who, until 1859, had been employed
as an "oculist with the former Health Committee."[124] He appears to have
continued practicing even after this date. I have some information on his
activities from the historian of medicine Pompei Samarian. He appears to
have started his career around 1830: from an application for tax exemption,
which he sent to the Treasury, we learn that he was involved in "commerce,"
but that he had also worked as an "eye doctor," in which capacity he had
cured over one hundred patients. His application was forwarded to the Physicians' Commission[125] and, luckily for him, the doctor appointed to verify
his skills was a fellow Greek, doctor Estioti. The latter wrote a glowing report in which he recommended that the applicant be granted the license
to practice. The application had a positive outcome, and Christea Ianotul
embarked on a successful career; he settled in Bucharest, where he practiced freely and held a paid position at the Committee for Quarantines until
1845.[126] His downfall came late in life, when his practice of over thirty years
was suddenly no longer tolerated. A complaint against him was sent to the
Health Authority by doctor Fiala, secondary doctor and oculist at Colţea
Hospital. Doctor Fiala complained that Ianotul "lacked all knowledge of the
anatomy and diseases of the eye, for which reason through his ill-advised

---

124 *Supliment la Monitorul Oficial*, July 14, 1860, no. 166, 778.
125 In Romanian: *Comisia doctoricească*.
126 Samarian, *Medicina şi farmacia în trecutul românesc*, 316–19.

procedures he appears to have harmed patients,"[127] and consequently he was banned from practicing. Interestingly, the rationale for the ban included an acknowledgement of the public service provided by empirics. The Health Authority recognized the usefulness of an empiric's activity as long as there were no specialized medical personnel: an empiric was better than nothing. But, once professional doctors became available, their empirical competitors had to accept that they had to withdraw without making a fuss.

It is noteworthy that the Health Authority only took an interest in cases where empirics claimed that they had found a treatment for hitherto incurable diseases such as rabies, epilepsy, insanity, etc. Those who made claims for conditions considered treatable by mainstream medicine were even less likely to succeed. Such was the case, for example, of Tudora, the wife of Nedelcu Slobozeanu from Călăraşi, in Ialomiţa district. She claimed to be able to cure "ragpicker's disease or sheep's scab."[128] Unluckily for her, the Medical Council considered that

> [...] the art of medicine possesses the medicinal and surgical means of combatting ragpicker's disease (Anthrax), and, as the district employed two doctors, the distr[ict] doctor and the city's doctor, sufferers could seek their competent services rather than resort to help of a doubtful quality from an empiric.[129]

By now, doctors had a full awareness of their professional monopoly over health care, and were no longer prepared to tolerate competition. A sustained witch-hunt was launched against empirics. To help in this campaign, the central health authorities gave new powers to the new borough doctors[130] and to district doctors. Among other roles, the borough doctor, a position created by Carol Davila in 1862, was supposed to "take measures against the spread of medical charlatan practices in his borough, and to communicate offenses to the district chief medical officer."[131] District doctors, too, had to make sure that "nobody practiced the medical or pharmaceutical arts and their sub-disciplines [...] without authorization from the General

127  *Supliment la Monitorul Oficial*, July 14, 1860, no. 166, 778.
128  In Romanian: "*dalacul sau buba oii.*"
129  ANIC, f. 78r.)
130  In Romanian: "*medici de arondisment.*"
131  *Monitorul. Jurnal Oficial al Principatelor-Unite*, April 2, 1862, no. 74, 309.

Directorate."[132] But these specifications for the two positions were no longer listed in the 1874 Health Act. Could this suggest that an armistice had been reached in the meantime?

Whereas doctors had acquired a monopoly on health care, pharmacists tried to obtain a monopoly on the preparation of medicines and the issuing of prescriptions. Their competitors were herbalists, chemists, and grocers. They had the doctors as their allies. However, their alliance with doctors was fraught with tensions of a financial nature: pharmacists were known to issue prescriptions signed by non-medics, a practice the Health Authority condemned in 1862.[133] The preparation of drugs and the issuing of prescriptions were bound to be at the forefront of modernization in the health system. The central administration, represented by the Minister of the Interior, Dimitrie Ghica, recommended the middle ground. Healers were not to be rejected "in an absolute manner" if they proposed remedies that proved effective in some cases. But "unfortunately, despite all recommendations, there are still individuals who, without special knowledge, administer medication without a second thought for compromising the lives of people who placed their trust in them."[134] These individuals were not to be tolerated.

The Health Authority and the central state administration mobilized themselves against the illegal medical practitioners. We do not know whether the threats they launched materialized into actual fines or prison sentences. Article 77 of the first modern Health Act (1874) stipulated that "anyone found to be practicing medicine, pharmacy, and veterinary medicine against the above legal norms will incur a fine of between 100 and 1,000 *lei* or a prison sentence of between 17 days and six months."[135] Slowly but steadily, the efforts of the Health Authority bore fruit: year after year, the number of trained doctors increased and that of empirics went down. Some of the specialized categories of empirics, such as oculists, disappeared altogether by the end of the nineteenth century.[136] At least that was the opinion of doctor Felix at the end of his career.

In conclusion, in the mid-nineteenth century the medicalization of the Romanian society was still in its early stages: the only section of the popu-

---

132 *Monitorul. Jurnal Oficial al Principatelor-Unite*, November 9, 1862, no. 248, 1030.

133 *Monitorul. Jurnal Oficial*, February 3, 1862, no. 25, 102.

134 *Monitorul. Jurnal Oficial al Ţării Româneşti*, October 2, 1860, no. 216, 853.

135 *Monitorul Oficial al României* 16, June 28, 1874, no. 131, 836.

136 Felix, "Alcoolismul poporaţiunei rurale în comparaţiune cu alcoolismul poporaţiunei urbane," 54.

lation that was thoroughly aware of the importance of national health was the top echelon of the medical profession. As we descend the social ladder, the degree of hygiene awareness decreases. Finally, in the eyes of the peasant, the doctor was just an exotic figure and a disloyal competitor to the rural healer. The rural world had yet to discover the benefits of the early modernization of the health system, as described by Lidia Trăușan-Matu.[137]

---

137 Trăușan-Matu, *De la leac la rețetă*, 395–98.

# CONCLUSIONS

One of the main questions that today's historian must address is the following: what is the relationship between representations of the peasant and the rural world in late nineteenth-century medical texts and the social realities they were supposed to reflect? This question arises from the powerful sense of otherness that the historian experiences from reading the narrative sources. As we have seen, the doctors' overall picture of the rural world was extremely negative. It comprised physical decline, poverty, a lack of education, disease, and death. Today, the author of this study lives and works in an ambient culture that looks at the peasant from a different perspective: far from being the "savage other" within, the peasant has turned into the archetypal good Romanian. This shift in perspective began in the period considered in this study, but not everybody was convinced at the time. Today, nobody can write about the peasant in the way some doctors did in 1880 without causing a furore. What has changed in the meantime? Another question ... But perhaps it is time to stop asking questions and attempt some affirmatives.

From my early contacts with the hygienist literature, I had a sense that there was something disingenuous about it. Or rather, I had the sense that the authors made sweeping negative generalizations about a reality that was in fact multiform and complex. But, I thought, trying to present the generic peasant, as doctors did, surely involved extracting the essentials from the average. Yet, there was a problem: from the multitude of peasants they encountered, doctors seemed to pick the most deprived among them for their narratives. In the medical literature of the late nineteenth century, the peasant world was quintessentially a world of social deprivation. This was a narrative choice that I wished to challenge. Doctors did not simply describe the factual reality as it presented itself: their gaze was selective, it foregrounded some figures while leaving others to hover vaguely on the margins of their discourse. Nowadays, we know that no gaze is innocent: describing social reality always involves a distortion. The doctors' descriptions were no exception.

The emergence of modernity in Romania was punctuated by the medical discourse about the peasant and the rural world. I discovered this fact when reading a recent study by Constanța Vintilă-Ghițulescu[1]: the medical discourse, multi-faceted and generous in the early of the nineteenth century, remained equally positive after 1860. But discourses evolve. Let's remember that all the themes analyzed in the second part of this study received a different treatment in 1880 and in 1900. It is true, however, that the conclusions remained the same, a sign that, although the form of the discourse changed, its rationale remained the same. Nevertheless, at least in some cases, the availability of statistical data eventually reduced the gap between representation and hard fact simply by placing facts in a long-term perspective. Think, for example, of descriptions of the peasant dwellings: until the early twentieth century, the imagery that doctors used was impressionistic and centered on the "hygienic ills" of the hovel. And yet, the hovel was not simply a "hole" in the ground, a "grave" for the living dead or a "den" adapted to the needs of its peasant inhabitants. The hovel was, in fact, a specific type of human habitation. And, while in the early twentieth century doctors started to recognize this, they continued to denigrate it. The census of 1912 contains a wide range of information on rural dwellings. It reveals something that the doctors should have known from their first-hand contacts with this environment: the peasant's dwellings were multiform structures that varied greatly in terms of building materials and techniques. Doctors did not document the extended hovel structure, which most probably existed, because their representations were fixated on the image of the hovel-as-human-grave.

In a similar way, other aspects of the rural habitat were marginalized or distorted. Doctors ended up by making improbable claims about the bodily hygiene of their co-nationals: in their opinion, peasants never washed their

---

[1]   Vintilă-Ghițulescu, *Evgheniți, ciocoi, mojici*, 297–327.

bodies, as they never washed their clothes. They did not always use soap, but they did use a lye-based laundry cleaner made from wood ashes. It is hard to believe that these doctors had not seen peasant women wash their laundry at the river or hanging it to dry on fences. But the discourse had to obey its own rules: once it became the established representation, a peasant world of suffering, squalor, and death did not square with images of tidy houses and peasants neatly dressed in their Sunday best. A separate discourse was created for this latter version of the rural world. In this discourse, the annual calendar of religious and "life-cycle" festivals was cited as evidence of our Latin origins, the peasant's miserable garments became picturesque ethnic costumes sported by elite ladies, and the squalid dwellings became museum displays of carved wood pillars and handmade embroideries. In this discourse, the paradigm of the gaze shifted, transforming the peasant from primitive other to native emblem of the nation.[2]

At the end of the nineteenth and the beginning of the twentieth century, these two competing representations coexisted in public discourse in Romania. Such contrasting imagery of the same object may surprise today's observer. The sustained way in which the dominant culture manipulated the image of the peasant was another facet of the "rural question" that haunted Romanian society in the second half of the nineteenth century.

Let's return to the medical discourse, which, as we have seen, marginalized certain aspects of social reality that might have, if not undermined it, at least added some nuances to it. I have always wondered why the period's set of images of the peasant world was so negative. How close to reality were doctors' representations of the peasant? My suspicions were confirmed quite quickly: while taking the peasant world as its starting point, the imagery generated by an algorithm proper to the medical discourse soon departed from it. As for the reasons why this should have happened, my first hypothesis prompted me to look at the rapport between author and intended readership. I hypothesized that doctors created an imagery specifically for the use of the political class: the social impact of the health and sanitary conditions in the rural environment was highlighted to alert this class to the needs of the huge rural masses in a country undergoing modernization. I was right to some extent. But, if this was the objective, the tone of

---

2   Mihăilescu, *Antropologie*, 263–330.

the medical narratives, which was often dismissive of the peasant's lifestyle, was hardly justified. The texts demonstrated compassion, it is true, but often they also revealed the barely concealed contempt doctors felt for these masses and their misery. Only rarely did doctors try to empathize with the peasant and understand his behavior.

Doctors, like other members of the elites, considered the peasant to be an 'inferior species', uneducated, stubborn, lazy, and malevolent. Problematically, as it represented 80 per cent of Romania's population, this population had to be transformed, modernized, civilized. There is significant evidence of the elites' deep incomprehension for the peasant way of life. I shall give two examples, both of a normative nature. We know that cattle were laboring animals for the peasant, therefore not to be slaughtered for food. It was only gradually, and much later, that beef, and especially veal, was accepted in the peasant diet. But the regulations of rural hospitals ignored this taboo, and beef was often served to patients.[3] I can only imagine the horror peasants felt upon learning that they had consumed beef while in hospital. This kind of cultural insensitivity must have done little to bolster the much-talked-about 'bridges' between peasants and the modern health service, which the medical profession claimed it was promoting.

The second example is the model of peasant dwelling the health authorities tried to impose by fiat in 1888: the regulations prescribed a separation between cooking areas and sleeping quarters,[4] which was not the structure traditionally used by peasants. Nobody, however, wanted to hear about the barbarous peasant habits. The elites tried to impose their norms, but they often failed. They deemed that the peasant had to be modernized and turned into a citizen. But the elite's modernizing projects were blocked by the often passive resistance of a reluctant peasantry. The peasantry had always been—and still is—a deeply anti-modern social group, justifiably so. After all, what did modernization mean for the rural world other than a deep transformation, which led to the total disruption of the peasants' way of life. It was synonymous with the disappearance of a traditional, pre-modern lifestyle. What type of community would not resist such a radical change? What were the benefits of modernization for the peasant world? Some would say

---

3    Șuta et al., 285–88.
4    Ibid., 296.

the allocation of land, which, starting with Alexandru Ioan Cuza's reforms, turned the serf into a landowner. It is a good argument, but not entirely convincing, because the reforms involved only a small section of the peasantry.

G. D. Creangă, an expert on the history of rural property in early twentieth-century Romania, argued that, despite a succession of land reforms between 1864 and 1905, the state failed to turn the new landowners into "well-off peasants, good citizens, brave soldiers, and law-abiding taxpayers."[5] It is quite possible that Mr Creangă was simply trying to discredit the social work promoted by the liberals because he had more conservative views. This may well be the case, but statistical data show that 291,771 heads of families, i.e. "31.68 per cent of the entire peasantry, now own[ed] small plots of 2 hectares," which meant that one third of peasants had "acreages which in the current circumstances are not sufficient to provide a peasant family with the *bare necessities of dry nourishment: bread and mămăligă*, not to mention the wherewithal to pay for meat, vegetables, clothes, taxes and other needs."[6] Bread? The same author considered that only peasants owning between seven and ten hectares of land were "relatively better-off and less dependent on landowners and leaseholders," but this category only amounted to 4.24 per cent of the rural population.[7]

In conclusion, when examined from the angle of landownership, the situation of the peasantry in 1905 appears disastrous. One third of peasants lived below subsistence levels, which suggests that doctors' descriptions of a peasant world of poverty, disease, and death is more accurate than I thought. Poverty was omnipresent and eclipsed the small group of peasants who enjoyed a measure of economic independence and even moderate affluence. Doctors were not interested in this group. One can only conclude that, in their majority, peasants benefitted very little, if at all, from the successive land reforms of the last decades of the nineteenth century. For these masses, modernization equaled a steady descent into even greater poverty, as suggested by the following testimonies from the early twentieth century. Ion Năbărogu was a ninety-year-old peasant from the village Poroschia in Teleorman County. He had his own views on the current developments. For him, pauperization had started in 1848:

5    Creangă, *Proprietatea rurală în România*, XXXVIII.
6    Ibid., LI.
7    Ibid., LV–LVI.

In the old days I had dairy cows, a hundred or two of sheep, some twenty bee-hives, and horses, as many as one could wish; and now I am as poor as a church mouse; no milk, no honey, there's nothing left, and this only because of the liberty [of 1848], when much bad was done, it is all bad now and it's not going to be good if the governors in Bucharest pay no heed.[8]

We might think that Ion Năbărogu was just a disillusioned old man looking back nostalgically upon his lost youth, but there are similar comments from younger peasants. Dandu Dina Duță from Mofleni, Dolj County, was only fifty-two, and he, too, had a negative view of the developments of the last four decades of the nineteenth century:

It was better in the times of the Turk, when I labored twelve days every year and gave a tithe in corn, nothing else. I spent the nights with the cattle in orchards 'til Saint George, and returned there when the fruit were back on the trees and nobody was bothered. I was in the field 'til mid-day and nobody asked where I was coming from or going. I carried wood back from the forest and still nobody asked. I mowed and ploughed where I wanted. And now, we are surrounded by the state everywhere, we can't move. The Turk kept his word, he was good, the poor Turk; he gave laws and kept them.[9]

Ioan Aurel Candrea, Ovid Densusianu, and Theodor Sperantia collected numerous such testimonies in the early years after 1900, and, luckily for the historian, they published them.

Returning to the explanations for the negative representations of the peasant world, I have considered the fact that this imagery was largely constructed with the aim of appealing to the political class. It is worth noting, however, that it also carried the imprint of the authors' own mind-sets. If the representations were so negative, it was because doctors perceived the peasant world in a negative light, something that today would be inconceivable.

At the end of the nineteenth century, Romania was a two-tiered country: it was inhabited by two "peoples," as doctor Vasile Sion called them, one rural and the other urban.[10] These two communities faced each other across

---

8    Candrea, Densusianu, and Sperantia, *Graiul nostru,* 142.
9    Ibid., 49.
10   Sion, "Asistența medicală în România rurală," 240.

a wide divide: one produced the "sacksful of grain,"[11] the foundation of Romania's modernity, the other consumed it; one governed, the other was governed; one was civilized, the other primitive. The only relations of reciprocity were based on hatred, a lack of trust, and disdain. In 1900, Romania was a country divided by a massive social landslide, a nation sitting astride two worlds: the world of the rural masses, which the state failed to modernize through a lack of means and political willpower, and the world of the urbanites, who, as the playwright I. L. Caragiale contended, have tried, ever since 1848, to mold Romania into a modern European country. The elites created modern Romania in their own image, but they failed to make this image acceptable to the broader sections of the nation. Hence the fragility of modern Romania's social body, so tragically demonstrated by the repressed peasant rebellion of 1907. I believe that, to understand the Romanian society during the latter half of the nineteenth century, today's historian must step across the chasm separating the two worlds and look at the peasant world with empathy and a readiness to explore its guiding life values and principles. Once this happens, the peasant will cease to be the doctors' 'barbarian' and become instead a human being of flesh and blood, with beliefs, habits, loves and hatreds—a person like all others, a human like us.

---

11  Zeletin, *Burghezia română. Originea și rolul ei istoric*, 107.

# BIBLIOGRAPHY

## Primary Sources

Agappi, V. I. *Cercetări demografice asupra populațiunii României și în special a districtului și orașului Iași* [Demographic studies on the population of Romania, with an emphasis on the district and city of Iași]. Bucharest: Tipografia Laboratorilor Romani, 1876.

Alesandrini, N. A. *Statistica României, de la Unirea Principatelor până în prezent* [The statistics of Romania from the union of the principalities to the present day], vol. I–II. Iași: Tipo-Litografia H. Goldner, 1895.

Antonescu, V. "Din raportul unui medic de circumscripție" ["Report of a district doctor"]. *Buletinul Direcțiunei Generale a Serviciului Sanitar*, year XXI, no. 14 (1909): 381–85.

Antoniu, I. *Cercetări asupra stărei țăranului român* [Studies on the condition of the Romanian peasant]. Bârlad: Tipografia George Cațafany, 1881.

Antoniu, I. *Traité de la pellagre*. Bucharest: Sotchek et C^ie Libraires-Éditeurs, 1887.

Apostoleanu, I. "Mortalitatea copiilor în România" ["Child mortality in Romania"]. *Buletinul Medical. Organ al Asociațiunei Generale a Medicilor din Țară*, year V, no. 25 (1902): 5–7, and no. 26, 3–4.

Augustin, I. "Raport general asupra serviciului sanitar din judetul Gorj, pe anul 1886, adresat direcțiunei serviciului sanitar" ["General report on the health services in Gorj county for 1886, addressed to the health directorate"]. *Monitorul Oficial*, October 10 (1887): 3602–6.

Aurelian, P. S. *Terra nostra. Schițe economice asupra României* [Terra Nostra: Essays on the economy of Romania], 2nd ed. Bucharest: Tipografia Academiei Române, 1880.

Babeș, A., and V. Bușilă. *Cercetări originale despre pelagra în România* [New studies on pellagra in Romania]. In *Publicațiunile Fondului Vasile Adamachi*, vol. VI, no. XXXIX. Bucharest: Librăriile Socec & Comp., C. Sfetea, Pavel Suru, 1915.

Babeș, Victor. *Regenerarea poporului român* [The regeneration of the Romanian nation]. Bucharest: Stabilimentul grafic I.V. Socec, 1901.

Babeș, Victor. "Raport asupra alimentațiunei României cu apă de băut" ["Report on the drinking water supply in Romania"]. *România medicală întrunită cu Presa medicală română*, year XI, nos. 15–16 (1906): 337–61.

Babeș, Victor. *Studii asupra pelagrei* [Studies on pellagra]. Bucharest: Librăria Socec & Comp., 1911.

Babeș, Victor. *Pelagra*. Bucharest: Editura "Cartea Românească," no date.

Baer, C. *Considerațiuni generale asupra locuințelor rurale în România* [General observations on rural dwellings in Romania]. Iași: Tip. Națională, 1897.

Bejan, V. "Raport asupra activității secțiunei a IV-a de ambulanță militară-rurală Botoșani-Dorohoi. De la 1 iunie până la 1 septembrie 1886" ["Report on the activities of Section IV of the military-rural ambulance service, Botoșani-Dorohoi, from June 1 to September 1, 1886"]. *Spitalul*, year VI, no. 11 (1886): 427–38, and no. 12, 480–90.

Bianu, V. "Serviciul sanitar al Plasei Bistriţa de Sus jud. Bacău de la 1 ianuarie până la 1 octombrie 1882" ["The health services of the district Bistriţa de Sus, Bacău, from January 1 to October 1, 1882"]. *Spitalul*, year II, no. XI (1882): 333–38, and no. XII, 365–69.

Bianu, V. "Spitalul rural Horezu. Raport sciinţific pe anul 1888" ["The rural hospital in Horezu. A scientific report for 1888"]. *Buletinul Direcţiunei Generale a Serviciului Sanitar*, no. 17 (1889): 275–82, no. 18, 289–97, no. 21, 343–47.

Bianu, Vasile. *Doctorul de casă sau dicţionarul sănătăţii* [The family doctor, or a medical dictionary]. Buzău: Imprimeria Al. Georgescu, 1910.

Bianu, Vasile. Însemnari din războiul României Mari [Notes from the war for greater Romania]. Vol. I, "De la mobilizare până la pacea de la Bucureşti" ["From mobilization to the peace of Bucharest"]. Cluj: Institutul de Arte Grafice "Ardealul," 1926.

Bibicescu, Ioan G. "Mişcarea poporaţiunii Capitalei în 1873" ["Population trends in the capital in 1873"]. *Românul*, year XVIII, December 23–24 (1874): 1128, and December 25–27, 1132.

Bibicescu, Ioan G. *Mişcarea poporaţiunii în România de la 1870 până la 1878* [Population trends in Romania from 1870 to 1878]. Bucharest: Tipografia "Românul," 1880.

Bordea, I. *Serviciul sanitar al României şi igiena publică între anii 1905–1922* [The health services in Romania and public health in 1905–1922]. Bucharest: Tip. "Cultura," 1924.

Bordea, I. *Zile trăite. Din amintirile unui fost medic rural* [A life as it was lived: The memoirs of a former rural doctor]. Bucharest: Institutul de Arte Grafice "Eminescu" S. A., 1938.

Burghele, N. *Amintiri din timpul războiului român-bulgar din 1913* [Souvenirs from the Romanian-Bulgarian war of 1913]. Bucharest: Noua Tipografie Profesională, Dimitrie C. Ionescu, 1913.

Buşilă, Vladimir. "Epidemia de febră tifoidă din Iaşi. Raport prezintat D-lui Ministru de Interne" ["The typhoid epidemic in Iaşi: A report to the home minister"]. *Buletinul Direcţiunei Generale a Serviciului Sanitar*, year XXI, no. 15 (1909): 409–15.

Candrea, I. A., Ov. Densuşianu, and Th. D. Speranţia. *Graiul nostru. Texte din toate părţile locuite de români* [Our language: Texts from all regions inhabited by the Romanians], vol. I, "România." Bucharest: Atelierele Grafice Socec & Co., 1906.

Carp, I. "Dare de seamă asupra stărei sanitare în Regimentul 1 Mehedinţi, no. 17 pe anul 1900–1901" ["Medical report for regiment I Mehedinţi no. 17 for the year 1900–1901"]. *Revista Sanitară Militară*, year V, nos. 6–7 (1902): 375–85.

Cazacu, P. "Locuinţele sătenilor" ["The villagers' dwellings"]. *Viaţa Românească*, year I, vol. III (bound volume) (1906): 540–51.

Călinescu, M. D. "Propunere de a se prevedea băi pe lângă toate noile clădiri şcolare rurale" ["A proposal for installing bathrooms in rural schools"]. *Spitalul*, year XXVII (bound volume) (1907): 205–7.

Cealic. "Nicolae Manolescu." *Spitalul*, year XXX (bound volume) (1910): 451–53.

Chernbah, Radu. "Alimentaţia bolnavilor în spitale" ["The diet of hospital patients"]. *Spitalul*, year XXV (bound volume) (1905): 401–4, 431–35.

Chernbach, Radu. "Câteva scurte observaţii practice asupra serviciului de spital comun general de provincie cu un singur serviciu" ["Practical observations on provincial one-department hospitals"]. *Spitalul*, year XXX (bound volume) (1910): 621–29.

Chintescu. "Raport general asupra serviciului sanitar din judeţul Dolj pe anul 1887, adresat direcţiunei generale a serviciului sanitar" ["General report on health services in Dolj county for 1887, addressed to the Health Directorate"]. *Monitorul Oficial*, August 2 (1888): 2404–5.

Ciobanoff, Christu R. *Despre pellagra* [About pellagra]. Bucharest: Tipografia "Svoboda," 1874.

Clement, E. "Raport ştiinţific asupra cazurilor constatate şi tratate precum şi despre modul funcţionării ambulanţei rurale Ilfov-Ialomiţa" ["Report on diagnosed and treated cases and the operation of the rural ambulance service in Ilfov-Ialomiţa"]. *Spitalul*, year VI, no. 8 (1886): 281–94.

Coridaly, Panteleon. "Studii phisice asupra districtului Ismail" ["Studies on the population of Ismail district"]. *Monitorul Medical*, year II, no. 23 (1863): 182–83, and no. 24, 186.

Colesco, Leonida. "Le mouvement de la population de la Roumanie en 1911." *Buletinul Statistic al României*, series III, nos. 26–27 (1912): 646–67.

Colesco, L. *La population de religion mosaïque en Roumanie. Etude statistique.* Bucharest: Imprimeries "Independența," 1915.

Colescu, L. *Statistica clădirilor și locuințelor din România întocmită pe baza recensământului general al populațiunii din 19 decembrie 1912/1 ianuarie 1913* [A statistic of buildings and dwellings in Romania based on the census of December 19, 1912/January 1, 1913]. Bucharest: Cartea Românească, 1920.

Constantinescu, C. *Contribuțiune la studiul pellagrei* [A contribution to the study of pellagra]. Bucharest: Tipo-Litografia Eduard Wiegard, 1887.

Crăiniceanu, Gheorghe. *Igiena țăranului român. Locuința, încălțămintea și îmbrăcămintea. Alimentațiunea în diferite regiuni al țării și în diferite timpuri ale anului* [The hygiene of the Romanian peasant: His dwelling, footwear and clothes; His alimentation in different regions by season]. Bucharest: Lito-tipografia Carol Göbl, 1895.

Crăiniceanu. "Dare de seamă asupra stărei sanitare a Regimentului Constanța, no. 34 pe anul 1897/8" ["Medical report on the regiment of Constanța, no. 34 for 1897/8"]. *Revista Sanitară Militară,* year III, no. 6 (1899): 358–64.

Crăiniceanu. "Raport General asupra stărei sanitare a Regimentului Prahova no. 7 de la 1 oct. 1901-1 octombre 1902 și a serviciului medical al garnizoanei Ploești" ["General medical report on the regiment of Prahova no. 67 for October 1, 1901 to October 1, 1902, and on the health service of the Ploiești Garrison"]. *Revista Sanitară Militară,* year VII, no. 1 (1905): 45–50, and no. 2, 101–6.

Crăinician, Gheorghe. *Literatura medicală românească. Biografii și bibliografie* [Romanian medical literature: Biographies and a bibliography]. Bucharest: Institutul de Arte Grafice "Progresul," 1907.

Creangă, G. D. *Proprietatea rurală în România* [Rural property in Romania]. Bucharest: Instit. De Arte Grafice "Carol Göbl," 1907.

Cruceanu, Mihail. "Dare de seamă asupra epidemiei de scarlatină care a bântuit în comunele Măgureni și Călinești, din județul Prahova" ["Report on the scarlet fever epidemic in the communes Măgureni and Călinești, Prahova County"]. *Buletinul Direcțiunei Generale a Serviciului Sanitar,* year XI, nos. 15 and 16 (1899): 240–43.

Cuza, A. C. *Monopolul alcoolului* [The monopoly on alcohol]. Bucharest: Imprimeria Statului, 1895.

Cuza, A. C. *Victimele alcoolului. Documente sociale* [The victims of alcohol: Social documents]. Iași: Tipografia Națională, 1899.

Dănescu, Ioan. *Încercări de demografie și geografie medicală* [Essays on medical demography and geography]. Bucharest: Tipografia Curții Regale, 1886.

Demostene, Atanasie. "Câteva cuvinte asupra apei cea de toate zilele" ["Observations on daily water"]. *Spitalul,* year XXIII (bound volume) (1903): 667–71.

Drăgescu, I. C. *Igiena poporană* [Popular hygiene]. Constanța: Tipografia Romana D. Nicolaescu, 1886.

Drăgescu, I.C. "Raportul D-lui medic primar al județului Dolj no. 1719 din 9 septembrie 1900, relativ la răspândirea culturii legumelor și fabricarea pânei la sate" ["Report of the Chief Medical Officer of Dolj County no. 1719 of September 9, 1900, on the spread of vegetable cultivation and bakeries in villages"]. *Buletinul Direcțiunei Generale a Serviciului Sanitar,* year XII, no. 9 (1900): 259–60.

Drăgoșescu, B. "Băile populare" ["The public baths"]. *Revista Științelor Medicale,* year IV, vol. I, no. 4 (1908): 397–404.

Drăgoșescu, B. "Puțuri igienice" ["Hygienic drinking wells"]. *Buletinul Direcțiunei Generale a Serviciului Sanitar,* year XXI, no. 12 (1909): 317–23.

Felix, I. "Despre nutrimentul țăranilor" ["On the nutrition of peasants"]. *Monitorul. Jurnal oficial al Principatelor-Unite,* no. 88, April 21 (1862): 365–66.

Felix, I. "Observațiuni asupra pellagri în județul Mușcel" ["Observations on pellagra in Mușcel County"]. *Monitorul Medical al României,* year I, no. 2 (1862): 16, and no. 3, 22–24.

Felix, I. *Servițiul sanitar al comunei Bucuresci. Raport general pe anul 1869* [The health services of the commune of Bucharest: General report for the year 1869]. Bucharest: Tipografia Ion Weiss, 1870.

Felix, I. *Tractat de hygiena publică și poliția sanitară*, partea I [A treatise on public hygiene and health policies, part one]. Bucharest: Tipografia Ion Weiss, 1870.

Felix, I. *Raport general pe anul 1875* [General report for the year 1875]. Bucharest: Typographia Curții (Lucrătorii Asociați), 1876.

Felix, I. *Raport general pe anul 1876* [General report for the year 1876]. Bucharest: Typographia Curții (Lucrătorii Asociați) F. Göbl, 1877.

Felix, I. "Mortalitatea în Capitală" [Mortality in the capital city]. *Revista Sciintifica*, year IX, no. 15 (1878): 225–27.

Felix, I. *Sur la prophylaxie de la pellagre. Rapport.* Geneva: Imprimerie de la "Tribune," 1882.

Felix, I. *Prophylaxia pelagrei* [The prevention of pellagra]. Bucharest: Tipografia Academiei Române (Laboratorii Români), 1883.

Felix, I. "Raportul D-lui I. Felix, membrul Consiliului Sanitar Superior, asupra inspecțiunei serviciului sanitar din circumscripția I a județelor Suceava, Dorohoi, Botoșani și Iași, în anul 1886, către D. Ministru de Interne" ["Report by Dr. I. Felix, member in the higher medical council, on the health inspection in the 1st circumscription of the counties Suceava, Dorohoi, Botoșani, and Iași in 1886, addressed to the home minister"]. *Monitorul Oficial*, May 28 (1887): 964–76.

Felix, I. *Tractat de Igiena publică și poliția sanitară*, partea a II-a [A treatise on public hygiene and health policies, part two]: "Boalele și Bolnavii" ["Illnesses and patients"]. Bucharest: Tipografia Academiei Române (Laboratorii Români), 1889.

Felix, I. *Raport general asupra igienei publice și asupra serviciului sanitar al Capitalei pe anul 1891* [General report on public health and the health services in the capital for 1891]. Bucharest: Lito-Tipografia Carol Gobl, 1892.

Felix, I. "Ordinul circular sub no. 10850 din 4 iulie 1892 către domnii medici primari de județe, de orașe și de spitale rurale" ["Circular no. 10850 of July 4, 1892, to the chief county doctors in urban and rural hospitals"]. *Buletinul Direcțiunei Generale a Serviciului Sanitar*, year IV, no. 13 (1892): 193–94.

Felix, I. "Raportul domnului doctor ~ , membru consiliului sanitar superior, asupra rezultatului inspecțiunii sanitare, făcute de d-nia. sa în județele Argeș, Dâmbovița, Prahova și Vlașca" ["Report by Dr. ~, a member of the higher medical council, on the results of the health inspection he conducted in the counties Argeș, Dâmbovița, Prahova, and Vlașca"]. *Buletinul Direcțiunei Generale a Serviciului Sanitar*, year IV, nos. 2–3 (1892): 17–25; no. 4, 41–57; no. 5, 65–77; no. 6, 82–93; no. 7, 97–105; no. 8, 113–21.

Felix, I. *Raport general despre igiena publică și despre serviciul sanitar ale Regatului României pe anul 1892* [General report on public hygiene and health services in the kingdom of Romania for the year 1892]. Bucharest: Imprimeria Statului, 1893.

Felix, Iacob, *Raport general upraise igienei publice și asupra serviciului sanitar al Regatului României pe anul 1894,* [General report on public hygiene and health services in the Kingdom of Romania for the year 1894]. Bucharest: Imprimeria Statului, 1895.

Felix, Iacob. *Raport general asupra igienei publice și asupra serviciului sanitar al Regatului României pe anul 1895* [General report on public hygiene and health services in the Kingdom of Romania for the year 1895]. Bucharest: Imprimeria Statului, 1897.

Felix, I. *Raport general asupra igienei publice și asupra serviciului sanitar al Regatului României pe anii 1896 și 1897* [General report on public hygiene and health services in the Kingdom of Romania for the years 1896 and 1897]. Bucharest: Imprimeria Statului, 1899.

Felix, I. *Istoria igienei în România în secolul al XIX-lea și starea ei la începutul secolului al XX-lea*, partea I [A history of hygiene in Romania in the nineteenth century and its state at the beginning of the twentieth century, part one]. Bucharest: Institutul de Arte Grafice "Carol Göbl," 1901.

Felix, I. "Alcoolismul poporațiunei rurale în comparațiune cu alcoolismul poporațiunei urbane" ["Alcoholism among the rural population compared to the urban population"]. *Antialcoolul*, year III, no. 1 (1902): 1–6.

Felix, I. "Pelagra în România" ["Pellagra in Romania"]. *Buletinul Medical. Organ al Asociațiunei Generale a Medicilor din Țară*, year V, 1902, no. 30 (1902): 2–4; no. 31, 2–4; no. 32, 2–3; no. 33, 3–4.

Felix, I. *Istoria igienei în România*, partea a II-a [A history of hygiene in Romania, part two], an extract from *Analele Academiei Române, Memoriile Secţiunii Ştiinţifice*, series II, vol. XXIV. Bucharest: Institutul de Arte Grafice "Carol Göbl," 1902.

Fialla, Ludovic. *Reminiscenţe din resbelul româno-ruso-turc al anului 1877 şi rolul Societăţii "Crucea-Roşie" în timp de pace şi de resbel* [Recollections of the Romanian-Russo-Turkish war of 1877 and the role of the Red Cross Society in times of peace and war]. Bucharest: Tipografia Ion Weiss, 1892.

Fialla, Ludovic. *Reminiscenţe din resbelul româno-ruso-turc anul 1877 şi rolul Societăţii "Crucea Roşie" în timp de pace şi de resbel*. Bucharest: Imprimeria şi librăria şcoalelor "C. Sfetea," 1906.

Flaişlen, G. *Consiliul de higienă şi salubritate publică din oraşul Iaşi. Raportul general pe anul 1875* [The council for public hygiene and health in the city of Iaşi: General report for the year 1875]. Iaşi: Tipografia Naţională, 1876.

Flor, P. "Azilul de pelagroşi 'Păuceşti-Dragomireşti' din judeţul Roman" ["The asylum for pellagra patients at Păuceşti-Dragomireşti in Roman county"]. *Spitalul*, year XVII (bound volume) (1897): 350–55, 405–7.

Flor, P. "Spitalul de pelagroşi Pănceşti-Dragomireşti. Dare de seamă de la 1896 mai până la 1899 mai, însoţită de câteva cercetări asupra etiologiei pelagrei" ["The hospital for pellagra at Pănceşti-Dragomireşti: Report from May 1896 to May 1899 with observations on the aetiology of pellagra"]. *Spitalul*, year XX (bound volume) (1900): 92–101, 115–19, 136–39.

Fotino, A. "Raportul D-lui dr. ~, membrul consiliului sanitar superior, asupra inspecţiunii serviciului sanitar din judeţele Buzău, Ilfov şi oraşul Bucureşti, în anul 1886, către D. ministru de interne" ["Report by Dr. ~, a member of the higher medical council, on the inspection of the health services in the counties of Buzău and Ilfov and the city of Bucharest, addressed to the Home Minister"]. *Monitorul Oficial*, June 4 (1887): 1126–39.

Fotino, A. "Raportul d-lui dr. Fotino, membru în consiliul sanitar superior, către d. Ministru de interne, asupra rezultatului inspecţiunei sanitare făcute de d-sa în anul 1891, în judeţele Brăila, Tulcea, Constanţa şi Ilfov" ["Report by Dr. Fotino on the health inspection he conducted in 1891 in the counties of Brăila, Tulcea, Constanţa, and Ilfov"]. *Buletinul Direcţiunei Generale a Serviciului Sanitar*, year IV, no. 21 (1892): 336–43.

Galian, D. "În cestiunea descreşterii populaţiunei oraşului Botoşani" ["On population decrease in the town of Botoşani"]. *Spitalul*, year XXX (bound volume) (1910): 473–81.

Georgescu, N. "Raportul d-lui medic-şef al Capitalei no. 2836 din 27 septembrie 1902, către direcţiunea generală a serviciului sanitar, relativ la cauzele febrei tifoide şi difteriei în Capitală" ["Report by the chief doctor of the capital no. 2836 of September 27, 1902, addressed to the general directorate of the health service on the causes of typhoid fever and diphtheria in the capital"]. *Buletinul Direcţiunei Generale a Serviciului Sanitar*, year XIV, no. 10 (1902): 298–300.

Gerota, Dimitrie. *Impresiuni şi aprecieri din timpul acţiunei militare în Bulgaria. 22 iunie–20 august 1913* [Impressions and comments on military action in Bulgaria, June 22–August 20, 1913]. Bucharest: Ed. Socec, 1913.

Grigoriu-Rigo, Gr. *Medicina poporului*, Memoriul II: Boalele vitelor [Popular medicine, memorandum II: The diseases of cattle], extract from *Analele Academiei Române, Memoriile Secţiunii Literare*, series II, vol. XXX. Bucharest: Institutul de Arte Grafice "Carol Göbl," 1907.

Gugea, Th. *Contribuţiune la studiul taliei soldatului român* [A contribution to the study of the body index of the Romanian soldier]. Bucharest: Tipo-Litografia Eduard Wiegand, 1888.

Haret, M. C. *Impozitul şi beuturile alcoolice în România* [The tax on alcoholic beverages in Romania]. Bucharest: Lito-Tipografia Carol Göbl, 1895.

Hârsu, M. "Fragmente din raportul unui medic de plasă. Notiţe asupra igienei şi demografiei circumscripţiei V, Muntele, din judeţul Suceava" ["Excerpts from the report of a district doctor: Notes on hygiene and demography in circumscription V, Muntele, Suceava County"]. *Buletinul Asociaţiunii Generale a Medicilor din Ţară*, year II, no. 7 (1899): 213–16; no. 8, 249–52; no. 9, 278–83; no. 10, 315–17.

Hintz, Robert. "Raport statistic de serviciul sanitar din Districtul Vlaşca pe anul 1864" ["Statistical report on the health services of Vlaşca District for the year 1864"]. *Monitorul Medical*, year IV, no. 15 (1865): 115.

Iacobovici, Iacob Melcon. "Cauzele mortalității primei copilării în România și mijloacele de a le combate" ["The causes of mortality in early infancy in Romania and its prevention"]. *Spitalul,* year XXII, supplement (1902): xx–xx.

Ionescu, Ion. *Agricultura romănă din judeţul Mehedinţi* [Romanian agriculture in Mehedinţi county]. Budapest: Imprimeria Statului, 1868.

Ionescu, N. T. "Pelagra în România în 1905" ["Pellagra in Romania in 1905"]. *Buletinul Direcţiunei Generale a Serviciului Sanitar,* year XVIII, nos. 23–24 (1906): 439–43.

Ionescu, N. T. *Medicii noştri. Portrete şi biografii* [Our doctors: Portraits and biographies], series I. Bucharest: Inst. de Arte Grafice "Carol Göbl," 1906.

Ionescu, N. T. "Pelagra în România în 1906" ["Pellagra in Romania in 1906"]. *Buletinul Direcţiunei Generale a Serviciului Sanitar,* year XX, no. 5 (1908): 110–17.

Ionescu-Trifan, I. "Dare de seamă asupra unui arondisment medical" ["Report on a medical borough"]. *Spitalul,* year XIV (bound volume) (1894): 553–60.

Istrati, C. I. "Expunere asupra băilor ieftine" ["A survey of cheap public baths"]. *Jurnalul Societăţii Sciinţelor Medicale din Bucureşti,* year I, no. 7 (1879): 106–16.

Istrati, C. I. "Despre locuinţa ţeranului" ["On the peasant's dwelling"]. *Jurnalul Societăţii Sciinţelor Medicale din Bucureşti,* year I, no. 19 (1879): 293–301.

Istrati, C. I. "Despre locuinţa ţăranului." *Românul,* year XXIII, November 4 (1879): 1016–17, and November 6, 1020–21.

Istrati, C. I. "Postul la români" ["Fasting among the Romanians"]. *Jurnalul Societăţii Stiinţelor Medicale din Bucureşti,* year I, no. 20 (1879): 309–18.

Istrati, C. I. *O pagină din istoria contimpurană a României din punctul de videre medical, economic şi national* [A page in the contemporary history of Romania from a medical, economic and national viewpoint]. Bucharest: Typografia Alesandru A. Grecescu, 1880.

Kopeţki, Ion. "Raport general a serviciului sanitar judeţului Tecuci în anul 1864" ["General report on health services in Tecuci county for the year 1864"]. *Monitorul Medical,* year IV, no. 13 (1865): 99–101, no. 14, 107–8.

Kretzulescu, Nicolae. *Amintiri istorice* [Historical recollections]. Bucharest: Tipografia şi fonderia de litere Thoma Basilescu, 1895.

Lapteş, N. "Mortalitatea copiilor la săteni. Comunicare făcută Congresului de Ştiinţe Sociale" ["Infant mortality among the peasantry: Paper presented at the congress of social sciences"]. *Revista ştiinţelor medicale,* year II, nos. 11–12 (1906): 431–40.

Lapteş, N. *Din nevoile satelor (note de igienă socială)* [Social hygiene in the countryside: An appraisal of needs]. Bucharest: Atelierele Grafice "Flacăra," 1914.

Laugier, Ch. "Intoxicaţie alimentară" ["Food poisoning"]. *Buletinul Direcţiunii Generale a Serviciului Sanitar,* year XVII, no. 1 (1905): 26–28.

Leon, N. *Istoria naturală medicală a poporului Român* [A History of natural medicine in Romania], extract from *Analele Academiei Române, Memoriile Secţiunii Ştiinţifice,* series II, vol. XXV. Bucharest: Institutul de Arte Grafice "Carol Göbl," 1903.

Leon, N. *Amintiri,* partea a III-a [Recollections, part three]. Iaşi: Viaţa Românească S. A., 1927.

Lupu, Nicolae. "Alimentaţia ţăranului" [The alimentation of the peasant]. *Viaţa Românească,* year I, vol. I, no. 2 (1906): 217–40.

Măldărescu, N. "Raportul d-lui doctor N. Măldărescu, membru consiliului sanitar superior, asupra rezultatului inspecţiunii sanitare, făcute de d-nia sa, în anul 1891, în judeţele Dolj, Gorj, Mehedinţi şi Vâlcea" ["Report by Dr. N. Măldărescu, a member of the higher medical Council on his health inspection of the Counties of Dolj, Gorj, Mehedinţi, and Vâlcea in 1891"]. *Buletinul Direcţiunii Generale a Serviciului Sanitar,* year IV, no. 10 (1892): 156–57; no. 11, 164–69; no. 12, 179–86; no. 13, 197–207; no. 14, 212–21; no. 18, 286–93.

Manicatide, Elena. *Contribuţiuni la studiul etiologiei pelagrei* [Contributions to the study of the aetiology of pellagra]. Bucharest: Tipografia şi Fonderia de litere Thoma Basilescu, 1900.

Manicea, G. V. *Consideraţiuni asupra mortalităţii generale în România* [Observations on general mortality in Romania]. Bucharest: Tipografia Alesandru A. Grecescu, 1880.

Manolescu, N. "Aparatul de încălzit camerele ţărăneşti în plaiul Buzău (distr. Buzău); cauze de boală" ["Heating installations in the district of Buzău: Its health hazards"]. *Românul*, year XXIII, June 11–12 (1879): 552–53; June 15, 564–65.

Manolescu, Nicolae. *Igiena țăranului. Locuința, iluminatul și încălzitul ei. Îmbrăcămintea, încălțămintea, alimentațiunea țăranului în deosebitele epoce ale anului și în deosebitele regiuni ale țării* [The hygiene of the peasant: his dwelling, its lighting and heating; clothes, footwear and alimentation by time of year and region]. Bucharest: Lito-tipografia Carol Göbl, 1895.

Manolescu, N. "Neputința organisațiunei actuale sanitare în apărarea populațiunei rurale contra boalelor" ["The failure of the current health organization in preventing disease"]. *Buletinul Asociațiunei Generale a Medicilor din Țară*, year I, no. 4 (1897): 99–105.

Manolescu, N. *Apărătorul sănătăței cuprinzător de cunoștințe de igienă și de medicină populară* [A companion to health: guide to popular hygiene and medicine]. Bucharest: Editura Institutului de Arte Grafice Carol Göbl, 1904.

Marțian, D. P. "Recensiunea din 1860" ["The census of 1860"]. *Annalele Statistice pentru cunoscința părții Muntene din România*, year I, nos. 3–4 (1860): 128–33.

Mendelssohn, S. *Câteva considerațiuni asupra mișcării populațiunii României* [Observations on population trends in Romania]. Bucharest: Tipografia Academiei Române, 1881.

Mendonini, I. S. *Contribuțiuni la demografia României* [Contributions to the demography of Romania]. Bucharest: Imprimeria Statului, 1892.

Michelstaedter, Solomon. "Raportul D-lui Michelstaedter, medicul primar districtului Brăila asupra stărei sanitare a districtului Brăila în anul 1865, înaintat Direcției Sanitare a Serviciului Sanitar" ["Report by Mr. Michelstaedter, chief doctor of the district of Brăila on public health in the district in 1865"]. *Monitorul Medical*, year V, no. 5 (1866): 35–37, and no. 6, 44–45.

Mileticiu, George. *Studii psihiatrice* [Studies on psychiatry]. Craiova: Tipo-Litografia Naționale Ralian și Ignat Samitca, 1895.

Mingareli, Mihail. "Raport general asupra serviciului sanitar din județul Mehedinți, pe anul 1887, adresat direcțiunei generale a serviciului sanitar" ["General report on the health services of Mehedinți country for the year 1887, addressed to the general health directorate]. *Monitorul Oficial*, August 9 (1888): 2521–23.

Neagoe, I. *Raportul d-rului I. Neagoe asupra misiunei sale în străinătate pentru a studia mijloacele de combatere a pelagrei din numitele țări* [Report by Dr. I. Neagoe on his mission abroad to study the means of combatting pellagra]. Bucharest: Imprimeria Statului, 1889.

Neagoe, I. *Pelagra în România* [Pellagra in Romania]. Bucharest: Tipografia "Dreptatea," 1899.

Neagoe, Ioan. "Studiu asupra pelagrei" ["A study on pellagra"]. In *Publicațiunile Fondului Vasilie Adamachi*, vol. I, 1898–1900, 279–527. Bucharest: Institutul de Arte Grafice Carol Göbl, 1900.

Neagoe, I. *Pelagra și administrația noastră* [Pellagra and our administration]. Bucharest: Tipografia "Munca," 1906.

Negrescu, Valerian George. *Contribuțiune la studiul pelagrei* [A contribution to the study of pellagra]. Bucharest: Tipografia Modernă, 1886.

Nicolăescu-Plopșor, C. S. "Bordeiul în Oltenia. Schiță antropogeografică" ["The hovel in oltenia: An anthropological-geographical essay"]. *Buletinul Societății Regale Române de Geografie*, year XLI (1922): 119–32.

Niculescu, D. D. *Alcoolismul în România* [Alcoholism in Romania]. Bucharest: Editura Librăriei Socec & Comp., 1895.

Niculescu, Ion. "Memoriu asupra stărei arondismentului Fundu din județul Roman," ["Memorandum on the borough Fundu in Roman county"]. *Monitorul Medical*, year III, no. 43 (1864): 381–84.

Obédénare, Georgiade. *Fièvres des marais (fièvres intermittentes). Petit guide à l'usage des gens du monde pour les localités où il n'y a pas de médecin.* Bucharest: Imprimerie de la Cour (Ouvriers Associés), 1871.

Obedenaru, Georgiade. *Despre friguri. Mic tractat potrivit pe înțelegerea poporului român pentru a servi în localitățile unde nu sunt medici* [On fevers: A short popular treatise for the use of localities without a doctor]. Bucharest: Imprimeria Statului, 1873.

Obedenaru, Georgiade. *Despre friguri. Mic tractat potrivit pe înțelegerea poporului român pentru a servi în localitățile unde nu sunt medici.* Bucharest: Tipografia Statului, 1883.

Obregia, Al. "Circulara no. 7.283 din 19 aprilie 1906, către D-nii medici ai spitalelor: Săveni, Târnăuca
și Darabani (Dorohoi); Sușița, Burdujeni și Ștefănești (Botoșani); Pășcani (Suceava); Rosnov
(Neamț); Parincea și Moinești (Bacău); Dămienești și Bâra (Roman); Răducăneni și Mălăești
(Fălciu); Florești (Tutova); Bujor și Pechea (Covurlui); Nifon și Pătârlage (Buzău); Urlați și
Văleni (Prahova); Cocoic și Poenari (Ilfov); Mozăceni (Argeș); Lădești (Vâlcea) și Vânju-Mare
(Mehedinți), relativă la instituirea unui serviciu de hrănire a bolnavilor de pellagra" ["Circular no.
7.283 of April 19, 1906, to the doctors of the hospitals in ~, concerning a new catering system for
patients"]. *Buletinul Direcțiunei Generale a Serviciului Sanitar,* year XVIII, no. 8 (1906): 142–43.

Obregia, Al. *Raport general asupra igienei publice și asupra serviciului sanitare al Regatului României
pe anii 1898-1904 inclusiv,* partea I [General report on public hygiene and the health services of
the kingdom of Romania for the years 1898–1904, part one]. Bucharest: "Minerva" Institut de
Arte Grafice și Editură, 1907.

Orleanu, C. Gh. *Raport general asupra igienei, stărei anitare precum și asupra serviciului sanitar al
Capitalei pe 1906* [General report on the hygiene, public health and health services in the capital for 1906]. Bucharest: "Minerva" Institut de Arte Grafice și Editură, 1907.

Pârvulescu, George. *Culegere de legile, regulamentele, instrucțiele, decretele și ver-ce alte dispozițiuni
sanitare civile și militare* [A collection of laws, regulations, instructions, decrees and other guidelines on civilian and military sanitation and health]. Bucharest: Tip. Alex. A. Grecescu, 1883.

Petrescu, Z. *O încercare de statistica medico-militară a României* [An essay towards a medico-mili-
tary statistic of Romania]. Bucharest: Imprimeria Statului, 1880.

Petrescu, G. Z. "Tocirea dinților la om" ["Tooth erosion in humans"]. *Revista Științelor Medicale,*
year I, vol. I, no. 2 (1905): 87–91.

Petrini (de Galatz), A. Mihail. *Despre amelioraţiunea rasei umane* [On the improvement of the
human race]. Bucharest: Tipografia D.A. Laurian, 1876.

Pitișteanu, Ion. "Raport general pe anul 1899. Starea sanitară a Plășei Snagov" ["General report for
the year 1899: Public health in Snagov district"]. *Buletinul Asociațiunii Generale a Medicilor din
Țară,* year III, nos. 10–11 (1900): 204–10.

Poenaru-Căplescu, C. *Alcool și Alcoolism* [Alcohol and alcoholism]. Bucharest: Institutul de Arte
Grafice "Eminescu," 1904.

Polyzu, A. Gheorghe. "Circulara D-lui Ministru de Interne no. 15.035 din 2 septembrie 1889, către
d-nii prefecți și medici primari de județe, relativă la alimentațiunea locuitorilor rurali la mun-
cile agricole" ["Circular of the Home Minister no 15.035 of September 2, 1889, to the prefects
and chief medical officers in counties concerning the alimentation of rural labourers"]. *Buletinul Direcțiunei Generale a Serviciului Sanitar,* year I, no. 19 (1889): 305–6.

Popescu, Constantin. *Contribuțiune la studiul stării higienice și sanitare a populațiunii rurale* [A
contribution to the study of hygiene and sanitation among the rural population]. Bucharest:
"Tipografia Nouă," 1896.

Popescu, Nicolae. *Pellagra. Observații în Vlașca și în special Neajlov-Glavacioc* [Pellagra: Observations for the region of Vlașca, with an emphasis on Neajlov-Glavacioc]. Bucharest: Tipografia
"Voința Națională," 1891.

Possa, St. "Ambulanța rurală Roman-Iași. Ochire generală asupra foloaselor ambulanțelor rurale"
[The Roman-Iași rural ambulance service: A general view on the uses of rural ambulances].
*Spitalul,* year VI, no. 10 (1886): 384–90.

Possa, St. "Alcoolismul." *Buletinul Asociațiunei Generale a Medicilor din Țară,* year IV, nos. 1–2
(1900): 4–24; nos. 3–4, 49–61; no. 5, 79–91.

Possa, St. "Alcoolismul înaintea Congresului Asociației Medicilor" ["Alcoholism: A presentation
to the congress of the medical association"]. *Antialcoolul,* year I (1900): no. 6, 81–87; no. 8, 113–
21; no. 9, 134–38; no. 10, 150–53; no. 11, 170–75; no. 12, 190–92; year II (1901): no. 1, 11–15;
nos. 2–3, 28–34; no. 7, 103–8; no. 8, 120–24; no. 12, 189–92.

Possa, St. "Mortalitatea copiilor" ["Infant mortality"]. *Buletinul Medical. Organ al Asociațiunei Generale a Medicilor din Țară,* year V, no. 24 (1902): 6–7.

Proca, G. "Cercetări asupra pelagrei" ["Studies on pellagra"]. *Spitalul,* year XXIII (bound volume)
(1903): 671–82.

Proca, G., and Gh. T. Kirileanu. "Cercetări asupra hranei țăranului. Înainte de Război" ["Studies on the peasant's nutrition: before the war"]. *Revista științelor medicale,* year XXVII, nos. 7–8 (1938): 607–23.

Raicevich, S. I. *Voyage en Valachie et en Moldavie.* Paris: Masson et Fils, 1822.

Rigani, Gheorghe. "Mersul serviciului sanitar al județului Mușcel în 1905" ["Developments in the health services of Mușcel county in 1905"]. *Buletinul Direcțiunei Generale a Serviciului Sanitar,* year XIX, no. 3 (1907): 78–84; no. 4, 97–113; no. 6, 153–64.

Rizu, E. *Schiță de igienă și medicină populară pentru școalele primare rurale* [An essay on hygiene and public health in rural primary schools]. Iași: Tip. Petru C. Popovici, 1891.

Romniceanu, Grigore. "Despre beuturi" ["On beverages"]. *Gazetta medico-chirurgicală,* year I, no. 4 (1870): 62–64; no. 5, 71–73; no. 6, 90–92; no. 7, 105–7; no. 8, 119–21.

Romniceanu, Grigore. "Despre băi" ["On baths"]. *Gazetta medico-chirurgicală a spitalelor,* year II, no. 12 (1871): 189–91.

Romniceanu, Grigore. "Igiena săteanului" ["The hygiene of the villager"]. *Revista contimporană. Litere-Arte-Științe,* year I, no. 1 (1873): 51–55; no. 2, 153–57.

Rosetti, C. A. "Adresa sub no. 14.757, a D-lui Ministru de interne, către D. director general al Serviciului sanitar, în privința mortalității din București" ["Memorandum no. 14.757 from the home minister to the director of the health service concerning mortality in Bucharest"]. *Monitorul Oficial al Romăniei,* August 31, no. 192 (1878): 5024–25.

Roth, M. *Memoriu asupra cauzelor mortalității populației romăno-creștine în raport cu cea de rit mosaic cu un proiect pentru ameliorarea relelor existente. Un studiu de hygienă comparată* [Memorandum on the causes of mortality among the Christian-Romanian population compared to the mosaic population, and a project for improvement: a study of comparative hygiene]. Bucharest: Tipografia Thiel & Weiss, 1880.

Sabin, Gh. "Raport general asupra serviciului sanitar al județului Vâlcea pe anul 1887, adresat Direcțiunei Generale a Serviciului Sanitar" ["General report on the health services of Vâlcea country in 1887, addressed to the general directorate of the health service"]. *Monitorul Oficial,* August 31 (1888): 2878–87.

Sabin, Gh. *Amintiri din războiul Independenței* [Recollections from the war for independence]. Bucharest: "Minerva" Institut de Arte Grafice și Editură, 1912.

Samarian, Pompei P. *O veche monografie sanitară a Munteniei "Topografia Țării Romănești" de dr. Constantin Caracaș (1800–1828)* [An old monograph on medicine in Muntenia: the topography of Țara Romănească by dr. Constantin Caracaș, 1800–1828]. Bucharest: Institutul de Arte Grafice "Bucovina" I. E. Toruțiu, 1937.

Samarian, Pompei Gh. *Medicina și farmacia în trecutul romănesc* [Medicine and pharmacy in Romanian history], vol. II, 1775–1834. Bucharest: Tipografia Cultura, 1938.

Scraba, G. D. *Starea socială a săteanului după ancheta privitoare anului 1905, îndeplinită cu ocaziunea Expozițiunei generale romăne din 1906 de către Secțiunea de economie socială* [Survey of the economic status of the peasant based on data collected in 1905 by the department of social economics for the Romanian general exhibition of 1906]. Bucharest: Inst. de arte Grafice "Carol Göbl," 1907.

Sergiu, Dimitrie. "Raportul D-lui dr. Sergiu, membru Consiliului Sanitar Superior asupra inspecțiunei serviciului sanitar din circumscripția V a județelor Brăila, Ialomița, Dâmbovița și Ploesci, în anul 1886, către D. Ministru de Interne" ["Report by Dr. Sergiu, member of the Higher Medical Council, on the health inspection of district V in the counties Brăila, Ialomița, Dâmbovița, and Ploesci in the year 1886, addressed to the Home Minister"]. *Monitorul Oficial,* June 11 (1887): 1304–19.

Sergiu, Dimitrie. "Pelagra. Lecțiune clinică a d-lui prof Sergiu culeasă de P. Adam, internul serviciului" ["Pellagra: minutes of a clinical lesson by Prof. Sergiu by P. Adam, intern at the department"]. *Spitalul,* year VII, no. 5 (1887): 178–86, and no. 6, 216–22.

Sergiu, Dimitrie. *Raport general asupra Pelagrei presintat domnului Ministru de interne* [General report on pellagra presented to the home hinister]. Bucharest: Imprimeria Statului, 1888.

Severeanu, C. D. *Din amintirile mele (1853–1928)* [From my recollections, 1853–1928], vol. I. Bucharest: Tipografia "Bucovina" I. E. Toruțiu, 1929.

Severeanu, C. D. *Din amintirile mele (1853–1929)*, vol. II. Bucharest: Tipografia "Voința," 1930.

Sion, V. "Referatul d-lui dr ~, asistent la institutul de patologie și de bacteriologie din București, despre cercetările făcute de d-sa asupra originii febrei tifoide la Galați" ["Report by Dr. ~, assistant doctor at the institute for pathology and bacteriology in Bucharest on the causes of typhoid fever in Galați"]. *Buletinul Direcțiunei Generale a Serviciului Sanitar*, year XI, nos. 17–18 (1899): 282–85.

Sion, V. "Asistența medicală în România rurală" ["Medical assistance in rural Romania"]. *Revistă de drept, sociologie și economie politică*, year VI, no. 4 (1904): 126–209, and no. 5, 239–56.

Soiu, Nicolae. *Valoarea perimetriei toracice în examenul recrutării* [The uses of thoracic measurements in conscription]. Bucharest: Tipografia "Românul," 1889.

Spiroiu, Al. "Ambulanța militară rurală din județul Mehedinți" ["The rural ambulance service in Mehedinți county"]. *Spitalul*, year V, no. 6 (1885): 193–98, and no. 7, 236–41.

Sufrin, S. *Câteva reflexiuni asupra etilogiei pelagrei* [Reflections on the aetiology of pellagra]. Bucharest: Tipografia "Dreptatea," 1899.

Sutzu, A. "Băuturile alcoolice și alcoolismul" ["Alcoholic beverages and alcoholism"]. *Gazetta medico-chirurgicală*, year III, no. 11 (1872): 172–76.

Sutzu, A. *Alienatul în fața societății și a științei* [Mental illness, society and science]. Bucharest: Noua Typographie a Laboratorilor Români, 1877.

Ștefănescu, I. V. "Raport asupra mișcării bolnavilor în Spitalul rural Horezu în cursul anului 1886" ["Report on patient statistics in the Horezu rural hospital in 1886"]. *Analele Medicale Române*, year VI, no. 9 (1887): 360–64, and no. 10, 376–88.

Ștefănescu, I. "Vindecarea beției ca remediu contra alcoolismului" ["Curing drunkenness as a remedy against alcoholism]. *Spitalul*, year XVI (bound volume) (1896): 341–47, 375–82, 405–10, 424–30, 451–57, 468–78.

Takeanu, N. "Raport general asupra serviciului sanitar din județul Covurlui, pe anul 1887, adresat direcțiunei generale a serviciului sanitar" ["General report on the health service in Covurlui county for the year 1887, addressed to the general directorate of the health service"]. *Monitorul Oficial*, August 2 (1888): 2400–3.

Teodori, I. "Raportul presintat D-lui Ministru de interne de către D. Dr. Iul. Teodori, membrul consiliului sanitar superior, asupra inspecțiunei făcută serviciului sanitar din circumscripțiunea II-a sanitară" ["Report presented to the home minister by Dr. Iul. Teodori, member of the higher medical council on the inspection of health services in district II"]. *Monitorul Oficial*, July 3 (1888): 1801–21.

Thomescu, N. C. "Asupra cauzelor mortalității în prima copilărie în țară și mijloacele de a le combate" ["On the causes of mortality in early infancy in our country and the means of combatting it"]. *Buletinul Medical. Organ al Asociațiunei generale a medicilor din Țară*, year V, no. 18 (1902): 4–6; no. 19, 1–3; no. 20, 1–3; no. 21, 1–4; no. 22, 3–7; no. 23, 2–4; no. 24, 1–5; no. 25, 3–5; no. 26, 4–6; no. 28, 2–5; no. 29, 2–4.

Urbeanu, A. *Țuica și basamacul. Studiu critic* [Plum brandy and basamac: A critical study]. Bucharest: Stabilimentul Grafic Albert Baer, 1900.

Urbeanu, A. *Îmbunătățirea alimentației țăranului român* [Improvements in the alimentation of the Romanian peasant]. Bucharest: Tipografia "Speranța," 1901.

Urbeanu, A. *Hrana săteanului în cei din urmă 40 de ani și îmbunătățirile de adus* [The villager's food in the last forty years and ways to improve it]. Bucharest: Imprimeria Statului, 1906.

Urechia. "Cercetări asupra alcoolizmului în România" ["Studies on alcoholism in Romania"]. *Spitalul*, year XXII (bound volume) (1902): 189–97.

Urechia. "Cercetări asupra alcoolismului în România." *Buletinul Medical. Organ al Asociațiunei Generale a Medicilor din Țară*, year V, no. 17 (1902): 1–4.

Vasiliu, A. "Mesele pelagroșilor" ["The pellagra lunches"]. *Buletinul Direcțiunei Generale a Serviciului Sanitar*, year XVIII, nos. 17–18 (1906): 335–36.

Vernav, Constantino Nob. *Rudimentum physiographiae Moldaviae*, Typis Regiae Scient. Budae: Universitatis Hungaricae, 1836.

Zorileanu. "Dare de seamă de rezultatul obținut cu tratarea bolnavilor de pelagră la stațiunea balneară Govora, în vara anului 1903" ["Report on the Outcomes of the Treatment of Pellagra in Govora Spa in the summer of 1903"]. *Buletinul Direcțiunei Generale a Serviciului Sanitar*, year XV, no. 9 (1903): 226–29.

Zosin, Panaite. *Calea unei vieți. Copilăria și adolescența – tinereța, virilitatea – maturitatea și bătrâneța. Mărturisiri, constatări, interpretări, aprecieri, învățături, povețe și îndemnuri pentru un copil de suflet, privind multiplele contingențe ale unei vieți* [A life journey. Childhood and adolescence, youth and manhood, maturity and old age. Confessions, reflections, interpretations, teachings and advice for an orphan, on the multiple contingencies of life]. Iași: Editura autorului [self-published], 1935.

Weissberg, Iosef. "Alcoolismul în Ialomița. Din cele raportate de un medic de plasă" ["Alcoholism in Ialomița: from the reports of a district doctor"]. *Buletinul Asociațiunei Generale a Medicilor din Țară*, year I, no. 11 (1898): 347–49.

## Secondary Literature

Albulescu, Gheorghe N., and Gheorghe Brătescu. *Însemnările unui medic din Războiul pentru Independență. Jurnalul de campanie al lui Zaharia Petrescu* [A doctor in the war of independence: The campaign diary of Zaharia Petrescu]. Bucharest: Editura Medicală, 1977.

Aries, Philippe. *Omul în fața morții* (The hour of our death). 2 vols. Bucharest: Editura Meridiane, 1996.

Atanasiu, Ion. "Activitatea științifică și socială a lui Dimitrie Gerota" ["The scientific and social activities of Dimitrie Gerota"]. In *Trecut și viitor in medicină. Studii și note* [Past and present in medicine: studies and notes], edited by G. Brătescu, 415–24. Bucharest: Ed. Medicală, 1981.

Bacalbașa, Constantin. *Bucurescii de altădată* [Bucharest of yesteryear], 5 vols. Bucharest: Ed. Albatros Corporation, 2007.

Băluță, Ionela. *La bourgeoise respectable. Réflexion sur la construction d'une nouvelle identité féminine dans la seconde moitié du XIXe siècle roumain.* Bucharest: Editura Universității din București, 2008.

Bărbulescu, Constantin. *Imaginarul corpului uman. Între cultura țărănească și cultura savantă (secolele XIX–XX)* [Representations of the human body between peasant culture and high culture, 19th–20th centuries]. Bucharest: Ed. Paideia, 2005.

Bărbulescu, Constantin, and Alin Ciupală (eds). *Medicine, Hygiene and Society from the Eighteenth to the Twentieth Centuries.* Cluj-Napoca: Ed. Mega, 2011.

Bărbulescu, Constantin, and Vlad Popovici (eds.). *Modernizarea lumii rurale din România în a doua jumătate a secolului al XIX-lea și la începutul secolului al XX-lea. Contribuții* [Contributions to the study of modernization in Romania in the second half of the nineteenth and the early twentieth century]. Cluj-Napoca: Ed. Accent, 2005.

Bărbulescu, Elena, Mihai Croitor, Ciprian Pavel Moldovan, and Alexandru Onojescu. *Țarani, boli și vindecători în perioada comunistă. Mărturii orale* [Peasants, illness and healers in the communist period: oral testimonies], vol. II, edited by Constantin Bărbulescu. Cluj-Napoca: Ed. Mega, 2011.

Bărbulescu, Elena. "At the edge of modernity: physicians, priests and healers (1940–1990)." *Philobiblon. Transylvanian Journal of Multidisciplinary Research in Humanities*, vol. XVI, no. 2 (2011): 549–61.

Bărbulescu, Constantin, Mihai Croitor, Ciprian Pavel Moldovan, Alexandru Onojescu, and Alina Ioana Șuta. *Țarani, boli și vindecători în perioada comunistă. Mărturii orale* [Peasants, illness and healers in the communist period: oral testimonies], vol. I, edited by Elena Bărbulescu. Cluj-Napoca: Ed. Mega, 2010.

Brătescu, G. *Doctorul Iacob Felix. Savantul și înfăptuitorul* [Doctor Iacob Felix: Scholar and founding father]. Bucharest: Ed. Viața Medicală Românească, 2004.

Bucur, Maria. *Eugenie și modernizare în România interbelică.* Iași: Ed. Polirom, 2005. First published as *Eugenics and Modernization in Interwar Romania.* Pittsburgh: University of Pittsburgh Press, 2002.

Buda, Octavian (ed.). *Despre regenerarea și … degenerarea unei națiuni. Discursurile inaugurale med-*

*icale în vremea lui Carol I, 1872–1912* [On the regeneration ... and degeneration of a nation: Doctors' induction speeches from the reign of Carol I, 1872–1912]. Bucharest: Ed. Tritonic, 2009.

Bulei, Ion. *Viața în vremea lui Carol I* [Daily life in the time of Carol I]. Bucharest: Ed. Tritonic, 2005.

Bynum, W. F. *Science and the Practice of Medicine in the Nineteenth Century*. Cambridge: Cambridge University Press, 1994.

Bynum, W. F. et al. *The Western Medical Tradition: 1800 to 2000*. Cambridge: Cambridge University Press, 2006.

Cernovodeanu, Paul (ed.). *Călători străini despre Țările Române în secolul al XIX-lea* [Foreign travellers' accounts of the Romanian lands in the nineteenth century], serie nouă [new series], vol. I (1801–1821). Bucharest: Editura Academiei Române, 2004.

Chamberlin, J. Edward, and Sander L. Gilman (eds.). *Degeneration: The Dark Side of Progress*. New York: Columbia University Press, 1985.

Claudian, Ion, and N. Gruia Ionescu. *Pelagra. Patologie. Sociologie* [Pellagra: pathology and sociology]. Ploieşti: Spitalul boli interne, 1944.

Corbin, Alain. *La miasme et la jonquille. L'odorat et l'imaginaire social. XVIIIe–XIXe siècles*. Paris: Flammarion, 1986. The study was published in English translation as *The Foul and the Fragrant: Odor and the French Social Imagination*. Leamington Spa: Berg, 1986.

Elias, Norbert. *Procesul civilizării. Cercetări sociogenetice şi psihogenetice*. 2 vols. Iaşi: Polirom, 2002. First published in 1939 and translated into English as *The Civilizing Process: Sociogenetic and Psychogenetic Investigations* (revised ed.) London: Blackwell, 2000.

Faure, Olivier. *Les Français et leur médecine au XIXe siècle*. Paris: Belin, 1993.

Focşa, Gheorghe. *Elemente decorative la bordeiele din sudul regiunii Craiova* [Decorative elements in the architecture of hovels in Southern Craiova]. Bucharest: Ed. Muzeului Satului, 1957.

Fochi, Adrian, and Datcu, Iordan, *Bibliografia generală a etnografiei şi folclorului românesc*, vol. 1 (1800-1891). Bucharest: Editura pentru Literatură, 1968. Gheorghiu, Emil. "'Memoria de taină' a lui Şt. V. Episcopescu" ["The 'secret memoir' of Şt. V. Episcopescu"]. In *Trecut şi viitor in medicină. Studii şi note*, edited by G. Brătescu, 303–20. Bucharest: Ed. Medicală, 1981.

Golescu, Dinicu. *Însemnare a călătoriei mele Constantin Radovici din Goleşti făcută în anul ,1824 1825 şi 1826* [Account of my travels, by Constantin Radovici of Goleşti in the years 1824, 1825 and 1826], edited by Mircea Iorgulescu. Bucharest: Ed. Minerva, 1977.

Gomoiu, V. *Istoria presei medicale în România* [A history of the medical press in Romania]. Bucharest: Tip. "Furnica," 1936.

Gomoiu, V., Gh. Gomoiu, and Maria V. Gomoiu. *Repertor de medici, farmacişti, veterinari (personalul sanitar) din ţinuturile româneşti*, vol. I (înainte de 1870) [An index of doctors, pharmacists, veterinary doctors (health personnel) from the Romanian lands], vol. 1 (before 1870). Brăila: Tip. "Presa," 1938.

Gomoiu, Victor. *Viața mea (memorii)* [My life (memoirs)], edited by Mihail Şcheau, 6 vols. Craiova, Editura Sitech, 2006.

Goubert, Jean-Pierre. *La conquête de l'eau. L'avènement de la santé à l'âge industriel*. Paris: Éditions Robert Lafont, 1986.

Goubert, Jean-Pierre. *Une histoire de l'hygiène. Eau et salubrité dans la France contemporaine*. Paris: Coll. "Pluriel," Hachette, 2008.

Gudin, Cristina, Oana Mihaela Tămaş, Mihaela Mehedinţi, Alin Ciupală, Constantin Bărbulescu, and Vlad Popovici. *Rapoarte sanitare în România modernă (1864–1906)* [Healthcare reports in modern Romania, 1864–1906]. Cluj-Napoca: Ed. Mega, 2010.

Gusti, Dimitrie, et al. *Cornova 1931*, edited by Marin Diaconu, Zoltán Rostás, and Vasile Şoimaru. Chişinău: Editura Quant, 2011.

Iancu, Carol. *Evreii din România (1866–1919). De la excludere la emancipare*. Bucharest: Ed. Hasefer, 2006. First published as *Jews in Romania, 1866–1919: From Exclusion to Emancipation* (Boulder, CO: East European Monographs, 1996).

Jackson, Mark (ed.). *The Oxford Handbook for the History of Medicine*. Oxford: Oxford University Press, 2011.

Jianu, I., and G. Vasiliu. *Dr. C. I. Istrati*. Bucharest: Ed. Ştiinţifică, 1966.

Jianu, Iancu, and C. I. Bercuş. *Constantin Severeanu. Epoca şi opera* [Constantin Severeanu: his time and work]. Craiova: Ed. "Scrisul Românesc," 1976.

Jorland, Gérard. *Une société à soigner. Hygiène et salubrité publiques en France au XIXe siècle*. Paris: Gallimard, 2010.

Karge, Heike, Friederike Kind-Kovács, and Sara Bernasconi (eds.). *From the Midwife's Bag to the Patient's File. Public Health in Eastern Europe*. Budapest and New York: Central European University Press, 2017.

Lejeune, Philippe. *Pactul autobiografic*. Bucharest: Editura Univers, 2000. First published as *Le pacte autobiographique*. Paris: Seuil, 1975.

Léonard, Jacques. *La France médicale. Médecins et malades au XIXe siècle*. Paris: Gallimard, 1978.

Lévi-Strauss, Claude. "Rasă şi istorie." In *Rasismul în faţa ştiinţei* [Racism vs. science], 3–47. Bucharest: Ed. Politică, 1982. First published as *Race et histoire* in 1952.

Livadă-Cadeschi, Ligia-Mihaela. *Discursul medico-social al igieniştilor români. Abordarea specificităţilor locale din perspectiva experienţelor occidentale europene, secolele XIX–XX* [The medico-social discourse of hygienists: the Romanian experience in European context, 19th–20th centuries]. Bucharest: Editura Muzeului Naţional al Literaturii Române, 2013.

Lungu, Traian P. *Viaţa politică în România la sfârşitul secolului al XIX-lea (1888–1899)* [Political life in Romania at the end of the nineteenth century, 1888–1899]. Bucharest: Editura Ştiinţifică, 1967.

Lupescu, Mihai. *Din bucătăria ţăranului* [On rural cuisine]. Bucharest: Ed. Paideia, 2000.

Mihăilescu, Vintilă. *Antropologie. Cinci introduceri* [Anthropology: five introductions]. Iaşi: Ed. Polirom, 2007.

Mihăilescu, Vintilă (ed.). *Etnografii urbane. Cotidianul văzut de aproape* [Urban ethnographies: the everyday in close-up]. Iaşi: Ed. Polirom, 2009.

Mitu, Sorin. *Transilvania mea. Istorii, mentalităţi, identităţi* [My Transylvania: histories, mentalities, identities]. Iaşi: Ed. Polirom, 2006.

Niculiţă-Voronca, Elena. *Datinele şi credinţele poporului român adunate şi aşezate în ordine mitologică* [The traditions and beliefs of the Romanians collected and presented in mythological order], vol. I. Iaşi: Polirom, 1998.

Nye, Robert A. *Crime, Madness and Politics in Modern France: The Medical Concept of National Decline*. Princeton: Princeton University Press, 1984.

Oişteanu, Andrei. *Imaginea evreului în cultura română. Studii de imagologie în context Est-Central european*. Bucharest: Ed. Humanitas, 2004. Published in English as *Inventing the Jew: Antisemitic Stereotypes in Romanian and Other Central-East European Cultures* (London: Lincoln, 2009).

Ornea, Z. *Poporanismul*. Bucharest: Ed. Minerva, 1972.

Ornea, Z. *Sămănătorismul*. 3rd revised ed. Bucharest: Ed. Fundaţiei Culturale Române, 1998.

Pick, Daniel. *Faces of Degeneration: A European Disorder, c. 1848–1918*. Cambridge: Cambridge University Press, 1989.

Platon, Alexandru-Florin. *Geneza burgheziei în Principatele Române (a doua jumătate a secolului al XVIII-lea- prima jumătate a secolului al XIX-lea). Preliminariile unei istorii* [The formation of the bourgeoisie in the Romanian principalities from the late eighteenth to the mid-nineteenth century: preliminaries for a history]. Iaşi: Ed. Universităţii "Alexandru Ioan Cuza," 1997.

Pop, Iulia. *Memorie şi suferinţă. Consideraţii asupra literaturii memorialistice a universului concentraţionar comunist* [Memory and suffering: observations on the life narratives of communist labour camp prisoners]. Cluj-Napoca: Ed. Argonaut, 2010.

Popovici, Vlad. *Istoriografia medicală românească (1813–2008)* [Research into the history of medicine in Romania, 1813–2008]. In *Hermeneutica Bibliothecaria: Antologie Philobiblon*, vol. V, 463–80. Cluj-Napoca: Editura Argonaut, 2011.

Porter, Roy. *Health for Sale: Quackery in England, 1660–1850*. Manchester: Manchester University Press, 1989.

Promitzer, Christian, Sevasti Trubeta, and Marius Turda (eds.). *Health, Hygiene and Eugenics in Southeastern Europe to 1945*. Budapest and New York: Central European University Press, 2011.

Ramsey, Matthew. *Professional and Popular Medicine in France, 1770–1830*. Cambridge: Cambridge University Press, 1988.

Săvulescu, Traian (ed.). *Porumbul. Studiu monographic* [Corn: a study]. Bucharest: Ed. Academiei Republicii Populare Române, 1957.

Selejan, Ana. *Adevăr și mistificare în jurnale și memorii apărute după 1989* [Truth and mystification in journals and memoirs published after 1989]. Bucharest: Editura Cartea Românească, 2011.

Sora, Andrei Florin. *Servir l'État Roumain. Le corps préfectoral, 1866–1940*. Bucharest: Editura Universității din București, 2011.

Șuta, Alina Ioana, Oana Mihaela Tămaș, Alin Ciupală, Constantin Bărbulescu, and Vlad Popovici (eds.). *Legislația sanitară în România modernă (1874–1910)* [Health legislation in modern Romania, 1874–1910]. Cluj-Napoca: Presa Universitară Clujeană, 2009.

Trăușan-Matu, Lidia. *De la leac la rețetă. Medicalizarea societății românești în veacul al XIX-lea (1831–1869)* [From remedy to prescription drug: the medicalization of Romanian society in the nineteenth century, 1831–1869]. Bucharest: Editura Universității din București, 2011.

Trăușan-Matu, Lidia. "The Doctor and the Patient: An Analysis of the Medical Profession in the Romanian society of the 19th Century (1831–1869)." *Transylvanian Review*, vol. XX, supplement no. 2, vol. 2 (2011): 465–74.

Tubiana, Maurice. *Histoire de la pensée médicale. Les chemins d'Esculape*. Paris: Flammarion, 1995.

Turda, Marius. *Eugenism și antropologie rasială în România. 1874–1944*. Bucharest: Editura Cuvântul, 2008.

Vigarello, Georges. *Histoire des pratiques de la santé. Le sain et le malsain depuis le Moyen Age*. Paris: Éditions du Seuil, 1999.

Vigarello, Georges (ed.). *Istoria corpului, vol. II: De la Revoluția Franceză la Primul Război Mondial*. Bucharest: Editura Art, 2008. First published as *Histoire du corps (XVIe-XXe siècle*, 3 vols., vol. II: *De la Révolution à la grande guerre* (Paris: Le Seuil, 2005–2006).

Vintilă-Ghițulescu, Constanța. *Evgheniți, mojici, ciocoi: despre "obrazele" primei modernități românești (1750–1860)* [The well-born, the arriviste, the plebs: characters of Romania's first modern age, 1750–1860]. Bucharest: Ed. Humanitas, 2013.

Vintilă-Ghițulescu, Constanța. "Primeneli și sulimanuri: despre igienă și modernitate" ["Clean laundry and beauty preparations: On hygiene and modernity"]. In *Introducere în sociologia corpului. Teme, perspective și experiențe întrupate* [An introduction to the sociology of the body: themes, perspectives and embodied experience], edited by Laura Grunberg, 199–223. Iași: Ed. Polirom, 2010.

Zeletin, Ștefan. *Burghezia română. Originea și rolul ei istoric* [The Romanian bourgeoisie: its origins and roles in history], 2nd ed. Bucharest: Ed. Humanitas, 1991.

Weber, Eugen. *La fin des terroirs: la modernisation de la France rurale (1870–1914)*. Paris: Le grand livre du mois, 1998.

# INDEX OF NAMES

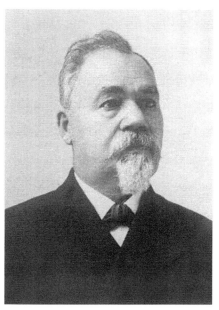

**Constantin Dimitrescu Severeanu**
(1840–1930)
From the Collection of Octavian Buda

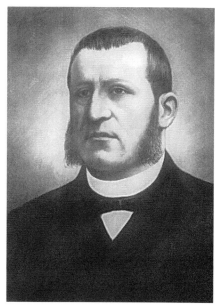

**Grigore Romniceanu**
(1845–1915)
From the Collection of Octavian Buda

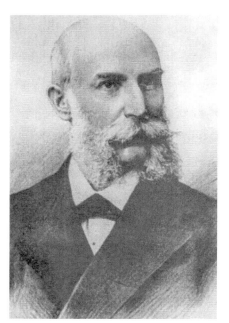

**Iacob Felix**
(1832–1905)
From the Collection of Octavian Buda

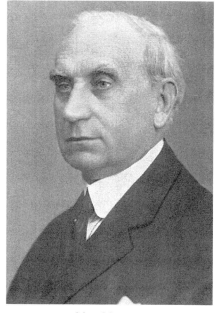

**Mina Minovici**
(1858–1933)
From the Collection of Octavian Buda

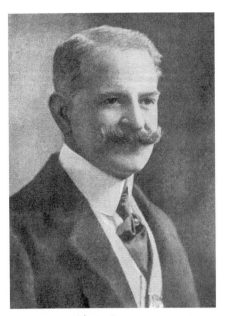

**Thoma Ionescu**
**(1860–1926)**
From the Collection of Octavian Buda

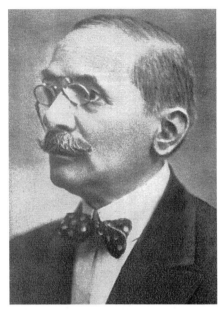

**Victor Babeş**
**(1854–1926)**
From the Collection of Octavian Buda

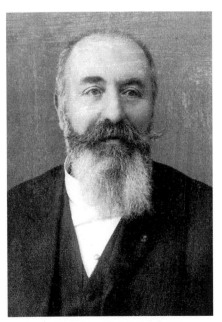

**C.I. Istrati (1850–1918)**
Courtesy of the "Lucian Blaga"
Central University Library, Cluj-Napoca

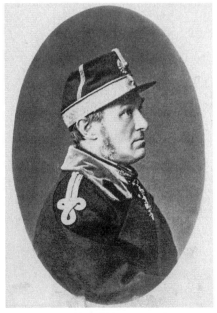

**Carol Davila (1828–1884)**
Courtesy of the "Lucian Blaga"
Central University Library, Cluj-Napoca

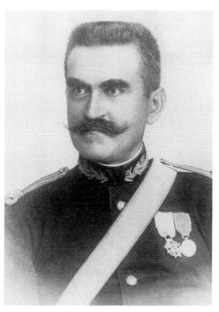

**Gheorghe Crăiniceanu (1853–1926)**
Courtesy of the "Lucian Blaga"
Central University Library, Cluj-Napoca

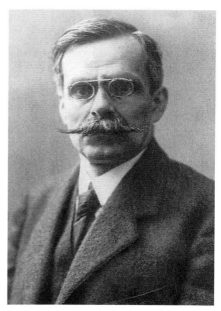

**Vasile Sion (1861–1921)**
Courtesy of the "Lucian Blaga"
Central University Library, Cluj-Napoca

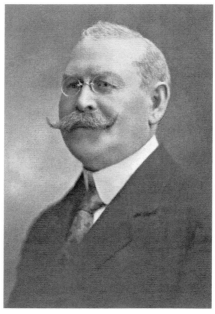

**Ştefan Possa (1857–?)**
Courtesy of the "Mihai Eminescu"
Central University Library, Iaşi